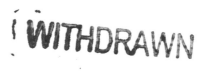

THE PSYCHOLOGICAL AND SOCIAL IMPACT OF DISABILITY

4th Edition

Robert P. Marinelli, EdD, CRC, is Professor and Coordinator of Rehabilitation Counselor Education in the Department of Counseling Psychology and Rehabilitation Counseling at West Virginia University College of Human Resources and Education. He received his master's and doctoral degrees in rehabilitation counseling from the Pennsylvania State University, the latter in 1971. A licensed psychologist and counselor, he has served on the faculties at Penn State and Boston University, as a consultant to rehabilitation agencies, mental health centers, and the Social Security Administration, and as a rehabilitation counselor. His professional activities have included national, regional, and state offices in rehabilitation associations and editorial board service to a variety of rehabilitation journals. His scholarly activities focus primarily on the psychological and career impact of disability and include coauthoring or coediting five books, and numerous book chapters and articles. He and Dr. Dell Orto coedited the first and only encyclopedic reference in the field, *Encyclopedia of Disability and Rehabilitation*. The Encyclopedia received the Excellence in Media Award by the National Rehabilitation Association as the outstanding rehabilitation publication in 1995.

Arthur E. Dell Orto, PhD, CRC, is Professor and Chairperson of the Department of Rehabilitation Counseling and Associate Executive Director of the Center for Psychiatric Rehabilitation at Boston University's Sargent College of Health and Rehabilitation Sciences. He was awarded his BA and MA from Seton Hall University, and his PhD from Michigan State University in 1970. Dr. Dell Orto is a licensed psychologist and certified rehabilitation counselor whose academic and clinical interests relate to the role of the family in the treatment and rehabilitation process. Dr. Dell Orto has given many presentations and workshops focusing on the needs of families living with illness and disability. He is coeditor or coauthor of eight books: *The Encyclopedia of Disability and Rehabilitation* (1995); *Head Injury and the Family: A Life and Living Approach* (1994); *The Psychological and Social Impact of Disability* (Springer Publishing, 1991); *Illness and Disability: Family Interventions Throughout the Life Span* (Springer Publishing, 1988); *The Psychological and Social Impact of Physical Disability* (Springer Publishing, 1977 & 1984), *Role of the Family in the Rehabilitation of the Physically Diabled* (1980); and *Group Counseling and Physical Disability*, (1979).

4th Edition

THE PSYCHOLOGICAL AND SOCIAL IMPACT OF DISABILITY

Robert P. Marinelli, EdD, CRC
Arthur E. Dell Orto, PhD, CRC
Editors

 Springer Publishing Company

Copyright © 1999 by Springer Publishing Company, Inc.

Springer Publishing Company, Inc.
536 Broadway
New York, NY 10012–3955

Cover design by Janet Joachim
Acquisition Editor: Helvi Gold
Production Editor: Helen Song

00 01 02 03 / 7 6 5 4

Library of Congress Cataloging-in-Publication Data

The psychological and social impact of disability / Robert P. Marinelli and
    Arthor E. Dell Orto, editors. — 4th ed.
        p.   cm.
    Includes bibliographical references and index.
    ISBN 0-8261-2213-2
    1. Handicapped—United States—Psychology. 2. Handicapped—
Rahabilitation—United States. 3. Handicapped—United States—
Family relationships. 4. Handicapped—United States—Sexual behavior.
5. Handicapped—United States—Public opinion. 6. Public opinion—
United States. I. Marinelli, Robert P., 1942–   . II. Dell Orto, Arthor E.,
1943–   .
HV1553.P75   1999
155.9'16—dc21
                                                                    98-42903
                                                                    CIP

CONTENTS

CONTRIBUTORS

Richard J. Beck, PhD
Southern Illinois University
Carbondale, IL

John J. Benshoff, PhD
Southern Illinois University
Carbondale, IL

Susan Buchanan
Freelance Writer and Consultant
on Disability Issues
Toronto, Ont.

Sandra S. Cole, PhD
University of Michigan Hospitals
Ann Arbor, MI

Theodore M. Cole, MD
University of Michigan Hospitals
Ann Arbor, MI

Larry Davidson. PhD
Yale University School of Medicine
New Haven, CT

Deb Ditillo, PhD
University of Arizona
Tucson, AZ

Albert Ellis, PhD
Institute for REBT
New York, NY

Sonja Feist-Price, PhD
University of Kentucky
Lexington, KY

Cheryl Gagne, MS
Doctoral Candidate
Boston University
Boston, MA

Robert L. Glueckauf, PhD
Indiana University-Purdue University
at Indianapolis
Indianapolis, IN

Harlan Hahn, PhD
Disability Forum
Santa Monica, CA

Ruth A. Huebner, PhD
University of Wisconsin-Madison
Madison, WI

Dale L. Johnson, PhD
University of Houston
Houston, TX

Kelly C. M-H. Keany, PhD
Indiana University-Purdue University
at Indianapolis
Indianapolis, IN

Susan D. M. Kelley, PhD
University of South Florida
Tampa, FL

Martin Koehler, BS
Boston University
Boston, MA

Nancy J. Lane, PhD
Minister
Elmira, NY

Karen G. Langer, PhD
New York University Medical Center
New York, NY

Ruth Torkelson Lynch, PhD
University of Wisconsin-Madison
Madison, WI

Diane T. Marsh, PhD
University of Pittsburgh at Greensburg
Greensburg, PA

Leslie C. McAllan, PhD
University of Arizona
Tucson, AZ

Henry McCarthy, PhD
Louisiana State University Medical
    Center
New Orleans, LA

Bruce D. Miller, MD
University of Rochester School of
    Medicine
Rochester, NY

Kim T. Mueser, PhD
Dartmouth Medical School
Concord, NH

Kenneth P. Nunn, PhD
New Children's Hospital
Parramatta, Australia

Barbara O'Rourke, MS
Doctoral Candidate, University
    of Iowa
Iowa City, IA

David Pfeiffer, PhD
Suffolk University
Boston, MA

John Schatzlein, MS
Senior Rehabilitation Consultant
Iowa City, IA

LeRoy Spaniol, PhD
Boston University
Boston, MA

David Stayner, PhD
Yale University, School of Medicine
New Haven, CT

Jay R. Stewart, PhD
Bowling Green State University
Bowling Green, OH

Edna Mora Szymanski, PhD
University of Wisconsin-Madison
Madison, WI

Kenneth R. Thomas, EdD
University of Wisconsin-Madison
Madison, WI

Roberta B. Trieschmann, PhD
Psychologist
Scottsdale, AZ

Henry T. Trueba, PhD
University of Houston
Houston, TX

Carolyn L. Vash, PhD
Psychologist
Attadena, CA

Dale Walsh, MA
Doctoral Candidate
Boston University
Boston, MA

Lee Ann Watson-Armstrong, MS
*Doctoral Candidate, University
  of Iowa*
Iowa City, IA

Stephen T. Wegener, PhD
*Johns Hopkins University, School
  of Medicine*
Baltimore, MD

Kathy Weingarten, PhD
Psychologist
Newton Centre, MA

Miranda Eve Weingarten Worthen
Consumer
Newton Centre, MA

FOREWORD

The study of rehabilitation is changing radically, if not rapidly. The eventual prospects of this movement are indeed revolutionary in view of the knowledge based on the lived experience of people with disabilities rather than professional expertise; a shift from the exploration of individual to social causes of endemic problems; and a quest for solutions through changes in laws and public policy instead of personal adjustment or motivation. But the transition is not yet complete. As a result, some of the most advanced research on rehabilitation currently embodies an unusual amalgam of divergent conceptual orientations. Students and others interested in this subject, therefore, need to understand several major sources of contrasting approaches to the investigation of disability.

The paradigm that has dominated research and practice in rehabilitation for many years emerged primarily from a theoretical construct in medicine that was highly successful in ameliorating physical maladies. This framework had often been joined with an economic formulation, which defines disability as an inability to work. From both vantage points, the focus of researchers seldom has exceeded a clinical examination of the human body or of occupational capacities and talents lodged within a single individual; and the search for remedies has concentrated on attempts either to enhance vocational skills or to "fix" supposed bodily defects or deficiencies. These views have tended to preclude the study of external phenomena including the effects of an inaccessibly and inhospitably built environment or the organization and structure of the economy, especially a system designed to provide services instead of agricultural or industrial labor. This combination of medical and economic perspectives, fundamentally founded on a notion of functional limitations or loss, treats disability as a physical or psychological deviation from the vague image of a "normal" or perfectible individual, an image that has never been fully or specifically delineated. Nonetheless, the implicit suppositions of this model are so strict that any person with a significant disability, who engages in common occupational or personal conduct, often is regarded paternalistically as an extraordinary "success story" and a source of inspiration rather than simply as another human being going about the routines of everyday life.

The peculiar blend of work and medical influences that formed rehabilitation surfaced most prominently after World War I and World War II. The economic dimension of the program developed first as a result of a growing interest in vocational education, the fear that unemployed disabled veterans would become ubiquitous beggars, a boundless optimism about the capacity of the American economy to generate an insatiable demand for employees, and a pattern of "creaming" that actually compelled rehabilitation officials to give the greatest help to the least disabled civilians. Despite these efforts, employers have continued to use disability as a means of sorting or discarding unwanted job applicants; and the unemployment rate for qualified adults with disabilities who want to work has persistently hovered around two thirds in almost all advanced industrialized nations.

The distinctively medical element of rehabilitation flourished after the Second World War under the aegis of Dr. Howard A. Rusk, Dr. Henry H. Kessler, Dr. Karl Menninger, and Mary Switzer. Since disability was equated with functional loss, physicians could not follow the conventional path of acute health care by focusing on the symptoms of an ailment in a particular part of the human body; instead, they borrowed crucial concepts from psychiatry, which is one of few medical specialties concerned with the whole organism instead of specific portions of it. The unstated assumption of many rehabilitationists is that the widespread poverty and unemployment of people with disabilities can be ascribed principally to psychological and emotional problems such as a lack of motivation or poor adjustment that impede them from "overcoming" the effects of their impairments. One difficulty, of course, is that the label of maladjustment has often been applied to the failure either to pursue a job opportunity successfully or to accept the restrictions of an impairment realistically. Most rehabilitationists appear to believe implicitly, however, that changing the personality of an individual with a disability offers the best means of their securing employment as well as mental and physical well-being. Most curricula in rehabilitation, therefore, include a relatively large number of courses or internships on psychological counseling, and a somewhat smaller amount of instruction on tests and measurement, medical diagnosis and vocabulary, and the administration of vocational rehabilitation programs. Only a few classes are usually devoted to the so-called "psychosocial" aspects of disability that should be among the most important parts of a program.

The principal alternative to the traditional model of research and teaching about disability and rehabilitation emerged from people with disabilities themselves who began to publicize the realization that their main problems stemmed from the architectural and attitudinal environment surrounding them rather than from their physical or psychological impairments. This sociopolitical definition of disability formed the basis for a "minority group" paradigm that identified discrimination, bias, and stigma or prejudice as the major barrier confronting citizens with disabilities and that supported the passage of crucial civil rights legislation such as the Americans With Disabilities Act. Some of the emerging issues and research topics implied by this alternative model are included in the fourth edition of *The Psychological and Social Impact of Disability*, which is enhanced by a rich selection of articles on various topics, autobiographical experiences, as well as study questions and disability awareness exercises. The content and focus of this material is a means to help understand and end the pervasive social isolation of people with disabilities and to facilitate an expanded critique of the excessive emphasis on physical attractiveness or perfection in modern society. Other articles explore and address similar concepts focusing on disability culture, legal issues, policy analysis, and the relation between disability and democratic values such as equality, freedom, and justice. The growing recognition of the social origins of disability in a disabling environment instead of organic flaws has relieved many persons of a sense of shame and enabled them to redefine their most salient bodily traits as a life-affirming source of personal and political identity. The onset of disability thus usually yields a different perspective that often is a valuable source of creativity—especially in coping with environmental obstacles that prominent specialists regard as a hallmark of intellectual skills and an essential prerequisite for many problem-solving jobs. In an era when permanent disabilities and chronic rather than acute conditions form America's most prevalent medical problems, positive lessons derived from lived experience with disability in a reformed academic curriculum could be the greatest resource available to physicians and other rehabilitation specialists. Many of them acknowledge the relative futility of heroic or therapeutic intervention but are not content simply to monitor or to ignore such difficulties. Both personal and social improvements can be achieved by embracing rather than overcoming the valuable contributions of life with a disability.

The fourth edition of *The Psychological and Social Impact of Disability* thus presents and addresses many of the issues related to a better understanding, awareness, and appreciation of people living with a disability and with the forces, policies, attitudes, and behaviors that impede or facilitate their options, quality of life, and empowerment.

Harlan Hahn
Santa Monica, California
1998

PREFACE TO THE FOURTH EDITION

THE CHALLENGE AND OPPORTUNITY OF DISABILITY

Disability is a challenge. Disability can also be an opportunity for all involved to better understand, respond to, and validate the totality of the human experience. Disability is not an alien experience that is strange and foreign to us all. It is a common ground that, in one form or another we, or those who are part of our lives, will have to travel for a short, or in some cases, a very long journey.

It is important to note that life's journey with a disability does not necessarily have to be better or worse than it would be without one. Unfortunately this journey is often made more difficult by the existence of negative forces that can frustrate, impede, and negate the goals of self-actualization, independence, recovery, and rehabilitation.

Although these forces such as ignorance, prejudice, negativism, and insensitivity exist in 1999, significant progress has been made toward their understanding, modification, and eradication since the first edition of this book in 1977. The goal of this edition is to present a realistic perspective on disability that validates those people who live with a disability and to explore the reality that our friend Irving Kenneth Zola so clearly stated, "we are all temporarily able bodied." These themes are poignantly presented in the articles but particularly in the ones ending each section that present a personal perspective on the disability experience.

The assumption that guided the earlier editions—disability affects different facets of a person's life—continues in this edition. During the past twenty-two years since the first edition, there has been an explosion of literature, particularly journals, which made the selection of the material for this edition very challenging but also very rewarding. Our goal was to select those articles that captured unique aspects of the psychological and social impact of disability which in turn created a tapestry of themes, issues, perspectives, concerns, and needs. One departure from the earlier editions was that we only included articles that appeared since 1993. Because this decision eliminated the inclusion of some of the classics, we selected those entries that captured more of the present and future issues in the field.

The developmental and social context in which disability occurs and which defines disability has received special emphasis in this edition. A major focus in this broadened definition of disability is on those persons who have physical, intellectual and emotional disabilities, as well as those who have a dual diagnosis. Regardless of the disabling condition, people share similar needs, dreams, aspirations, concerns, and the desire for independence and a reasonable quality of life.

This book is the reflection of the work of others and we want to thank the authors and their publishers for permission to reprint their articles.

We are pleased that Dr. Harlan Hahn, who is a visionary in the field of disability, wrote the Foreword to this book, however, we are saddened by the loss of our mutual friend Irv Zola who wrote the foreword to the second and third editions and to whom this book is dedicated.

We would like to thank Candy Long at West Virginia University for the valuable assistance she provided in manuscript preparation as well as Jeff Dulko and Bethanne Jacobson, PhD candidate at West Virginia University, who assisted with the literature review.

We also gratefully acknowledge the support of Dr. Ursula Springer who has encouraged us to do this fourth edition as well as of Helvi Gold, our editor, who kept us focused during this process.

RPM
ADO
1998

Part I

Perspective on Disability and Consumers

D
isability impacts at many levels. At the personal level various life functions are affected. At the interpersonal level relationships with other individuals typically change. Responses to disability at the social and cultural
levels have resulted in legislative change and improved services and rights. The
effects of disability—personal, interpersonal, and cultural—therefore have significant implications for persons with disabilities, rehabilitation professionals, the
rehabilitation and health system, and our society. The purpose of Part I is to sensitize the reader to these issues by providing both professional and consumer perspectives about disability.

Hahn, in chapter 1, compares the "functional limitations" paradigm, which
forms the basis for the traditional medical and economic definitions of disability
with the newer "minority group" model which is the basis of the sociopolitical
perspective. The latter has contributed to antidiscrimination legislation for persons with disabilities. In a thoughtful and thorough analysis Professor Hahn discusses the principal dimensions of the medical, economic, and sociopolitical
definitions and concludes that there is a need for further investigations of the
sociopolitical model by both disability activists and researchers who are committed to this model.

In chapter 2, Pfeiffer details state laws (past and present) that discriminate
against people with disabilities in the area of domestic relations. He further discusses the Eugenics Movement, which was and continues to be the driving force
behind these laws. His purpose is to enlighten those, including academics, who
do not believe that such discrimination exists, with a hoped for goal of improving the lives of persons with disabilities.

In her discussion of the energy model in chapter 3, Trieschman presents the
conceptual framework and the strategies of the energy model. This model
assumes that happiness leads to physical health and therefore, our beliefs, the
meaning we attach to daily events, and the emotional reaction to these beliefs are
crucial to physical health and well-being. This paradigm is contrasted with the
medical model, which assumes that physical health produces happiness and,

1

therefore, emotional reactions, meaning of life and belief systems are secondary to one's physical health and the practice of medicine. Strategies designed to empower both the professional and the person with the disability to transcend the hopelessness and helplessness that often accompany the disability experience are provided.

Ethical issues and values are integral to the decisions made by rehabilitation professionals and the persons they serve. In chapter 4, Wegener presents an evolving set of ethical models developed to elucidate key issues and facilitate decision making. He presents the deliberative model as a means to prevent and resolve ethical dilemmas. This model emphasizes both providers and consumers acting with empathy and in community.

Walsh, a survivor of long-term psychiatric disability and the mental health system, has also worked in the field of mental health for about 20 years. In chapter 5, she presents her personal path toward recovery and her beliefs regarding that which is necessary to support the recovery process. She believes that significant changes are needed in language, treatment models, power, decision making, and environmental supports to improve the quality of life for persons with disabilities.

1

The Political Implications of Disability Definitions and Data

Harlan Hahn

One of the most significant recent developments in the study of disability is the emergence of a *minority-group* model (Gliedman & Roth, 1980; Hahn, 1985b) as a prominent challenge to what has been called the *functional-limitations* paradigm which traditionally guided the compilation of statistics about this subject (Hahn, 1982, 1985a, 1987). The principal proponents of this new model include people with permanent disabilities who find that earlier research has seemingly had little relevance to their own experience and who argue that policies based on these investigations have not resulted in significant improvements in their lives. Like many other nascent models that have sought to replace conventional paradigms in the physical sciences (Kuhn, 1962), the minority-group concept has encountered covert—and sometimes public—resistance from established professionals who have exerted a dominant influence on disability research. As a result, prior studies have not developed the theoretical implications of the minority-group view to permit the formulation of empirical measures that could be used in the collection of data to test the value of this approach; and, of course, the minority-group perspective has not yet been accepted as a substitute for the functional-limitations paradigm in disability research. Nonetheless, while the traditional theoretical orientation furnished the implicit or explicit foundation for earlier programs, including vocational rehabilitation, Social Security Disability Insurance (SSDI), and Supplemental Security Income (SSI), the minority-group model provided the basis for new antidiscrimination laws such as section 504 of the Rehabilitation Act of 1973, the Civil Rights Restoration Act, and the Americans with Disabilities Act of 1990.

The purpose of this study is to compare the conceptual, operational, and policy implications of the different definitions of disability that have supported the minority-group and functional-limitations paradigms. To avoid unnecessary

From *Journal of Disability Policy Studies,* 4(2) (1993), 41–52. Reprinted with permission.

misunderstandings and controversy, perhaps it is appropriate to note that the ideas presented here encompass both experiential and systematic studies; they are derived from my training as a social scientist who has concentrated on disability research for more than 10 years and from my everyday life as a person who has used crutches and braces or a wheelchair since the age of 6. Thus, this analysis reflects not only an attempt to examine the ramifications of these definitions but also to amplify the theoretical foundations of the minority-group model; the latter effort should facilitate the continuing struggle to introduce this approach for serious consideration by other researchers engaged in the study of disability.

While the functional-limitations model is supported by prevailing *medical* and *economic* understandings of disability, the minority-group paradigm is based on a new *sociopolitical* definition of this phenomenon. Each of these concepts reflects different emphases in Nagi's (1979) classic definition of disability as "an inability or limitation in performing roles and tasks expected of an individual within a social environment." Whereas the medical perspective focuses on inabilities or limitations, the economic notion centers on the performance of (especially vocational) roles and tasks, and the sociopolitical concept stresses the social environment. From the final vantage point, the crucial determination of what can be expected of human beings is shaped primarily by modifications of the environment instead of modifying the individual.

THE MEDICAL VIEW

Perhaps the most commonly accepted meaning of disability in popular understandings of this subject is represented by the medical view which is closely aligned with the notion of impairment or organic pathology. Although the postulates of the *medical model* have been described generally more often than they have been defined specifically, they seem to embrace both sociological and philosophical rather than strictly scientific elements. The former dimension includes the concept of *Aesculapian,* or benevolent, authority (Siegler & Osmond, 1974) and Parson's (1964) analysis of "the sick role," which exempts individuals from ordinary social obligations provided that they submit to professional direction or control until they achieve the ultimate goal of full recovery. Since disabilities represent chronic conditions that cannot be cured through therapeutic intervention, this viewpoint seems to have little direct relevance to the development of theories or policies concerning permanent physical characteristics.

In addition, an important part of the philosophical dimension of the medical model is represented by the principle of etiology, or the study of causation, which has yielded diagnostic categorizations based on causes rather than consequences. Although these classifications have been used for definitional purposes in some programs involving developmental disabilities, the potential usefulness of the medical orientation as a basis for the formulation of disability policy is significantly reduced by the inability to extrapolate functional or other characteristics from these categories. Hence, the use of diagnostic criteria in disability determinations has failed to produce universal or consistent rules (Stone, 1984). The major policy implications of the emphasis on causation in the medical perspective seem to imply an almost exclusive focus on prevention, or the eradication of disabling conditions, that may be interpreted by persons who have already acquired these disabilities as threatening or as an indication of neglect of their problems.

Moreover, the clinical focus on the individual as the unit of analysis has precluded the diagnosis of architectural or other environmental barriers in the treatment of permanent impairments. The operational measurement of the medical understanding of disability in surveys conducted by the National Center for Health Statistics (NCHS) and related studies focuses on the capacity to perform certain routine tasks or *major life activities*. Some of these activities have been included as criteria, along with self-definitional and labeling concepts, in the definition of disability adopted in antidiscrimination laws such as the Americans with Disabilities Act (ADA). Although several of the items in an index derived from NCHS surveys reflect the influence of environmental constraints, analyses have not attempted to draw a clear distinction between limitations that result from physical impairments and difficulties that stem from environmental obstacles. Instead, medical assessments are based on a combined measure that reinforces the impression, which is being increasingly challenged by disabled activists, that disability is a trait lodged within a person rather than a construct of external surroundings.

THE ECONOMIC APPROACH

The definition of disability most widely adopted in public policy is founded on an economic viewpoint that seems to reflect the prevalent tendency in an industrialized society to stipulate physical capabilities as occupational requirements. Hence, ubiquitous questions about disability on application forms, or physical examinations, have been used for many years to facilitate the difficult process of making personnel decisions by screening out individuals who lack the physical attributes that employers deem necessary to perform a job. Prompted in part by a commitment to veterans benefits, vocational training, and economic growth, however, rehabilitation legislation was adopted early in the twentieth century to encourage the employment of persons with disabilities; those programs, however, did not directly challenge the presumed connection between physical capabilities and job qualifications. Disability was not included in the Social Security Act of 1935 in part because of definitional difficulties (Witte, 1963). Federal government benefits for disabled persons deemed unable to engage in "substantial gainful activity" were extended after the war, first, through Social Security Disability Insurance primarily to middle-aged employees considered too old to retrain when they became disabled and, later, to younger individuals with a work history, and then to other individuals with disabilities in a means-tested program that eventually became known as Supplemental Security Income (Erlanger & Roth, 1985).

Significantly, economists have tended to neglect the "industrial reserve army" of housewives and disabled workers who ordinarily act as a buffer on the competitive pressures for jobs in a capitalistic economy; they were hired during World War II, however, when personnel barriers such as physical exams were waived only to be fired again when young nondisabled males returned to the labor force, and these restrictions were reinstated. Moreover, vocational rehabilitation programs have retained a clinical focus on matching unadapted job requirements with the interests and skills of disabled individuals, even though empirical research has documented a correlation between awards as well as applications for disability benefits and geographic areas experiencing economic recession (Howards, Brehm, & Nagi, 1980). These programs have been augmented by public-relations and educational activities sponsored by a presidential committee to "hire the handicapped" and by affirmative action policies, which have never been enforced. America has generally relied on voluntary measures to promote the employment of disabled persons instead of the quotas adopted in several European nations that have not been effectively implemented again in part because of definitional problems (Hahn, 1984).

Thus more than two-thirds of disabled adults of working age do not have jobs; and the tendency to treat disability and unemployability as equivalent terms at least in some welfare policies remained relatively undisturbed until the passage of antidiscrimination laws. The operational measure of the economic definition of disability is any "limitations on the amount or kind of work" that a person can perform. (The relative nature of this standard is perhaps best illustrated by an exchange with a graduate student who reacted to my negative answer to this issue on a questionnaire by saying, "But, after all, you couldn't be quarterback for the Los Angeles Rams." Without hesitation, I replied, "But neither could you.") Along with medical assessments, economic measures do not seem to provide a clear, consistent, or universal standard for evaluating the link between disability and various sorts of vocational or other capabilities.

THE SOCIOPOLITICAL PERSPECTIVE

The sociopolitical definition of disability, which is the foundation of the minority-group model, concentrates on interactions between individuals and the environment. This approach also focuses primarily on the social or attitudinal environment rather than the present configuration of natural or built surroundings. Thus, the appropriate standard of assessment is the as-yet-unrealized ideal of a totally nondiscriminatory habitat adapted to the needs of everybody, which seems to lie within the reach of technological feasibility, even if it is not yet within the grasp of human imagination. Departures from these guidelines, such as architectural or communications barriers which imply that an unspecified level of functional proficiency is needed to master the existing context of everyday life, may be regarded as forms of discrimination that can ultimately be ascribed to attitudes signifying a desire for social and physical separation from persons with disabilities. Although the environmental criteria of the sociopolitical approach are still necessarily abstract, significant progress has already been made in developing specific operational applications of this definition.

Perhaps the principal difference between the sociopolitical perspective and the medical or economic definitions of disability is the focus on public attitudes rather than physical limitations as the primary source of the difficulties facing disabled people. Other postulates of the minority-group model specify that all facets of the environment are molded by public policy and that government policies reflect widespread social attitudes or values (Hahn, 1986); as a result, existing features of architectural design, job requirements, and daily life that have a discriminatory impact on disabled citizens cannot be viewed merely as happenstance or coincidence. On the contrary, they seem to signify conscious or unconscious sentiments supporting a hierarchy of dominance and subordination between nondisabled and disabled segments of the population that is fundamentally incompatible with legal principles of freedom and equality. The logical implications of these propositions have not yet been fully explored; but constitutional standards do not appear to be satisfied, for example, by architectural restraints that deny citizens in wheelchairs equal access to public facilities or freedom of movement in their own neighborhoods, by communication barriers that inhibit free speech for persons with vision or hearing impairments, or by the requirements that place disabled employees at a competitive disadvantage by compelling them to expend extraordinary amounts of time and effort simply to perform routine personal or work activities.

One might interpret the interactive connection between persons and the environment embodied in the sociopolitical definition as indicating the need for a social theory that presupposes an indissoluble link between subject and object and that would preclude empirical measurement. However, the emphasis in the definition on the attitudes elicited by people with disabilities provides a method of assessing the problems of disabled citizens from a sociopolitical vantage point. Whereas the effects of a disabling environment are the penultimate origins of the restrictions encountered by persons with disabilities, an even more fundamental source of their difficulties can be located; it is the social attitudes of the nondisabled majority that may finally be responsible for virtually all types of environmental restraints. Thus, from a sociopolitical perspective, people with disabilities have been subjected to prejudice and discrimination on the basis of visible or labeled physical differences.

These embodied characteristics usually are revealed by personal appearance or by information reported in job applications or other records; hence, attitudinal discrimination reflects unfavorable perceptions that exist in the minds of employers or other observers instead of the inherent attributes of disabled individuals. Consequently, people with disabilities are a minority group because they have been the objects of prejudice and discrimination. Coleman (1986) has speculated that these manifestations of stigma may have originated from infant "stranger anxiety" and from the childhood effort to form a self-identity by differentiating what is "like me" and "not like me." And the early propensity to fear and to retreat from persons who are perceived as alien or significantly different is, of course, reinforced by the subsequent process of socialization and by social structures that institutionalize the separation of disabled and nondisabled portions of the population in a manner similar to the segregation imposed on other minority groups.

Principal Dimensions

While the extensive ramifications of a sociopolitical approach to research on attitudes toward persons with disabilities have not yet been thoroughly investigated, preliminary hypotheses have proposed that the principal dimensions of such perceptions may reflect a division between so-called *existential anxiety*, which is closely associated with the functional-limitations paradigm, and what has been termed *aesthetic anxiety*, which seems to be implied by the minority-group model (Hahn, 1988). While the former concept seems to embody projected fears or apprehensions about human mortality and about the prospect that physical impairments could interfere with a preferred lifestyle, the latter phrase refers not only to the extraordinary stress concentrated on culturally defined ideals of corporeal beauty or attractiveness, but also to the overwhelming insecurities that may prompt nondisabled women and men to shun or to avoid others who are viewed as unattractive or unappealing. Aesthetic worries are founded not only on the enormous cultural social importance of physical appearance (Hatfield & Sprecher, 1986), but also on the common proclivity to seek social acceptance by striving for conformity with perceived similarities among human beings and by evading contact with those who are physically different.

The essential elements of the sociopolitical viewpoint on disability are represented by the concepts of *visibility* and *labeling*, which can be operationalized and measured in survey research. Whereas visibility could be assessed not only by direct observation but also by questions about whether a person has a disability that is immediately obvious to others or whether it would become known only through close scrutiny and extensive familiarity, the impact of labeling might be appraised by queries about the extent to which people have never been compelled to affix the badge of disability to themselves on an application form or on other records. The former question is somewhat similar to the item adopted in the Harris (1986) survey of disabled Americans, which asked whether or not most people would "consider you a disabled or handicapped person" either "at a first meeting" or after they had gotten to know you "fairly well." But the use of the rather evaluative term *consider*, instead of a more empirical word such as *see* or *recognize*, may have allowed some disabled persons to indulge in a sort of psychological denial about the possible effects of their most salient physical characteristics on the reactions of others. Clearly, in the context of a cultural propensity to confuse disability and inability, for example, many persons displaying the conspicuous marks of a disability naturally might deny that other people would consider them disabled.

There is surprisingly little, if any, available evidence regarding the correlation between the visible or labeled attributes of a disability and the prevalence or incidence of discrimination. Nor is there presently any extensive information concerning the association between these variables and other demographic indicators such as socioeconomic status, family ties, unemployment rates, and related social problems. Obviously, since discrimination cannot occur without visual or written knowledge of a stigmatizing trait such as a disability, these studies could disclose potentially valuable statistics for the administration of antidiscrimination policies such as the Americans with Disabilities Act. At a minimum, government officials might want to know the potential size of the group affected by discrimination as well as the possible magnitude of the problems they could encounter. There is an imperative need, then, to secure the studies and the funding necessary to examine these issues by granting the minority-group paradigm and the sociopolitical definition parity or attention comparable to the vast amount of survey and other research founded on medical and economic views of disability.

Political Identity

There is, however, another crucial aspect of the sociopolitical understanding of disability that has major political implications for future methods of seeking to ameliorate this problem. By ascribing the meaning of disability to external rather than internal sources and to a disabling environment instead of personal flaws or deficiencies, the sociopolitical viewpoint has permitted disabled citizens to engage in the process of translating formerly discredited bodily attributes into a dynamic sense of political identity. For some disabled individuals, including the leadership of the social and political movement of people with disabilities, the effects of this change have been profoundly liberating. As Anspach (1979) noted, this transformation also has allowed women and men with disabilities to develop a positive feeling of self-esteem and a critical appraisal of society as a dual foundation for political activism. But the legislative victories of the disability rights movement have been achieved without the support of a massive constituency of disabled voters capable of exerting a decisive impact on government programs. Ironically, perhaps one of the major reasons for their relative lack of political strength can be attributed to the same sense of stigma that has been a primary determinant of the subordinate role of disabled persons in modern society. Most individuals with disabilities usually have attempted to gain social acceptance by "passing," or denying, their status as disabled persons. As a prominent cultural symbol of shame, disability has customarily yielded a reluctance to identify openly with this salient corporeal feature, especially among men and women with relatively imperceptible physical disabilities or chronic health conditions. Yet, as research on ethnicity has revealed (Lieberson & Waters, 1986; Waters,

1990), self-identification is one of the most valid, if not necessarily consistent or reliable, measures of group membership. In fact, since disability as well as ethnicity and even age or gender are fundamentally social or cultural constructs rather than organic or inherent characteristics, changes in the willingness to identify with these groups might be a valuable index of the electoral influence of different segments of the population. Although data based on self-identification seem more relevant to political than to policy issues, the questionable use of ethnic measures to create immigration quotas as well as the tendency to equate disability with unemployability or physiological defects underscore the desirability of ensuring that statistics fulfill the interests of those from whom they are collected instead of the exclusive ambitions of politicians or experts who might be more concerned about the survival or growth of favorite government programs than about the needs of the group they are supposed to serve.

CONCLUSION

The definitions employed in gathering information frequently are shaped more by the theoretical orientation of dominant research paradigms, as well as the primary objectives of policymakers and professionals, than by the group which is the subject of interest. In disability studies, this hegemonic position long has been occupied by medical and economic definitions that share comparable assumptions about the priority of functional limitations. Despite the struggle by some researchers and by disabled people themselves to introduce the minority-group paradigm and the sociopolitical definition of disability, the understandable delay in acquiring the support of established professionals for these innovative approaches has meant that pioneering laws based on the new perspectives were approved even before basic data founded on these understandings had been collected. The two as-yet-unanswered questions that seem to be most compatible with these trends revolve around visibility or labeling and self-identification. To restore a sense of balance in the study of disability policy, there is a need for increased support of investigations that reflect the interests and objectives both of disabled activists who precipitated and sustained this shift in conceptual paradigms and of researchers who are committed to increased exploration of the implications of the minority-group model.

REFERENCES

Anspach, R. R. (1979). From stigma to identity politics: Political activism among the physically disabled and former mental patients. *Social Science and Medicine, 13A* 765–773.

Coleman, L. M. (1986). Stigma: An enigma demystified. In S. C. Ainlay, G. Becker, & L. M. Coleman (Eds.), *The dilemma of difference: A multidisciplinary view of stigma* (pp. 211–232). New York: Plenum Press.

Erlanger, H. S., & Roth, W. (1985). Disability policy: The parts and the whole. *American Behavioral Scientist, 28,* 319–345.

Gliedman, J., & Roth, W. (1980). *The unexpected minority.* New York: Harcourt Brace Jovanovich.

Hahn, H. (1982). Disability and rehabilitation policy: Is paternalistic neglect really benign? *Public Administration Review, 42*(4), 385–389.

Hahn, H. (1984). *The issue of equality: European perceptions of employment policy for disabled persons.* New York: World Rehabilitation Fund.

Hahn, H. (1985a). Changing perceptions of disability and the future of rehabilitation. In L. G. Perlman & G. F. Austin (Eds.), *Societal influences in rehabilitation planning: A blueprint for the 21st century* (pp. 53–64). Alexandria, VA: National Rehabilitation Association.

Hahn, H. (1985b). Toward a politics of disability: Definitions, disciplines, and policies. *The Social Science Journal, 22(4),* 87–105.

Hahn, H. (1986). Disability and the urban environment: A perspective on Los Angeles. *Society and Space, 4,* 273–288.

Hahn, H .(1987). Civil rights for disabled Americans: The foundations of a political agenda. In A. Gartner & T. Joe (Eds.), *Images of the disabled/disabling images* (pp. 181–203). New York: Praeger.

Hahn, H. (1988). The politics of physical differences: Disability and discrimination. *Journal of Social Issues, 44*(1), 39–48.

Harris, L. (1986). *The ICD survey of disabled Americans: Bringing disabled Americans into the mainstream.* New York: International Center for the Disabled.

Hatfield, E., & Sprecher, S. (1986). *Mirror, mirror . . .: The importance of looks in everyday life.* Albany: State University of New York Press.

Howards, I., Brehm, H. P., & Nagi, S. Z. (1980). *Disability: From social problem to federal program.* New York: Praeger.

Kuhn, T. S. (1962). *The structure of scientific revolutions.* Chicago: University of Chicago Press.

Lieberson, S., & Waters, M. C. (1986). Ethnic groups influx: The changing ethnic responses of American whites. *The Annals of the American Academy of Political and Social Sciences, 487,* 79–91.

Nagi, S. Z. (1979). The concept and measurement of disability. In E. D. Berkowitz (Ed.), *Disability policies and government programs* (pp. 1–25). New York: Praeger.

Parsons, T. (1964). *Social structure and personality.* New York: The Free Press.

Siegler, M., & Osmond, H. (1975). *Models of medicine, models of madness.* New York: Macmillan.

Stone, D. A. (1984). *The disabled state.* Philadelphia, PA: Temple University Press.

Waters, M. C. (1990). *Ethnic options: Choosing identities in America.* Berkeley: University of California Press.

Witte, E. (1963). *The development of the Social Security Act.* Madison: University of Wisconsin Press.

2

Eugenics and Disability Discrimination

David Pfeiffer

INTRODUCTION

At the weekly luncheon of a service club in Massachusetts two men—one a local federal official who is well known for his civil rights work and who is black, the other an advocate for disabled people and who is disabled and the author of this piece—were invited to give short presentations about civil rights. The federal official made the comment that blacks were the only group whose civil rights had been limited by statute. When the disability advocate demurred, the federal official became very incensed. Like many persons the official was unaware of the many statutory ways in which the civil rights of disabled people were and still are violated through state and local government laws in the US.

This same misconception is widespread in the academic community. Recently an anonymous reviewer wrote, as a reason for rejecting an article similar to the present piece, that "developmentally disabled persons were always treated differently". It is not known what definition of developmental disabilities the reviewer held, but the point of the article was that all people with disabilities were either treated as developmentally disabled persons who were not legally competent or else lived with the real possibility that they would be treated in such a way. That is, there was a real possibility that a person with a disability would be institutionalized, sterilized, and be denied all parental rights. Seemingly, for the anonymous reviewer, it was all right to treat developmentally disabled persons that way, but other persons with a disability would never be so treated.

The purpose of this piece is to present evidence that both the federal official and the reviewer were wrong. People with disabilities, any disability, had their rights limited in the immediate past in the US and still do so today by existing state statutes and the courts' incorrect interpretation of other statutes. They are constantly faced with the possibility of being deprived of fundamental rights that

From *Disability & Society,* 9(4) (1994), 481–499. Reprinted with permission.

non-disabled persons enjoy. The great interest today in discovering which genes cause inherited impairments only accentuates the problem. As Rothstein (1992) points out, the Americans with Disabilities Act is only a first step toward fundamental changes necessary to avoid widespread discrimination based upon genetic testing.

The view of many scholars is represented in a law review article by Robert and Marcia Burgdorf entitled "The wicked witch is almost dead" (Burgdorf & Burgdorf, 1977). It discussed the problems of US Supreme Court Justice Oliver Wendell Holmes' opinion in Buck v. Bell, 274 US 200 (1927), in which a woman labelled feebleminded was sterilized against her will. Calling Holmes' opinion embarrassing, the authors (p. 1033) concluded:

> . . . the decision was incorrect on its facts, was based on now discredited scientific theories, relied upon inaccurate analogies, applied inappropriate constitutional standards, and was in conflict with many philosophical principles of the American governmental system.

The Burgdorfs called for an end to compulsory sterilization laws in this country and concluded their article with the sentence: "Fifty years of Buck v. Bell is enough." This ending was a reference to Holmes' infamous phrase in the end of his opinion: "Three generations of imbeciles are enough." Nevertheless, contrary to what many persons believe, it was never overruled and is still the law of the land in the US.

DOMESTIC RELATIONS

The right to have children, to marry, and to raise one's children are taken for granted by most US citizens. These rights are not automatic for disabled persons. As will be recounted below, the Eugenics Movement greatly influenced public laws regarding domestic relations in this country over the last century.

Sterilization

During the nineteenth century and into the twentieth century sterilization was a common remedy for 'feeblemindedness', as most disabilities were called. Before 1900 castration by removal of ovaries or testicles was the only method available for sterilization. During the third quarter of the nineteenth century the superintendent of the Winfield Kansas State Home for the Feebleminded castrated 44 boys and 14 girls before being forced to stop for medical (not legal) reasons. However, around 1900 Dr Harry Sharpe of the Indiana State Reformatory developed the procedure of vasectomy which is simple and cheap. About the same time in Europe the procedure of salpingectomy for women was developed. Sterilization on a large scale was then begun even though there was no legal basis for it. Dr Sharpe alone sterilized 600–700 hundred boys in the Indiana State Reformatory (Burgdorf, 1980, p. 860).

In Indiana in 1907 the first involuntary sterilization law in the country was enacted. By 1911 Washington, California, Connecticut, and New Jersey enacted involuntary sterilization laws. By 1930 a total of 33 states had enacted such laws although in three states—New Jersey in 1913, New York in 1918, and Indiana in 1921—the laws were struck down as unconstitutional. In Michigan a law was enacted, but struck down in 1918. Seven years later a version of the Michigan statute was accepted by the courts as constitutionally valid. The US Supreme Court then upheld involuntary sterilization laws in 1927 in Buck v. Bell, 274 US 200.

Even though Buck v. Bell has never been overruled by the US Supreme Court, some scholars (Burgdorf, 1980, p. 857) say that the reasoning used by Holmes was rejected in Skinner v. Oklahoma, 316 US 535 (1942), and is therefore no longer governing. In the case of Skinner v. Oklahoma a person who was convicted of larceny, stealing a chicken, was sentenced, as the law provided, to be sterilized because of prior convictions. The involuntary sterilization law would not have been applied if the crime had been another crime such as embezzlement. The Supreme Court struck down the Oklahoma law on the basis of equal protection. The Court said that the difference between the two crimes of theft and embezzlement could not be supported. As the Court wrote (Skinner v. Oklahoma, 316 US 535 at 542):

> Oklahoma makes no attempt to say that he who commits larceny by trespass [the chicken theft] or trick or fraud has biologically inheritable traits which he who commits embezzlement lacks. . . . We have not the slightest basis for inferring . . . that the inheritability of criminal traits follows the neat legal distinctions which the law has marked between those two offenses.

The US Supreme Court in the Skinner Case found that the contention of inheritable criminal traits was sound. The law was struck down because it violated the principle of equal protection. This principle guaranteed to the chicken thief equal treatment which other criminals committing similar crimes would receive. Since an embezzler would not face the same punishment of forced sterilization, the Supreme Court struck down the law. Buck v. Bell remained the law of the land.

It is also widely argued that in Roe v. Wade, 410 US 113 (1973), the US Supreme Court established a fundamental right of privacy which would prevent compulsory sterilization. The Roe Case, however, was decided by a 5–4 vote. There is considerable sentiment in the Courts, in the legal profession, and in public opinion that Roe should be overturned. If it were to be overturned, this protection against compulsory sterilization would vanish. Even if it is not overturned, the right of privacy is limited in the US Supreme Court's June 1986 decision in Bowers v. Hardwick. In the Bowers Case the Supreme Court upheld the right of a state, in this case Georgia, to invade the privacy of the bedroom to observe if sodomy was being performed. The right of privacy is not a sufficient shield.

Another argument that Buck v. Bell is no longer the law of the land is the fact that in it the Court relied upon the police power of the state to uphold

Virginia's compulsory sterilization law. The police power gives the state the right to act to protect the public health, safety, and welfare. While it is probably true that an argument based solely upon the police power would not be accepted by the Court, it is by no means certain. And in many cases the Supreme Court has agreed that the police power along with other powers of the state can be used to uphold a law or an action.

Nevertheless, there are more persuasive arguments today for the legality of involuntary sterilization than the ones used by Holmes. In upholding the Virginia statute Holmes used the 'rational basis' test. This test provides that if a rational basis for a statute can be established and that there are no other problems, the courts should not invalidate the act. The Court found a rational basis and therefore did not strike down the law. Scholars today (Murdock, 1974) contend that more than a rational basis would be needed to uphold a compulsory sterilization law for disabled people. While their argument may be correct, it is not relevant. The defense of involuntary sterilizations today is based upon the doctrine of *parens patriae* which means, in a loose way, 'father power'. That is, fathers—both biological and legal—know what is in the best interest of the 'child' and can force the 'child' to comply even if the 'child' is an adult who happens to have a disability.

A 1975 North Carolina statute (General Statutes 35-50) which provided for the sterilization of mentally defective persons was successfully defended under the doctrine of *parens patriae.* The statute gives the following definition of a mentally defective person (General Statutes 35-1.1):

> A 'mental defective' shall mean a person who is not mentally ill, but whose mental development is so retarded that he has not acquired enough self-control, judgment, and discretion to manage himself and his affairs, and for whose own welfare or that of others, supervision, guidance, care, or control is necessary or advisable. The term shall be construed to include 'feeble-minded', 'idiot', and 'imbecile'.

All that is necessary for sterilization of such a person is for the superintendent of an institution or a county director of social services to obtain a court order for it. In fact, it is the duty of the superintendent or county director to initiate such proceedings whenever the official feels it is in the person's best interest or the public's interest. If a superintendent or county director can convince a judge that a person with a disability can not manage day-to-day affairs, needs guidance, and would 'benefit' from the sterilization, then the judge can order that it be done.

With some procedural modifications, the statute was upheld in NCARC v. North Carolina, 420 F. Supp. 451 (1976). In 22 states a similar law exists including Arizona (Revised Statutes 36-532 ff.), California (Penal Code 2670), Connecticut (General Laws 17-19), Delaware (16 Code 5701 ff.), Indiana (Statutes 1973, 16-13-13-1 ff.), Maine (Revised Statutes 34-2461 ff.), Michigan (Statutes 14.381 ff.), Minnesota (Statutes 252A.13), New Hampshire (Revised Statutes 1 74:1 ff.), South Carolina (Code 44-47-10 ff.), and Virginia (Code 37.1-1 56-71). Involuntary sterilization is specifically authorized in 14 states: Arkansas, Colorado, Connecticut, Delaware, Maine, Minnesota, Mississippi, North

Carolina, New Jersey, Oklahoma, Oregon, South Carolina, Utah, Virginia, and West Virginia. (Brakel *et al.,* 1985, pp. 523–524) Epilepsy is still included as a permissible reason for compulsory sterilization in Delaware, Mississippi, and South Carolina. Most states base the action on the person's or society's 'best' interest, but nine states still base it on an eugenic argument. Even in the absence of a law authorizing sterilization, courts can and do compel persons with disabilities to undergo compulsory sterilization with no regard of the disabled person's view of his or her 'best' interest. It is a threat to all disabled persons in the US (Brantlinger, 1992; Elkins & Anderson, 1992; Ferguson & Ferguson, 1992; Fredericks, 1992; Kaeser, 1992; Macklin & Gaylin, 1981).

Marriage

The right to marry is an important one which most people take for granted. This right is subject to regulation by the states because, in part, it establishes a contract and governs inheritance and ownership of real property. State legislation which appears to limit this right receives close examination by the US Supreme Court in the context of the Fourteenth Amendment as a result of Meyer v. Nebraska, 262 US 390 (1923). In the Meyer case the Court declared the right to marry to be a fundamental right under the US Constitution. Any limitation of this right must respect the principles of equal protection and due process. The Court struck down a state statute which prohibited interracial marriage as a violation of these principles in Loving v. Virginia, 388 US 1 (1967). However, the Court never struck down a state statute which limited marriage by or to a disabled person even when equal protection was clearly violated.

For example, Connecticut had a statute which prohibited any man who was ". . . epileptic, imbecile, or feeble-minded" from marrying a woman under 45 years of age, the presumed limit of child-bearing. A woman under 45 years of age who was ". . . epileptic, imbecile, or feeble-minded" could not marry regardless of the man's age. In Gould v. Gould, 61 A. 604 (1905), this statute was upheld by the Connecticut courts. While acknowledging that under the Connecticut constitution marriage is a fundamental right, the court refused to strike down the statute. It said that the legislature also had constitutionally set a minimum age to marry and had prohibited persons related by blood from marrying. One of the persons in this case had epilepsy and the court wrote:

> That epilepsy is a disease of a peculiarly serious and revolting character, tending to weaken mental force, and often descending from parent to child, or entailing upon the offspring of the sufferer some other grave form of nervous malady, is a matter of common knowledge, of which courts will take judicial notice. . . . One mode of guarding against the perpetuation of epilepsy obviously is to forbid sexual intercourse with those afflicted by it, and to preclude such opportunities for sexual intercourse as marriage furnishes. To impose such a restriction . . . is no invasion of the equality of all men before the law, if it applies equally to all . . . who belong to a certain class of persons. . . .

The class of persons included all those with epilepsy so, the Connecticut court reasoned, there was no denial of equal protection or any other right. Members of the class of people with epilepsy, by implication, do not share the equal rights of the class of US citizens. Similar laws also existed, at that time, in Michigan, Minnesota, Kansas, and Ohio. The Connecticut act was not repealed until 1969.

A 1953 statute in Pennsylvania (48 Statutes 1-1 ff.) prohibits a marriage certificate from being issued to a person who has epilepsy, is "weakminded, insane, or . . . of unsound mind" except under a court order. In Washington (26 Revised Code 26.04.030) marriage is prohibited if either party:

. . . is a common drunkard, habitual criminal, imbecile, feeble-minded person, idiot or insane person, or person who has theretofore been afflicted with hereditary insanity, . . . unless it is established that procreation is not possible by the couple intending to marry.

The Massachusetts prohibition (General Laws 207, section 5) reads:

An insane person, an idiot, or a feeble-minded person under commitment to an institution for the feeble-minded, to the custody or supervision of the department of mental health, or to an institution for medical defectives, shall be incapable of contracting marriage.

Thirty eight states and the District of Columbia either ban or closely restrict the right of a mentally retarded person to marry. (Wells, 1983) This basic right is not guaranteed to disabled people.

Parenting

The right to parent, to raise your biological children, is also recognized as a fundamental right by the US Supreme Court. However, it can be overridden on the grounds of the health or safety of the child (Bernstein, 1991; Sackett, 1991). Even though it has little relationship to these grounds, the common basis for removing children from disabled parents is parental IQ. (State ex rel. Paul v. Department of Public Welfare, 170 So.2d 549 (1965), Louisiana Court of Appeals; In re McDonald, 201 N.W.2d 447 (1972), Iowa Supreme Court; Sexton v. J.E.H., 355 N.W.2d 828 (1984), North Dakota Supreme Court; and In re G.C.P., 680 S.W.2d 429 (1984), Missouri Court of Appeals) Research shows that IQ tests are biased and limited (McCall, 1984; Sternberg & Gardner, 1984) a fact recognized by the courts in education cases (Larry P. v. Riles, 495 F. Supp. 926 (1979), N.D. California; PASE v. Hannon, 506 F. Supp. 831 (1980), N.D. Illinois). Nevertheless, disabled parents must prove their ability to parent to a degree beyond that of non-disabled parents. A couple in California who were hearing and speech impaired, but quite capable of parenting, were prevented from adopting a child in Adoption of Richardson, 59 Cal. Rptr. 323 (1967).

Recent cases may indicate a new trend. A California trial court judge had removed two children from a father's custody because he was a quadriplegic. The trial court judge had concluded that the father could never be a 'good' parent because he could not, for example, play catch with his son. The California Supreme Court, In re Marriage of Carney, 598 P.2d 36 (1979), sharply rebuked the trial judge and overturned his decision. A district court judge in Idaho had refused a mother custody of her two children because she had epilepsy. The Idaho Supreme Court reversed the decision in Moye v. Moye, 627 P.2d 799 (1981). In Michigan the Michigan Court of Appeals, in Department of Social Services v. McDuel, 369 N.W.2d 912 (1985), overturned a lower court decision because it had improperly interpreted 'mental illness' to be the same as 'physical illness'. And in Johnson v. J.K.C., Sr., 841 S.W.2d 198 (Mo. Ct. App. 1992), the Missouri Court of Appeals reinstated the parental rights of a 'mildly mentally retarded' couple in regard to their 9-year-old son because there was a bonding between son and father and because the child's advanced age meant that the parents could provide for his care. However, it upheld the termination of parental rights in regard to a five-year-old daughter because of her age and the fact that she had never lived with her parents.

From the viewpoint of the child, California (Civil Code 227b) is the only state in the union which allows a parent to petition to have an adoption decree annulled on the basis of a disability in the child. The statute provides that if within 5 years of the final decree the child gives evidence of a developmental disability which is so severe that the child would be considered not adoptable, that the disability was the result of pre-adoption conditions, and that the parents did not know of the condition, then the adoptive parents can ask the court to annul the adoption (*The Legal Rights of Persons with Epilepsy*, 1985, p. 107). That occurred in Christopher C. v. Kay C., 278 Cal. Rptr. 907, when the California Court of Appeals affirmed a lower court decision to grant a petition to set aside an adoption because the child had an undisclosed mental illness.

Perhaps the courts are changing their view of persons with disabilities who are parents. At the same time they seem to be making it easier for involuntary sterilization to occur. Once sterilized a person with a disability no longer has the chance to have biological children and so the problem involving parenting will not arise since it is also all but impossible for them to adopt a child.

STEREOTYPES AND DISABILITY

These laws and court cases are based upon common stereotypes of disability and disabled persons. They are based upon several inaccurate assumptions about disabled people. (Bogdan & Biklen, 1977; Bogdan & Taylor, 1987, 1989; Dearing, 1981; Longmore, 1985; Wright, 1985). The first one is the assumption of general maladjustment of disabled persons.

There are numerous studies which purport to show that disabled people are maladjusted, but the studies suffer from grave methodological problems involving the instruments used. Just as bias exists in IQ tests, there are biases in instruments used to gauge adjustment. In addition, if the researcher expects maladjustment in disabled persons, that is what will be found, a self-fulfilling prophecy. Furthermore, there is a strong tendency in these studies to attribute any deviation from the norm to the existence of a disability: if a person is disabled, then the person must be maladjusted. The truth is that the assumption of general maladjustment is a gross over simplification of the facts conditioned by prejudice as careful analysis of these studies show.

The second assumption is that of tragedy. Non-disabled persons can not imagine how disabled persons can bear their lives. The existence of a disability appears to them to be an overwhelming tragedy, a life filled with suffering and frustration. It is true that disabled persons suffer and become frustrated, but so do non-disabled persons. There are many carefully done studies which show that things like divorce or death cause more pain, suffering, and tragedy in the lives of disabled persons than the existence of a disability.

The next assumption is closely related to the first two and that is the assumption of excessive frustration. It is simply not correct that disabled people experience more frustration than other people. Perhaps disabled persons are more aware of frustrating, unnecessary barriers placed before them, but non-disabled persons also experience excessive frustration. If a researcher expects to find excessive frustration, it will be found just like general maladjustment will be found. But the way to overcome frustration for both disabled and non-disabled persons is to remove the frustrating barriers, not to counsel more adjustment.

These assumptions are all based upon yet another incorrect assumption: the assumption of disability as a personal attribute. A disability is a central part of the life and identity of a disabled person, but it is not simply a personal attribute. It is rooted firmly in the environment. In certain environments particular disabilities are not noticed while in other environments they are very noticeable. A disability is often a limitation because of an environmental barrier which is unnecessary, unneeded, largely unwanted, but there because of someone's unthinking.

The final assumption is the myth of sin. That is, the cause of a disability must be someone's sin or wrong doing: the disabled person, the parents, the physician, the drunk-driver, and so on. Perhaps the disability can be traced to a specific event, but the reason for that event is certainly not sin on the part of someone who ends up with a disability. Frequently, people in society attempt to locate the blame or reason for everything perceived as 'bad'. When nothing else can be blamed, sin is the obvious alternative explanation.

The stereotypes resulting from these false assumptions are influential and this influence is magnified by language. The power of language to shape policy and influence views of reality is great (Edelman, 1985). The terms 'nigger' and 'chick' are evocative as is the term 'cripple'. While the first two terms are rarely used today in the media, the third term is commonly used as a verb (to cripple), as an adjective (crippled), and as an adverb (crippling) (Longmore, 1985; Zola,

1985). It is not surprising that the stereotypes are deeply influential upon public policy in this society (Crispell & Gomez, 1988; Hahn, 1985a; Handberg, 1989; Higgins, 1980). These stereotypes influence friendships (Kleck & DeJong, 1983), govern success (Beuf, 1990; Bordieri *et al.*, 1983), and determine how disabled people are viewed by the professionals who seek to help them (Barnett, 1986; Nixon, 1985; Owen, 1985; Scott, 1981; Westbrook & Nordholm, 1986). They are widely found today and throughout history.

In the US disabled persons were stereotyped from colonial times as defective and thus not being able to participate as citizens. Not until the nineteenth century did disabled people attempt in any numbers to participate in civic matters. When they tried to do so, they were usually barred. The 1872 civil procedure code of the County of Los Angeles prevented persons who were deaf, blind, and physically handicapped from serving on juries. The reason was that such persons were considered, according to the code, to be "decrepit and lacking in all their natural faculties". When the Los Angeles County Supervisors were considering a measure to repeal this provision in 1976, it was opposed by two county judges because ". . . the blind would have difficulty in determining the credibility of witnesses since they could not observe witnesses' demeanor" (Los Angeles to Decide . . ., 1976) Such stereotypes about blind persons are common (Chevigny, 1946; Criddle, 1953; Scott, 1981) as they are about disabled persons in general.

The legal impact of these stereotypes upon the lives of people with disabilities did not happen by accident. It was the result of an identifiable social movement whose purpose was to make society better in all ways.

THE EUGENICS MOVEMENT

The reason for the impact of the stereotypes and the resulting discriminatory laws can be found in the values and prejudices of people in society (Brown, 1988; Caplan, 1989; Proctor, 1988; Weindling, 1989; Weiss, 1987). One of the primary sources of these prejudicial attitudes which led to the laws is the Eugenics Movement which has its roots in nineteenth century biology, especially the work of Charles Darwin (Mazumdar, 1992; Stepan, 1992). The evolutionary ideas of Darwin are not necessarily supportive of the goals of the Eugenics Movement, but they led to the work in genetics which gave rise to the movement.

It is not accidental that a certain pessimism can be read into Darwin because he took his central idea from Thomas Malthus' work *Essay on Population,* first published in 1798 (Dampier, 1952, chap. 7). Malthus wrote that the human race would always grow in numbers until it has insufficient means for survival. Then war, famine, or disease would trim back the number of people. Unnecessary individuals would die. This pessimistic view of history influenced Darwin. As he wrote (quoted in Dampier, 1952, p. 276):

> In October 1838 I happened to read for amusement Malthus on Population, and being well prepared to appreciate the struggle for existence which everywhere goes on from long continued observation of the habits of animals and plants, it at once struck

me that under these circumstances favourable variations would tend to be preserved, and unfavourable ones to be destroyed. The result of this would be the formation of new species. Here than I had a theory by which to work.

For the next 20 years Darwin collected data and conducted experiments. In November 1859 his *Origin of Species* was published.

Ideas of evolution were not unknown during the nineteenth and previous centuries. Toward the end of his life Charles Darwin acknowledged the influence that his grandfather, Erasmus Darwin, had on his ideas. Erasmus Darwin was one of a number of writers who had advanced the idea of evolution, but in a different form (Colp, 1986). Unlike earlier works, Charles Darwin's *Origin of Species* established evolution on a firm basis because it was accompanied by extensive facts based on his observations and experiments. Thomas Huxley, the chief expositor of Darwin's theory, describes it as a flash of lightning in the dark (Dampier, 1952, pp. 279–280). It was not a flash appreciated by all persons because there was intense opposition to Darwin's theory over the next twenty years. Only toward the end of his life did the opposition begin to subside.

Out of the controversy generated by *The Origin of Species* came the field known today as genetics. Unlike most fields, genetics can be said to have a birth month, although not exactly a birth day. In April 1900 three different plant breeders rediscovered and/or republished what Gregory Mendel had published in 1866. Mendel's ideas encompassed a statistical rule by which plant characteristics could be predicted from one generation to another (Waddington, 1972). Such a statistical approach was championed in Great Britain by W.F.R. Weldon, Karl Pearson, and Francis Galton. Pearson, the statistician who developed the product moment correlation coefficient as well as other statistical tools, founded the journal *Biometrika* with Weldon. Galton, who had turned his attention to the genetic improvement of people, coined the term eugenics for his work. Another contributor to this movement was the statistician G. Udny Yule who developed the definition of statistical independence used today with the Chi Square statistic. Finally, there was the statistician Ronald Fisher, known for his work with statistical tests of significance, who reconciled early objections raised by Weldon and Pearson to the Mendel approach.

Fisher was very concerned that previous civilizations had collapsed because the 'better' classes had failed to reproduce a sufficient number of offspring. In 1912 he addressed the second annual meeting of the Cambridge University Eugenics Society and stressed the need for careful breeding among the 'better' classes. A year later in an address to the Eugenics Education Society he repeated his concern and said (as quoted in Box, 1978, p. 32):

> We do not dub ourselves knights of a new order. But necessarily, inevitably, it might be unconsciously, we are the agents of a new phase of evolution. Eugenists will on the whole marry better than other people, [they will have] higher ability, richer health, greater beauty. They will, on the whole, have more children than other people.

Although Fisher might have repudiated much of what later happened in the name of eugenics, by 1929 he was actively engaged in a campaign to legalize sterilization (Box, 1978, pp. 196–203). His public position was always that the sterilization must be voluntary and must be viewed as a right. He firmly believed that if viewed in this way sterilization would become widespread and would reduce the number of 'defectives' being born.

Fisher's views were not shared by all members of the Eugenics Movement. During the nineteenth century and on into the twentieth century there was considerable sentiment that certain racial or ethnic groups were superior in terms of intelligence and moral character. Such reasoning is the foundation for the doctrine of Manifest Destiny in the United States which justified the genocide of Native Americans and the conquest of Puerto Rico and the Philippines. Within the American society, the argument went, the lower classes were intellectually and morally inferior. In order to preserve civilization and social order, the lower classes must be restrained. Unionization of American industry was opposed on the grounds that the common worker could not know what was best for him/herself much less for the entire nation.

Like Fisher, many persons in the US were concerned that civilization was doomed unless 'defective' persons were kept from multiplying. Lothrop Stoddard wrote in 1922 (quoted in Smith, 1985, p. 3) that "the stern processes of natural selection" had kept down the number of "defective" people in the past, but now "modern society and philanthropy have protected them and thus favored their rapid multiplication".

Arguments in the abortion debates often contain premises of the Eugenics Movement (Heifetz, 1989; Hollander, 1989; Merrick, 1989; Wertz & Fletcher, 1989; Wolfensberger, 1989). Equating the availability of abortion with the encouragement of promiscuity, David Wilson (1986) states that mature, educated married couples who "conscientiously practice contraception" sometimes conceive children. The probability that unmarried teenage girls, he writes, will become pregnant is close to certainty if abortion continues to be available.

> The process is negatively self-selective. The most responsible, educated, economically self-sufficient, genetically and culturally endowed are the least likely in any age cohort actually to produce offspring. What abortion is producing instead . . . is male irresponsibility and a dysgenic reproductive pattern in which those less prepared to cope with the multitudinous challenges of advanced technocracies are outbreeding those whose capacities may be expected to be superior.

The 'better' classes will obtain abortions while the 'inferior' classes will multiply. This concern is the same one voiced at the beginning of the century by Fisher, but not only will the 'better' classes produce fewer children, the 'inferior' classes will produce 'defective', i.e. disabled children.

In the nineteenth century due (in part) to the Eugenics Movement, there was social policy implemented to deal with the 'defective' and disabled members of society. The earliest institution for 'defectives' and 'feebleminded' persons in the

US was established in Boston by Samuel Howe in 1849. It was Howe's intent to educate the 'defectives' so that they could return to society. However, he was so successful in removing unwanted persons from the streets and from public sight that families and communities refused to have them back. Although he warned against permanent segregation, no one listened. All that public leaders could see was that persons whom they associated with poverty, crime, insanity, prostitution, alcoholism, and general immorality were being removed from society. As Massachusetts Governor Benjamin Butler said in his 1883 address to the state legislature (Butler, 1883):

> When the state shall have sufficiently educated every bright child . . . it will be time enough to undertake the education of the idiotic and feeble-minded. I submit that this attempt to reverse the irrevocable decree as to the survival of the fittest is not even kindness to the poor creatures who are at this school. . . . none of the pupils have become self-supporting. . . . a well cared-for idiot is a happy creature. An idiot awakened to his condition is a miserable one.

Howe had been too successful.

A few years before Butler's address, R.L. Dugdale published his famous study *The Jukes* in 1877. In his book Dugdale described what he called the degeneracy of the Jukes family. His work stimulated the publication of a large number of family histories (Rafter, 1988). Although Dugdale said it was caused by the social environment, an increasing number of these family histories, as a result of the influence of the Eugenics Movement, ascribed the degeneracy to hereditary factors. The most influential of all of these works appeared in 1912 and was authored by Henry Goddard (Goddard, 1912). It was entitled *The Kallikak Family: a study in the heredity of feeble-mindedness.*

Like Darwin's *Origin of Species,* Goddard's work was immediately accepted as scientific proof of a theory. It was a theory which ascribed almost all social ills to a particular class, the feebleminded. Henry Goddard was, in all senses of the word, an academic. He was well educated with a bachelor's and master's degree from Haverford College. In between his two degrees from Haverford, he taught for a year at the University of Southern California in 1888. For 8 years he worked as a secondary school principal and then entered Clark University to study psychology. He received his PhD from Clark in 1899 and went to teach at the Pennsylvania State Normal School in West Chester (Smith, 1985, p. 39). In 1906 he went to the Training School for Feeble-Minded Boys and Girls in Vineland, New Jersey, as director of research. As an empirically minded scientist he wanted to do research into the causes and hopefully the cure of one of society's major problems, as he saw it.

While traveling in Europe he met Alfred Binet and returned with his intelligence test which was to become the cornerstone of Goddard's research. The Binet test was to be used by Goddard and future generations to detect mental defectives. As late as 1981, 92% of the state vocational rehabilitation agencies in the United States were using some form of an IQ test to diagnose mental retardation and in 80% of the states no formal adaptive behavior assessment was used to validate the conclusions based on the test results (Sheldon, 1982). For example, Rhode Island (General Laws, 40.1-22-3 (5)) defines a mentally retarded person as one "with significant subaverage general intellectual functioning two (2) standard deviations below the normal. . . .". Even though IQ tests give questionable results, 'experts' place great reliance upon them even today (Snyderman & Rothman, 1989).

After establishing (to his satisfaction) that feeblemindedness was inherited, Goddard turned to the policy question of how to combat the many social ills which the feebleminded brought to society. He focused on the slums where, he said, most of the crime, poverty, and immorality existed. As he wrote (quoted by Smith, 1985, p. 18):

> If all of the slum districts of our cities were removed tomorrow and model tenements built in their places, we would still have slums in a week's time because we have these mentally defective people who can never be taught to live otherwise than as they have been living. Not until we take care of this class and see to it that their lives are guided by intelligent people, shall we remove these sores from our social life.

Of course, Goddard and others would be the 'intelligent people' who guided the 'mentally defective people'. How would he undertake to remove the 'sores'? Sterilization was advanced as a temporary measure, but segregation into institutions as the final solution. Again, as Goddard wrote (quoted by Smith, 1985, p. 19):

> Such colonies [institutions] would save an annual loss in property and life, due to the action of these irresponsible people, sufficient to nearly, or quite, offset the expense of the new plant . . . Segregation through colonization seems in the present state of our knowledge to be the ideal and perfectly satisfactory method.

People with disabilities were to be segregated and sterilized for the betterment of society.

Although Goddard's work was soundly criticized by some for its abysmal methodology and its faulty genetics, it was widely praised by others. Each criticism received a reply from either Goddard or from a defender of Eugenics (Meile *et al.* 1989). Persons made their academic career by writing about this country's moral degradation and proposals for ridding the country of this scourge of feeble mindedness.

But Goddard was not the only person who advocated sterilization and segregation and who was heard. Havelock Ellis, a leader in the struggle for human rights and especially women's rights, begins his work *The Task of Social Hygiene* with attention to the problem of feeblemindedness (to use his words). Citing the work of Goddard and others, Ellis (1927, p. 35) writes:

> The feeble-minded have no forethought and no self-restraint. They are not adequately capable of resisting their own impulses or the solicitations of others, and they are unable to understand adequately the motives which guide the conduct of ordinary people.

Not only are they presently a menace, wrote Ellis, but they are ". . . the reservoir from which the predatory classes are recruited" (Ellis, 1927, p. 38). They are "an evil that is unmitigated", a "poison to the race", and their "very existence is itself an impediment" to civilization (Ellis, 1927, p. 43). But Ellis stopped short of Goddard's methods of sterilization and segregation. Instead, Ellis wanted the ideals of Eugenics to become part of the civic religion so that civilization would work to rid itself of the "defectives" using various public policies including statutory law.

Other persons in the Eugenics Movement were not as reticent as Ellis to recommend Goddard's methods. Walter Fernald, a successor to Howe, was quite blunt (Fernald, 1912, p. 92).

> The feebleminded are a parasitic, predatory class, never capable of self-support or of managing their own affairs. The great majority ultimately become public charges in some form. . . . It has been truly said that feeblemindedness is the mother of crime, pauperism and degeneracy. . . . The most important point is that feeblemindedness is highly hereditary. . . . No feebleminded person should be allowed to marry or become a parent. . . . Certain families should become extinct. Parenthood is not for all.

The only question remaining was how to implement this policy. Extermination was hinted, but not openly used (Lusthaus, 1985). Instead, segregation into institutions and sterilization was the answer.

Goddard's influence spread. He was invited to Ellis Island to help identify and thus exclude feebleminded immigrants. Using the Binet test, Goddard found that 79% of all Italian immigrants, 80% of all Hungarian immigrants, 83% of all Jewish immigrants (the only group not listed by nationality), and 87% of all Russian immigrants were feebleminded (Smith, 1985, pp. 119–120). Goddard concluded that if the American people wanted feebleminded immigrants barred then they had better let Congress know. In 1924 Congress passed the Immigration Restriction Act limiting the number of immigrants from Southern and Eastern Europe.

During World War I army recruits were given the Binet test. Goddard's interpretation of the results were that half the country had the intelligence of a 13-year-old or less. His conclusions (Smith, 1985, pp. 128–130) were that it argued against democracy. No society, he said, could exist with decisions being made by the average, much less the lowest, in intelligence. About half of the country should be disenfranchised so that the more intelligent citizens could guide public policy makers.

Numerous other studies appeared after Goddard's which found 'defectives' to be the source of most social evils (Smith, 1985, chap. 9). Similar policy recommendations were put forth by these writers. One of the more zealous followers of Eugenics was Harry Laughlin who drew up a model sterilization law in 1922. His model law would require the sterilization of the following 'defective' classes (Laughlin, 1922, pp. 446–447):

. . . (1) feebleminded; (2) insane (including the psychopathic); (3) criminalistic (including the delinquent and wayward); (4) epileptic; (5) inebriate (including drug habitues); (6) diseased (including the tuberculous, the syphilitic, the leprous, and others with chronic infectious, and legally segregable diseases); (7) blind (including those with seriously impaired vision); (8) deaf (including those with seriously impaired hearing); (9) deformed (including the crippled); and (10) dependent (including orphans, ne'er-do-wells, the homeless, tramps, and paupers).

It is interesting to note (Smith, 1985, p. 138) that Laughlin himself was a person with epilepsy. Although married, he had no children.

By 1938, 33 states had a sterilization law and nation wide over 27 000 compulsory operations were performed (Smith, 1985, p. 139). The California law required the sterilization not only of the "feebleminded" and anyone with "inherited mental diseases or diseases of a syphilitic nature", but also anyone in a state hospital who showed evidence of "perversion or marked departures from normal mentality" (Berns, 1953, p. 770). By 1951 over 19,000 persons had been sterilized under the California law. In Virginia, in the institution where Carrie Buck had lived, over 4000 had been sterilized (Smith, 1985, p. 150). Even though the law under which she was sterilized was repealed in 1968 (Burgdorf & Burgdorf, 1977), the practice in Virginia was not stopped until 1972. According to Ferster (1966), over 63,000 persons were involuntarily sterilized in the US for genetically related reasons from 1921 to 1964.

CONCLUSION

The laws discussed earlier were based on the hard science of the day as well as the attitudes of the public toward disabled persons. There was no small clique which secretly promulgated the sterilization and segregation laws which were applied to disabled persons and which still operate today (Bell, 1962; Berns, 1953; Forman & Hetznecker, 1982; Haller, 1963; Hahn, 1982, 1983; Pfeiffer, 1985, 1987; Wolfensberger, 1975, 1981). It was (and is) public opinion as articulated by public leaders and scientific opinion as articulated by professionals which gave these laws impetus for their passage and for their implementation. It is this public and scientific opinion which still supports them today (Barnett, 1986; Bell, 1986; Bock, 1983; Bosk, 1992; Gochros & Gochros, 1977; Gould, 1985; Holtzman, 1989; Lusthaus, 1985; Mehan, Hertweck, & Meihls, 1986; Melnick, 1985; Miringoff, 1991; Sanderson, 1990; Starr, 1982). Although in 1985 the Governor of Texas signed legislation which removed from Texas laws such terms as idiot, feeble-minded, crippled, and deformed, the terms remain in the statutes of most states. The prejudicial attitudes still exist in public law.

Physicians and hospital administrators routinely allow newly born disabled infants to die. They disconnect the life sustaining apparatus of elderly persons because their quality of life is too meager. Parents who discover that the mother is carrying a 'defective' fetus are counselled to obtain an abortion (Miringoff,

1989, 1991). Wolfensberger (cited in Herr, 1984, p. 8) estimates that some 200,000 abortions a year are for this reason.

Disabled children who are allowed to live receive second-rate or worse education in public schools. Some disabled children, especially if the child has AIDS, receive no education at all. Disabled people today are fired or not hired in the first place because of their disability. Health care is denied to persons with disabilities. Although many municipalities supply, at taxpayers' expense, services such as parks and airports, personal assistants who would allow disabled persons to work and be taxpayers are curtailed for budget reasons. Many public transit systems, paid for and subsidized by the tax moneys of disabled persons, can not be used by persons with mobility and sensory disabilities.

In a number of states former residents in state schools and hospitals are reinstitutionalized because there is not sufficient funds appropriated for community centers. Public housing is constructed to be not accessible and tenants who behave in a peculiar way are evicted. Citizens with hearing and vision impairments are denied access to public documents. Other disabled persons who are judged not able to manage daily tasks are sterilized for their own 'benefit'. They are also prohibited from marrying or from parenting their own children.

Disabled persons are also the outcasts of academia. It was public attitudes which allowed the oppressive laws to be promulgated and implemented, but it was academia which gave justification for those laws (Allen, 1986; Blackford, 1993; Gelb, 1989; Hahn, 1985b; Mazumdar, 1992; Meile *et al.*, 1989; Nelkin & Tancredi, 1989; Weiss, 1987; Wingart, 1989). To counter this threat to the civil rights of people with disabilities, public and private agencies (including academia) must mount an effective drive to educate the public in regard to the facts about disabilities and the legal rights of disabled persons.

The passage of the Americans with Disabilities Act (P.L. 101-336) is a step toward dealing with the discriminatory state laws and practices. It is time that even more be done. State laws which discriminate against a person with a disability must be struck down. Prior decisions which allow such discrimination must be overruled. State and federal regulations implementing laws must be revised.

Persons with disabilities are capable of managing their affairs, of being responsible, tax paying citizens, and of being lovers and parents. If people with disabilities have the right to exist in this society, then they have the right to ways to make that existence meaningful and effective. Through education and political action this end can be achieved.

REFERENCES

Allen, G. (1986) The Eugenics Record Office at Cold Spring Harbor, 1910–1940, *Osiris,* 2d Series, 2, pp. 5 –42.

Barnett, W. (1986) The transition from public residential schools for retarded people to custodial facilities: an economic explanation. *Disability, Handicap & Society,* 1, pp. 53–71.

Bell, A. (1962) Attitudes of selected rehabilitation workers and other hospital employees toward the physically disabled, *Psychological Reports,* 10, pp. 183–186.

Bell, T. (1986) Education policy development in the Reagan administration, *Phi Delta Kappan,* 67, pp. 487–493.

Berns, W. (1953) *Buck v. Bell:* Due process of law?, *Western Political Quarterly,* 6, pp. 762–775.

Bernstein, P. (1991) Termination of parental rights on the basis of mental disability: a problem in policy and interpretation, *Pacific Law Journal,* 22, pp. 1155–1185.

Beuf, A. (1990) *Beauty is the Beast* (Philadelphia, University of Pennsylvania Press).

Blackford, K. (1993) Erasing mothers with disabilities through Canadian family-related policy, *Disability, Handicap & Society,* 8, pp. 281–294.

Bock, G. (1983) Racism and sexism in Nazi Germany: motherhood, compulsory sterilization, and the state, *Signs: Journal of Women in Culture and Society,* 8, pp. 400–421.

Bogdan, R. & Biklen, D. (1977) Handicapism, *Social Policy,* March/April, pp. 14–19.

Bogdan, R. & Taylor, S. (1987) Toward a sociology of acceptance: the other side of the study of deviance, *Social Policy,* Fall, pp. 34–39.

Bogdan, R. & Taylor, S. (1989) Relationships with severely disabled people: the social construction of humanness, *Social Problems,* 36, pp. 135–148.

Bordieri, J., Sotolongo, M. & Wilson, M. (1983) Physical attractiveness and attributions for disability, *Rehabilitation Psychology,* 28, pp. 207–215.

Bosk, C. (1992) *All God's Mistakes: genetic counseling in a pediatric hospital* (Chicago, University of Chicago Press).

Box, J. (1978) *R.A. Fisher: the life of a scientist* (New York: Wiley).

Brakel, S., Parry, J. & Weiner, B. (1985) *The Mentally Disabled and the Law,* 3rd edn (Chicago, American Bar Foundation).

Brantlinger, E. (1992) Professionals' attitudes toward the sterilization of people with disabilities, *The Journal of The Association for Persons with Severe Handicaps,* 17, pp. 4–18.

Brown, R. (Ed.) (1988) *Quality of Life for Handicapped People* (London, Croom Helm).

Burgdorf, R. (Ed.) (1980) *The Legal Rights of Handicapped Persons* (Baltimore, Paul H. Brookes).

Burgdorf, R. & Burgdorf, M. (1977) The wicked witch is almost dead: *Buck v. Bell* and the sterilization of handicapped persons, *Temple Law Quarterly,* 50, pp. 995–1034.

Butler, B. (1883) Address to the Great and General Court of Massachusetts.

Caplan, A. (198) The meaning of the holocaust for bioethics, *Hastings Center Report,* July/August, 19(4), pp. 2–3.

Chevigny, H. (1946) *My Eyes Have a Cold Nose* (New Haven, Yale University Press).

Colp, R. (1986) The relationship of Charles Darwin to the ideas of his grandfather, Dr. Erasmus Darwin, *Biography,* 9, pp. 1–24.

Criddle, R. (1953) *Love Is Not Blind* (New York, W.W. Norton).

Crispell, K. & Gomez, C. (1988) *Hidden Illness in the White House* (Durham, Duke University Press).

Dampier, W. (1952) *A History of Science and Its Relations with Philosophy & Religion* 4th cdn (Cambridge, Cambridge University Press).

Dearing, B. (1981) Literary images as stereotypes, in: D. Biklen & L. Bailey (Eds) *Rudely Stamp'd: imaginal disability and prejudice* (Washington, DC, University Press of America).

Edelman, M. (1985) Political language and political reality, *PS,* 18, pp. 10–19.

Elkins, T. & Andersen, H. (1992) Sterilization of persons with mental retardation, *The Journal of The Association for Persons with Severe Handicaps,* 17, pp. 19–26.

Ellis, H. (1927) *The Task of Social Hygiene,* 2nd edn (Boston, Houghton Mifflin).

Ferguson, P. & Ferguson, D. (1992) Sex, sexuality, and disability, *The Journal of The Association for Persons with Severe handicaps,* 17, pp. 27–28.

Fernald, W. (1912) The burden of feeblemindedness, *Journal of Psychoasthenics,* 18, pp. 90–98.

Ferster, E. (1966) Eliminating the unfit—is sterilization the answer?, *Ohio State Law Journal,* 27, pp. 591–633.

Forman, M. & Hetznecker, W. (1982) Physician and the handicapped child: dilemmas of care, *The Journal of the American Medical Association,* 247, pp. 3325–3326.

Fredericks, B. (1992) A parents' view of sterilization, *The Journal of The Association for Persons with Severe Handicaps,* 17, pp. 29–30.

Gelb, S. (1989) Not simply bad and incorrigible: science, morality, and intellectual deficiency, *History of Education Quarterly,* 29, pp. 359–379.

Gochros, H. & Gochros, J. (Eds) (1977) *The Sexually Oppressed* (New York, Association Press).

Goddard, H. (1912) *The Kallikak Family: a study in the heredity of feeble-mindedness* (New York, Macmillan).

Gould, S. (1985) *The Flamingo's Smile: reflections in natural history* (New York, W.W. Norton).

Hahn, H. (1982) Disability and rehabilitation policy: is paternalistic neglect really benign?, *Public Administration Review,* 73, pp. 385–389.

Hahn, H. (1983) Paternalism and public policy, *Society,* March/April, pp. 36–46.

Hahn, H. (1985a) Disability policy and the problem of discrimination, *American Behavioral Scientist,* 28, pp. 293–318.

Hahn, H. (1985b) Toward a politics of disability definitions, disciplines, and policies, *The Social Science Journal,* 22, pp. 87–105.

Haller, M. (1963) *Eugenics: hereditarian attitudes in American thought* (New Brunswick, Rutgers University Press).

Handberg, R. (1989) Talking about the unspeakable in a secretive institution: health and disability among supreme court justices, *Politics and the Life Sciences,* 8, pp. 70–73.

Heifetz, L. (1989) From Munchausen to Cassandra: a critique of Hollander's "euthanasia and mental retardation", *Mental Retardation,* 27(2), pp. 67–70.

Herr, S. (1984) *Issues in Human Rights* (New York, Young Adult Institute).

Higgins, P. (1980) *Outsiders in a Hearing World: a sociology of deafness* (Beverly Hills, Sage).

Hollander, R. (1989) Euthanasia and mental retardation: suggesting the unthinkable, *Mental Retardation,* 27(2), pp. 53–262.

Holtzman, N. (1989) *Proceed with Caution: predicting genetic risks in the recombinant DNA era* (Baltimore, Johns Hopkins University Press).

Hubbard, R. (1990) *The Politics of Women's Biology* (New Brunswick, Rutgers University Press).

Kaeser, F. (1992) Can people with severe mental retardation consent to mutual sex?, *Sexuality and Disability,* 10, pp. 38–42.

Kleck, R. & Dejong, W. (1983) Physical disability, physical attractiveness, and social outcomes in children's small groups, *Rehabilitation Psychology,* 28, pp. 79–91.

Laughlin, H. (1922) *Eugenical Sterilization in the United States* (Chicago, Psychopathic Laboratory o the Municipal Court of Chicago).

The Legal Rights of Persons with Epilepsy (1985) 5th edn (Landover, MD, Epilepsy Foundation of America).

Longmore, P. (1985) Screening stereotypes: images of disabled people, *Social Policy,* Summer, pp. 31–37.

Los Angeles to decide on letting blind and handicapped on juries (1976) *The New York Times,* 18 October, p. 53.

Lusthaus, E. (1985) 'Euthanasia' of persons with severe handicaps: refuting the rationalizations, *Journal of the Association on Severe Handicaps,* 10, pp. 87–94.

Macklin, R. & Gaylin, W. (Eds) (1981) *Mental Retardation and Sterilization: a problem of competency and paternalism* (New York, Plenum Press).

Mazumdar, P. (1992) *Eugenics, Human Genetics, and Human Failings: the Eugenics Society, its sources and its critics in Britain* (New York, Routledge).

Mehan, H., Hertweck, A. & Meihls, J. (1986) *Handicapping the Handicapped: decision making in students' educational careers* (Stanford, Stanford University Press).

McCall, R. (1984) Developmental changes in mental performance: the effect of the birth of a sibling, *Child Development,* 55, pp. 1317–1321.

Meile, R., Shanks-Meile, S. & Spurgin, M. (1989) Changes in the care and treatment of 'feeble-mindedness': a political-economic interpretation, paper delivered at the *Meeting of the Society for Disability Studies,* Washington, DC, June.

Melnick, R. (1985) The politics of partnership, *Public Administration Review,* 45, pp. 653–660.

Merrick, J. (1989) Federal intervention in the treatment of handicapped newborns: Baby Doe regulations and the 1984 child abuse amendments, *Policy Studies Review,* 8, pp. 405–419.

Miringoff, M. (1989) Genetic intervention and the problem of stigma, *Policy Studies Review,* 8, pp. 389–404.

Miringoff, M. (1991) *The Social Costs of Genetic Welfare* (New Brunswick, Rutgers University Press).

Murdock, C. (1974) Sterilization of the retarded: a problem or a solution?, *California Law Review,* 62, pp. 917–945.

Nelkin, D. & Tancredi, L. (1998) *Dangerous Diagnostics: the social power of biological information* (New York, Basic Books).

Nixon, H. (1985) Organizational subversion in voluntary rehabilitation associations for disabled people, *American Behavioral Scientist,* 28, pp. 3437–366.

Owen, M. (1985) A view of disability in current social work literature, *American Behavioral Scientist,* 28, pp. 397–403.

Pfeiffer, D. (1985) Affirmative action and the unemployment of disabled persons, *Proceedings of the 1985 AHSSPPE Conference,* pp. 254–256.

Pfeiffer, D. (1987) Civil rights with clout: the disabled citizen in Massachusetts, in: S. Hey, G. Kiger & J. Seidel (Eds) *Impaired and Disabled People in Society: structure, processes and the individual* (Salem, OR, The Society for Disability Studies and Willamette University).

Proctor, R. (1988) *Racial Hygiene: medicine under the Nazis* (Cambridge, MA, Harvard University Press).

Rafter, N. (1988) *White Trash: the eugenics family studies, 1877–1919* (Boston, Northeastern University Press).

Rothstein, M. (1992) Genetic discrimination in employment and the Americans with Disabilities Act, *Houston Law Review,* 29, pp. 23–42

Sackett, R. (1991) Terminating parental rights of the handicapped, *Family Law Quarterly,* 25, pp. 253–273.

Sanderson, S. (1990) *Social Evolutionism: a critical history* (Cambridge, Basil Blackwell).

Scott, R. (1981) *The Making of Blind Men: a study of adult socialization* (New Brunswick, Transaction Books).

Sheldon, K. (1982) Communication to vocational rehabilitation colleagues, December.

Smith, J. (1985) *Minds Made Feeble: the myth and legacy of the Kallikaks* (Rockville, MD, Aspen Systems Corporation).

Snyderman, M. & Rothman, S. (1988) *The IQ Controversy, the Media, and Public Policy* (New Brunswick, Transaction).

Starr, R. (1982) Wheels of misfortune, *Harper's,* January, pp. 7–15.

Stepan, N. (1992) *"The Hour of Eugenics": race, gender, and nation in Latin America* (Ithaca, Cornell University Press).

Sternberg, R. & Gardner, H. (1984) Testing intelligence without IQ scores, *Phi Delta Kappan,* 65, pp. 694–698.

Waddington, C. (1972) Biology, in : C.B. Cox & A.E Dyson (Eds) *The Twentieth Century Mind,* Vol. 1, chap. 10 (London, Oxford University Press).

Wendling, P. (1998) *Health, Race, and German Politics Between national Unification and Nazism, 1870–1945* (New York, Cambridge University Press).

Weingart, P. (1989) German eugenics between Science and politics, *Osiris,* 2d Series, 5, pp. 260–282.

Weiss, S. (1987) The race hygiene movement in Germany, *Osiris,* 2d Series, 3, pp. 193–236.

Wells, K. (1983) As laws and attitudes change, the retarded are entering society, *The Wall Street Journal,* 15 February, pp. 1, 20.

Wertz, D. & Fletcher, J. (1989) Fatal knowledge? Prenatal diagnosis and sex selection, *Hastings Center Report,* May/June, pp. 21–27.

Westbrook, M. & Nordholm, L. (1986) Effects of diagnosis on reactions to patient optimism and depression, *Rehabilitation Psychology,* 31, pp. 79–94.

Wilson, D. (1986) The high human price to pay for abortion, *The Boston Globe,* 29 June, p. A23.

Wolfensberger, W. (1975) *The Origin and Nature of Our Institutional Models* (Syracuse, Human Policy Press).

Wolfensberger, W. (1981) The extermination of handicapped people in World War II Germany, *Mental Retardation,* 19, pp. 1–7.

Wolfensberger, W. (1989) The killing thought in the eugenic era and today: a commentary on Hollander's essay, *Mental Retardation,* 27(2), pp. 63–66.

Wright, B. (1985) *Disabling Myths About Disability* (Chicago, National Easter Seals Society).

Zola, I. (1985) Depictions of disability—metaphor, message, and medium in the media: a research and political agenda, *The Social Science Journal,* 22, pp. 5–17.

3

The Energy Model: A New Approach to Rehabilitation

Roberta B. Trieschmann

Rehabilitation has always emphasized the importance of dealing with the whole person, herein defined as an amalgamation of the personality, the body, and also the environment. The interaction of the personality and body with the environment not only establishes the nature of the disability but also becomes the focus of much of the stress in the disabled person's life. Management of stress and learning to work well with the environment are major tasks throughout the life of all people, but especially for those with significant physical impairments. Anger, anxiety, and depression are frequently a part of life with a disability and learning to cope with these emotions is a necessary part of rehabilitation and integration into the community.

Much of the current research in psychoneuroimmunology reveals the powerful relationship between emotional reactions and health status. Unfortunately, knowledge of this relationship has not been translated into a health care policy which provides increased resources for psychological and rehabilitation counseling services to people with disabilities. Rather, in a misguided attempt to control costs, a strictly physical approach to rehabilitation is increasingly the modus operandi of third party payors, and current trends within the health care system do not suggest any reversal of this policy as long as the medical model of health care is dominant.

In my 29 years of experience as a clinical psychologist who works with people who have major physical disabilities, I have become increasingly dissatisfied with the conceptual models of traditional western medicine and psychology because they do not offer me comfortable viewpoints or strategies that are really helpful in teaching people to find happiness. When people do find happiness, it derives from a re-evaluation of what is important in their lives, usually accompanied by a deepening of their spirituality, and usually accomplished by themselves without help from professionals.

From *Rehabilitation Education, 9*(2) (1995), 217–227. Reprinted with permission.

Thus, for the past 14 years, I have been searching for other ways to understand the issues of medical illness and physical disability. This odyssey led me to oriental medicine and eastern philosophy because these sources of wisdom clearly have merits that have been unrecognized and unexplored by our traditional medical establishment. Both a program of independent study of the literature from these fields as well as personal training and practice in the eastern traditions have permitted me to blend many of the ideas from oriental philosophy into my approach to people who come to me for counseling. In this philosophy, the health of the body is a direct reflection of the quality of the spirit (energy), and therefore, spirituality is an integral feature of any health care program.

In my experience, my patients and clients have been very receptive to this approach which honors the human as more than a body, so much more than a brain. In my opinion, spirituality can and must come back into health care, and especially rehabilitation, without being tied to any particular religious tradition or dogma. But this requires a shift in paradigms of health care, from a strictly medical (physical) model of function to an energy model of human function. Psychoneuroimmunology and alternative medicine approaches represent a transition between these two models, but they will be truly effective in improving health care and function only to the extent that they shift their focus from the physical to the emotional, from the mechanical to the spiritual (quality of energy).

In order to understand the nature of the transition that is required from medical model to energy model, it is essential to understand the origin of many of our beliefs and assumptions. These have shaped not only western science and health care but also each western person's expectations of how the world operates and the approaches that are necessary to understand this world.

THE MEDICAL MODEL

Thomas Kuhn, in his classic book, *The Structure of Scientific Revolutions* (1970), indicated that paradigms (models) play a powerful role in determining which issues become legitimate questions for research in any given field and which methodologies are considered acceptable for studying a problem. In health care, the dominant paradigm, the medical model, states, essentially, that the body is a physical mechanism which is capable of study and understanding using the methods of the physical sciences. The implicit assumption is made that quantitative measurement of physiological function will be sufficient to diagnose the cause of sickness and that treatment, as well, can be accomplished at a strictly physical level. Subjective data, emotional reactions, and psychological concepts are viewed as contaminating variables, at best, or irrelevant, at worst, and they need to be controlled, i.e., excluded, so that they do not hinder progress in the medical sciences.

The evidence is growing, however, that emotional reactions and psychological processes are not irrelevant but rather integral to the homeostasis and healthy functioning of the human body. Hans Selye pioneered the study of stress, described the physiology of the stress response, and showed how long-term stress produced numerous physical disorders, such as ulcers, arthritis, and hypertension. More recently, the psychobiology of stress and its effect on the immune system has become a major research endeavor called psychoneuroimmunology. We now know that emotional reactions have a direct and immediate physiological correlate in the human body and there is ample research to demonstrate this relationship. Unfortunately, the health care system as a whole is not structured to use these results to assist people to feel better and to reduce their stress because these data do not fit into the medical model of human function. Although a patient may be referred to a psychologist for treatment, the paradigm which gives primacy to physical treatments of the body remains intact. Psychological services are not considered integral to the recovery of the person but rather are viewed as an adjunct service which can easily be eliminated if funding is limited or a schedule conflict prevails.

Unfortunately, the medical paradigm is based on the concept of reductionism which fractionates the human body into its component parts for study and treatment. This strictly physical approach ignores the systems interactions of the various physical parts because there is no coherent philosophy of health which unites all human functioning at the core of this model. The mind, the feelings, and the soul are extraneous to the focus of the medical system although all good medical healers have never ignored these aspects in their patient care.

Our current medical paradigm has prevailed for only a couple of centuries. Prior to this, a religious paradigm of physical function dominated in which health and wellness were viewed within a grander cosmic scheme which included God, nature, and humanity's relationship to nature and to God. Illness was often viewed as punishment from God. The Church was the locus of most education and most books were hand copied by monks in monasteries. Scientific investigation was dependent upon Church support and any results which interfered with the church's teachings were banned. In this climate, superstition and misinformation were difficult to challenge and scientific explorations were often deemed dangerous to the church's authority.

In order to free science from the church, Rene Descartes devised an ingenious solution which set the stage for the scientific revolution of the last 300 years. He proposed to separate the body of man from God. He suggested that the body, much like a clock or machine, could be understood as a complex physical mechanism and studied through physical principles, using mathematics as the major method of describing the results of investigations. Thus, the body would be the province of science whereas the mind and the soul would belong to the Church. In reality he knew that body and mind could not be separated but his proposal of the body-mind split became an intellectual contrivance which allowed for a division of power intellectually between the church and science.

Isaac Newton developed the laws of gravity and expanded the idea of applying physical measurements to material objects, the planets, and eventually to all of the universe. Mathematics became the language of this new science in which subjective data were suspect. If it could not be measured physically, then it was presumed not to exist. Francis Bacon elaborated on these concepts and developed the scientific method which emphasized standardized procedures, control of extraneous variable (viewed as errors), quantitative measurement, and reproducibility of results.

In essence this political solution worked. The paradigm of western science investigation was based upon the concept of reductionism; analysis of something into its component parts was seen to produce greater understanding of how it worked. Quantification of data became a cornerstone of the scientific methodology as well as reproducibility of the results through control of extraneous variables and standardized procedures of investigation. Objective, quantifiable data were the means to achieve the goal of control over nature in order to influence it in the direction desired by man.

The physical sciences prospered under this approach and the industrial revolution fueled the belief that this paradigm guaranteed success and, consequently, the well being of a person would be assured. Well being was synonymous with material comfort and wealth, however, and it was assumed that the Church would take care of the soul. The medical sciences followed this quantitative, reductionistic model, as did the science of psychology.

Psychology Within the Medical Model

Originally, psychology and the field of philosophy were one. Some individuals, however, chose to view the mind as open to the same mode of investigation as the hard sciences, using quantitative measurement techniques. Thus, psychophysiological studies initially characterized the new field of psychology as the sensory inputs to the brain were measured and described. When it came to behavior, however, there was a further split into two camps. One group followed Freud and the field of psychoanalysis was born, while the other followed Watson, and the field of behaviorism was created. The latter field emphasized reductionism and quantification of measures and evolved into the field of experimental psychology. The former field of psychoanalysis created a theory of human behavior and a specific methodology for treating behavioral problems. But many disagreed with certain aspects of psychoanalytic theory and moved beyond it to create other theories of personality functioning and other treatment techniques, primarily psychotherapy. The field of clinical psychology descended from this latter branch of psychology's evolution.

However, the modern clinical psychologist (for the last 40 years) has become a hybrid of these branches of psychology in an attempt to create the clinician-scientist. There has been an emphasis on providing quantitative measures of human behavior (primarily through psychological tests) and a large variety of intervention strategies which provide qualitative and quantitative measures of results. Psychotherapy and meditation are examples of the former and biofeedback and classic behavior therapy are examples of the latter. Thus, the field of psychology has been trying to respond to the actual needs of the public at large while trying to maintain credibility within the professional community in which the medical and western science model dominates.

In the last half of this century, the field of medicine has produced a wealth of data on body function, invented phenomenal technology to diagnose and treat illness, and developed a series of powerful chemicals to influence body function. The desired outcome was the removal of the symptoms of sickness with the ultimate intention of curing all disease. Descartes' intellectual convenience of 300 years ago, however, gradually evolved into the assumption that mind and body were separate. And the requirement that all data must be physically quantifiable and objective reinforced the belief that a phenomenon was not important if it could not be measured. Unfortunately, these intellectual assumptions and the methodology of western science have created an unreal view of life by providing a distorted perception of the nature of the world and the nature of human beings.

The Shift to Alternative Medicine

In the last 20 years, however, the separation between mind and body is being challenged by data from the field of psychoneuroimmunology. Emotional reactions have direct and immediate consequences at the cellular level; they do influence body states; and they do lead to organ system dysfunction. Simultaneously, the American public is increasingly disenchanted with traditional medical interventions which are perceived to be invasive and often more destructive than helpful. Thus, the field of alternative medicine is gaining favor with an increasing number of Americans who are seeking such treatments and paying for services out of pocket. These interventions include meditation, acupuncture, massage, rolfing, jin shin jyutsu, reiki, tai chi, yoga, qi gong, naturopathy, homeopathy, and the use of vitamins and herbs, to name just a few. The aversion to invasive and destructive interventions is fueling a movement for natural healing alternatives which are gentle and health promoting. A core theme of these alternative strategies is that they link mind and soul to body and health.

Many of these interventions from the field of alternative medicine do make people feel much better, at least for a while. But results depend upon the number of treatments, the ability of the practitioner, and ultimately the willingness of the person to make the life style changes necessary to alter the factors which led to the malaise in the first place. These treatments usually are delivered by a practitioner who integrates the mind and emotions with the body which accounts for the positive reception by the American public. But here also, the specific treatment approach to the problem is often unifocal and in many cases still focuses primarily on physical interventions to the person.

Thus, the medical paradigm that well being results from a strictly physical approach to health problems is crumbling. It is time for a new paradigm to take its place. Kuhn (1970) indicates that the operational paradigm of any scientific area will be strongly defended and adhered to until the sheer weight of evidence which cannot be handled by the old paradigm leads to the introduction of a new paradigm which does account for the conflicting data. Such a paradigm (model) does exist, the energy model.

THE ENERGY MODEL

The Role of Energy

The energy model integrates the body, mind, emotions, and soul into a philosophy of health and wellness which returns humanity to a linkage with nature. This has been the core of oriental philosophy and medicine for 500 years (Reid, 1994). In this model, energy is the foundation of all functioning in the world. The universe **is** energy and all physical material, including living beings, are a **product** of that energy. While the exterior appearance and even the internal structure of all matter may be different, the basis in energy is the unifying concept. Thus, all parts of the universe are linked and consequently interdependent. There are rhythms to the universe and the flow of energy which promote life, account for change, and involve natural cycles that repeat themselves. Birth, growth, death, decay, rebirth, the diurnal cycle, and seasonal changes are all examples of the natural rhythms of the universe.

The energy model also states that there is a natural harmony and balance among all types of matter, if not altered by the actions of man. This natural harmony and balance leads to peace, happiness, health, and well being when one is in alignment with the natural rhythms of the universe. Our health is inextricably linked to the health of the environment as well as to the health of the universe.

The field of physics deals with the concept of energy and Einstein's equation, $E = MC^2$, that energy equals matter times the speed of light, has been taught in high school for years. The technological advances of our Western civilization are based upon the use of electrical energy, fossil fuel energy, and nuclear energy; yet human energy is not mentioned in the field of medicine except in terms of fatigue (the decline of energy) as a symptom of illness. Clearly energy and its role in human physical functioning are not considered to be important in Western medicine. Yet what is the source of the heart beat? What is it that causes a sperm and egg to unite? What causes the fertilized ovum to divide and multiply to produce an embryo, then a fetus, and then an infant? What prompts the birth process signaled by contractions of the uterus? What is the difference between a live body and a corpse? The answer to all of these questions is the universal life force which we call energy. Quantum physics has been dealing with the concept of energy as the basis for universal functioning for almost a century and has concluded that the laws of Newtonian physics do not apply at the quantum (energy) or systems level. Yet human beings are systems and the attempts to understand this system by using the principles of Newtonian science has reached its limit. Thus the stage has been set for medical science and the healing arts to follow the lead of quantum physics just as medical science originally followed the lead of Newtonian physics.

Clearly, the human body is a very complex system but our medical paradigm seldom looks at the systems of human function but remains preoccupied with increasingly smaller units of physiological function in isolation from the world in which the organism lives. In contrast, the energy model is based on the concept of a universal system which includes all planets, all parts of the planet earth, all who live on it, and all aspects of these living creatures—body, mind, emotions, and soul.

Energy, the Emotions, and Health

Any disturbance to the harmony and balance of energy in the system leads to repercussions within the entire system. Within the energy model, one of the main disruptions to the balance of energy in the human system is emotional reactions. All emotional reactions involve an activation of the sympathetic nervous system and a resolution of this emotion with return to balance is fostered by the parasympathetic nervous system. Thus, calm, ease, peace, and feeling good are natural and normal states of the organism. This is the state of balance, harmony, homeostasis.

Emotional disturbance and reactions are destructive to the human system because they drain energy. When an emotional reaction occurs, attention should be paid to restoring the energy balance and to replenishing the energy that has been drained away. If emotional disturbance continues for an extended period of time, the energy in the human system will remain out of balance. Essentially, energy will gradually be drained away since replenishment of the energy is not occurring while the system remains out of balance. Over a period of time, a continued state of energy imbalance will eventually lead to dysfunctions at the physical level. As a signal of energy imbalance, physical symptoms occur, such as headaches, sleep disturbances, pain, allergies, infections, and eventually immune system disturbances and organ system failures. Major medical illnesses—such as cancer, heart disease and arthritis—occur after many years of energy imbalance.

A schematic representation of the above is as follows:

HEALTHY: Emotional Calm → Balanced Energy → Happiness → Optimal Physical Function → Emotional Calm → Etc.

UNHEALTHY: Emotional Arousal → Unbalanced Energy → Unhappiness Physical Symptoms → Emotional Arousal → Etc.

In this system, energy balance is achieved through control of emotional reactions so as to maintain a state of calmness and peace across the day. Health, happiness, and contentment are the outcome, and energy is available for productive and creative efforts of all kinds.

Within this paradigm, a person is born with a certain amount of energy, called "prenatal energy," acquired from one's parents. Over the lifetime one expends this energy, either quickly or slowly depending upon the lifestyle of the individual. Energy depletion occurs as the result of emotional arousal and an inattention to the natural rhythms of the body (in harmony with the rhythms of the universe) so that energy is not replenished through a proper and healthy life style. Many years of living in an aroused emotional state (stressed state) and non-replenishment of expended energy sets the stage for problems at the physical level.

The early warning signs are fatigue, headache, disturbed sleep, muscle tension, aches and pains. Treatment of these symptoms with caffeine, pain pills, and relaxants only masks the symptoms and allows one to avoid looking at the real problem, a disordered life style and improper approach to emotions. Consequently, the energy imbalance continues, as does the energy depletion, which leads to the next stage, more serious physical disorders such as immune system disturbances, cancer, heart disease, etc.

At the point that body system problems appear, the energy imbalance has existed for many years. Unfortunately, the diagnostic procedures of the medical model look strictly at the physical level and totally ignore the real cause, disordered patterns of energy within the human system. Treatments are focused strictly at the physical level as well and do not address the energy problem either.

The real solution to the problem is to replenish the energy and restore the balance of energy within the system. While one gets a supply of prenatal energy from one's parents, one can access the universal supply of prenatal energy in order to replenish oneself through meditation, through a variety of qi gong and tai chi exercises, and through Shen Qi, an advanced form of qi gong recently developed by the Chinese Qi Gong Master, Aiping Wang.

In Shen Qi training, the student becomes reacquainted with the feel of the natural rhythms of the universe within the body, learns to sense the energy flow in daily life, learns to become nonreactive to emotionally provocative stimuli, learns to eliminate those influences in life which drain energy, and learns to access prenatal universal energy to replenish the body supply which had been depleted in previous years of stress-filled life. During the course of training, the superficial symptoms of stress wane first and over time the more serious symptoms of bodily dysfunction wane as well. Lifestyle change, however, is essential because it is emotional reactions to the stress-filled lifestyle which lead to the energy imbalance in the first place.

Consequently, within the energy model, in order to produce relief in physical symptoms, reduction in emotional reactions and alteration of behavior are necessary. In contrast to the medical model, a clear mind, happy emotions, and peaceful soul are the **cause** of physical health, not the result of physical health. Likewise, a cluttered mind, a disturbed emotional state, and an unhappy soul are the cause of physical sickness, not the result of physical sickness.

Spirituality, in this context then, is the process of living life in harmony with the natural flow of events, the utilization of a quiescent approach to life in which emotional reactions are minimal, and the presence of openness, happiness, and flexibility in the face of challenges and changes. Such an approach allows one to touch the nature of God, no matter what particular religion one belongs to, and to live life with great spirit and soul.

Relevance of the Energy Model to Psychology and Rehabilitation

A review of the work of Hans Selye, particularly his book, *The Stress of Life* (1976), reveals that this scientist who devoted his life to analyzing the physiology of stress came to essentially the same conclusions as outlined above in the energy paradigm. As a physiologist his focus was primarily at the physical level, yet the last sections of his book espouse a similar philosophy as presented here. Mihaly Csikszentmihalyi has written two works which espouse similar points, *Flow: The Psychology of Optimal Experience* (1990) and *The Evolving Self: A Psychology for the Third Millennium* (1993). Happiness, he believes is not only the key to psychological health and physical health, but also necessary to resolve the social disasters of the late 20th century. Happiness is contingent, however, not on finding optimal external circumstances, but in gaining control over one's mind in order to shape one's reaction to external events rather than be bludgeoned by these reactions.

The psychology and self-help sections of all bookstores are replete with volumes which offer advice an strategies to cope with general and specific types of stressors in daily life. To dismiss such material as "pop psychology" ignores the tremendous need of the public for help in feeling better and the recognition that material success does not provide happiness. People are yearning for answers to the basic questions of the meaning of life, and finding that the traditional health care professionals and the churches do not provide satisfying assistance. These books do provide assistance and set the stage for eventual work with a teacher who is experienced in these methods, if that is desired. Yoga teachers, Taoist masters, Zen Buddhist roshis, Tibetan Buddhist lamas and tulkus are teaching in the West and do provide powerful training which improves a person's overall ability to handle stress in daily life. Many American teachers also provide good training, many of whom have studied themselves with great teachers. In my experience, reading could take me only so far. At a certain point I had to begin to practice some of the techniques described in the books, and I found that meditation groups and teachers of many of these alternative strategies provided feedback and input which supplemented my reading invaluably.

For all people and especially those with physical impairments, the external world is full of challenges and changes to which we need to respond. Whether or not these challenges and changes are defined as problems or obstacles depends upon the belief system of the person and this belief system profoundly influences the tendency to react emotionally to life events. I try to help people to accept challenges and changes in their lives as "what is," just the natural flow of life, and not to view them automatically as obstacles and problems. When something is viewed as a problem, then we begin to react emotionally, whereas if we view an event as just what is, then we have the choice to not react emotionally but rather to work with or work around "what is."

In my own professional practice, I educate people with physical disabilities about the energy model and shift the emphasis away from looking exclusively at their physical function and from analyzing their feelings toward challenges and changes in their lives to learning to feel the fluctuations in energy across the day and from day to day. Learning to identify which approaches to life's events enhance energy and which ones deplete energy is facilitated by training the client to meditate. I provide people with a simple strategy for meditation which, if followed, will reduce the ambient level of stress (emotional arousal) and make the person more sensitive to which events trigger the emotional reaction leading to the depletion of energy. By altering one's method of handling the life event, energy can be conserved and enhanced. But the real challenge is to learn to feel how emotional reactions deplete energy. Then one learns to be less emotionally responsive by interrupting the thought-emotion feedback loop by applying the techniques learned in meditation. By consistently applying this approach to daily life, equanimity and well being can occur in the presence of the environmental constraints which the person may face as the result of the disability. I am not suggesting that people with disabilities stop advocating for change to promote justice and dignity for all people and just accommodate to discriminatory practices in the environment. My goal is to provide a methodology that allows us to live more comfortably with "what is" in this world of ours at any moment so that we do not burn ourselves up with sustained emotional reactions which lead to malaise and further physical problems, which according to the energy model can be prevented.

The external events of daily existence are increasingly stressful for everyone. However, for people with physical disabilities, the toll is much greater because of the additional physical, emotional, and financial pressures of daily life. Trieschmann (1987) emphasized the role that stress plays in accelerating the aging process in people with disabilities but research is yet in its infancy to pursue this issue in depth. In 1988, Trieschmann outlined the parameters of the physical, emotional, and financial stresses of living with a spinal cord injury but the psychosocial and counseling services in rehabilitation continue to be underfunded because of the priorities inherent in the assumptions of the medical model.

A switch to the energy model from the medical model has made my professional life much easier, more fun, and more personally rewarding. My patients benefit to the extent that they continue to apply the techniques that I have taught them after ceasing therapy. But most importantly, a switch to the energy model truly empowers both the professional and the person with the disability to shift the focus from helpless victim of unfair circumstances to active agent in transcending difficulties in life.

Rehabilitation has always been concerned with the whole person, has always emphasized the importance of the environment in daily function, has always acknowledged the role of stress and emotion in response to the disability state.

Thus, the energy model provides a philosophical foundation and a set of principles which can give rehabilitation the stability it needs and the credibility it deserves.

REFERENCES

Csikszentmihalyi, M. (1990). *Flow: The psychology of optimal experience.* New York: Harper Perennial.

Csikszentmihalyi, M. (1993). *The evolving self: A psychology for the third millennium.* New York: Harper Perennial.

Kuhn, T. (1970). *The structure of scientific revolutions* (2nd ed.). Chicago: University of Chicago Press.

Reid, D. (1994). *The complete book of Chinese health and healing.* Boston: Shambhala.

Selye, H. (1976). *The stress of life.* New York: McGraw Hill.

Trieschmann, R. (1987). *Aging with a disability.* New York: Demos.

Trieschmann, R. (1988). *Spinal cord injuries: Psychological, social, and vocational rehabilitation.* New York: Demos.

4

The Rehabilitation
Ethic and Ethics

Stephen T. Wegener

D ue to the slow growth of rehabilitation medicine and the high-profile
decisions engendered by acute care medicine, ethical dilemmas in rehabilitation settings are only recently receiving careful consideration. It
may be here, in the arena of rehabilitation and chronic illness, that ethical and
human choices are most fully realized. The nature of the medical conditions, the
setting in which treatment takes place and changes in our society all are factors
in this realization.

While values may play only a small role in defining what constitutes treatment in acute care medicine, the nature of the medical conditions encountered in
rehabilitation necessitates that values play a large role in determining not only
what constitutes treatment but what constitutes a treatable problem. Here the
patients and providers play a key role in determining the treatable problem and
the extent to which this problem is a disability. The goal of acute medical care is
clear in both parties: cure. In rehabilitation the goals are defined by values and
what constitutes "quality of life." Differences in goals can develop between, or
among, staff, patients, families, and, increasingly, third-party payers.

The rehabilitation setting differs from the acute setting in terms of treatment
duration, demand characteristics and the number of health care providers
involved. The extended length of the rehabilitation/chronic illness process allows
for the development of close relationships between provider and patient. These
emotional connections and this affectively charged interaction provide a unique
context for the development of ethical dilemmas.

Hartke (1991), speaking to the predicament of older adults entering the rehabilitation setting, posits that these patients encounter a situation with specific

*I thank Ann Deaton, Ph.D. and the anonymous reviewer for helpful comments on an
earlier draft of this article.*
From *Rehabilitation Psychology, 41*(1) (1996), 5–17. Reprinted with permission.

expectations and demand characteristics. This rehabilitation ethic reflects, and is the medical counterpart of, the Protestant work ethic. In this setting, independence, effort, accepting pain, and maximizing functional ability are valued at the expense of comfort and potential nurturance. Gunther (1987) has identified values evidenced by the rehabilitation environment and workers that reflect this rehabilitation ethic. There is an emphasis on performance-oriented goal attainment where activity, cooperation, and independence are highly valued. These values may reflect the general youth of rehabilitation workers as well as the emphasis by the current health care environment on speed and outcome measurement to justify expense. The rehabilitation experience is presented in a scholastic atmosphere characterized by classes, discussions and requirements for learning health care information. Here rehabilitation professionals, due to their advanced education, are likely to be comfortable while those whose background has not emphasized educational activity may find the role of patient or student equally uncomfortable. These observations may be no less true of younger individuals who find themselves in the rehabilitation setting.

The complexity of quality of life issues may be lost in the focus on performance, outcome and cooperation. Patients who do not reflect these values may engender defensive, angry or labeling responses from staff. The number of professionals involved in the rehabilitation process complicates the decision process. The task brings together a group of people who must work together with considerable trust and loyalty, but who may adhere to different moral teachings and values. The psychologist may be consulted to evaluate the patient's suitability or motivation for rehabilitation when the patient does not conform to the characteristics of the rehabilitation team or environment. It may be equally appropriate for the psychologist to evaluate the adequacy of the team's response to patients' wishes, autonomy or values. These conditions all contribute to increased risk for the development of conflicts regarding treatment protocols and goals.

Beginning with the independent living movement in the mid-1960s, and culminating in the passage of the Americans with Disabilities Act and the Self-Determination Act of 1991, there have been changes in our society toward greater individual autonomy. There has also been increased recognition, at least in the legal system, of people with impairments and illness as individuals with rights who are disabled by environmental (economic, mobility, lack of personal care assistance) and social barriers. Other social developments such as consumerism, the civil rights movement, trends toward deinstitutionalization of persons with medical needs, and the demystification of medical professionals contribute to recognition of the rights of patients (DeJong, 1979). These developments, in conjunction with other aspects of the rehabilitation environment, set the stage for determining human values in one of their most profound forms. Psychologists need to consider the basic assumptions underlying their behavior in the rehabilitation setting and become knowledgeable of ethical models that may provide guidance in resolving potential ethical dilemmas.

ETHICAL DILEMMAS IN CHRONIC ILLNESS AND REHABILITATION

Ethical issues and values play an integral role in decisions made by both staff and patients. While patient refusal of treatment garners our attention and concern, staff decisions regarding admission and termination of rehabilitation treatment are equally fraught with ethical issues. There are few data to guide admission and discharge decisions which are often not recognized as decisions informed by ethical issues. Patients are usually not consulted on the terms of admission to rehabilitation and often they are not aware of the criteria leading to termination of treatment. Decisions for termination are often based on patients "plateauing" in treatment, i.e., leveling out in their rate of progress or degree of progress. These decisions are made by staff, and increasingly third-party decision makers, whose values, morals and view of the world are critical to the determination. Further, the patient and family may not be aware of the influence third-party payers and financial issues play in the decision. The larger role of third parties in decision making requires psychologists attend to their responsibility to recommend and advocate for the most appropriate rehabilitation service for their patients.

To date the most careful studies in treatment refusal have focused on the area of patients or their surrogate seeking termination of life support, medication, or food and water. A number of recent cases have brought to our attention the issue of refusal of treatment in rehabilitation, primarily in right to die situations such as David Rivlin in Michigan, Elizabeth Bouvia in California, Larry McAfee in Georgia, and Kenneth Bergstedt in Nevada (Batavia, 1991; Longmore, 1991; Reidy, Crozier, Caplan, Kutys, & Sinnott, 1992). Treatment refusals may arise in a number of areas: (1) utilization of life support, (2) medically necessary care to prevent life-threatening illness, and (3) rehabilitation to improve level of functioning/quality of life. While these later two events are thought to be common, no data exist on their frequency. This attention on treatment refusal by patients may not be warranted by the number of cases involved, particularly in comparison to the number of cases where nonlife-sustaining treatment is withdrawn by staff.

Treatment refusal by patients raises the issue of noncompliance with its connotations of deviance as described in Talcott Parson's classic view of the doctor-patient relationship and the sick role (Parsons, 1951). There are often assumptions that refusal is due to psychopathology, notably depression. These assumptions persist in spite of evidence that depression may not be as widespread as initially thought, particularly in the spinal cord injury population (Frank, Elliott, Corcoran, & Wonderlich, 1987). There are also data to suggest that the extent and severity of these emotional reactions are overestimated by the rehabilitation staff (Cushman & Dijkers, 1990; Tucker, 1980). Wright (1988, 1993) has identified and reiterated the continuing "fundamental negative bias" that perpetuates "disabling myths" regarding those with disability. Patients who exercise their rights of self-determination may threaten the treatment team in a number of ways. This act raises doubts as to the importance of rehabilitation professionals' work and may challenge their views regarding quality of life.

Ethical Models

What guidelines are available to assist us in addressing these ethical issues? The American Psychological Association (APA) Code of Ethics provides only the broadest guidelines, speaking to the issue of patient autonomy in the "General Principles" and in a number of sections. Principle D focuses on respect for "Peoples' Rights and Dignity" requiring psychologists to "accord appropriate respect to the fundamental rights, dignity, and worth of all people" such that they are ". . . aware of cultural, individual, and role differences, including those due to . . . disability . . . and do not knowingly participate or condone unfair discriminatory practices" (pp. 1599–1600). Notable also are Section 1.09, Respecting Others, requiring psychologists to "respect the rights of others to hold values, attitudes, and opinions that differ from their own." Section 7.06 further notes "In forensic matters psychologists are required to be familiar with rules governing their roles." (This section would surely encompass familiarity with the ADA and Self-Determination Act of 1991.) Section 2.04, Use of Assessment in General and with Special Population, requires that psychologists make adjustments in interpretation of evaluation instruments because of factors such as disability (American Psychological Association, 1992).

These guidelines provide broad principles to inform behavior but do not specifically address the issues encountered in the practice of rehabilitation psychology. The ethical literature presents an evolving set of models to illuminate key issues and provide guidance in approaching these decisions. These models reflect varying emphasis on the two primary principles underlying ethical decision making—beneficence and autonomy. The ethical models are the paternalistic model, contractual model, educational model, and deliberative model. The roles, goals, and ethical principles inherent in each of the models are summarized in Table 4.1.

The Paternalistic Model

The paternalistic model casts the provider in the role of decision maker. According to this model, providers, due to their specialized training and expertise determine what treatment is necessary, as well as the course and goals of that treatment. The provider is the active party and the patient is the passive recipient of care. The patient may, or may not, be informed of treatment decisions, the underlying rationale or the implications based on the provider's beliefs about how this information may impact the patient. The predominant ethical principle guiding this model of interaction is beneficence. Decisions are made in the patient's best interest with the provider as the primary decision maker who is thought to be in the best position to determine what interventions are indicated.

An example of this model in practice is that of a health care provider deciding for a patient who has experienced a T-12 spinal cord injury that it will be too difficult to attempt brace walking and that the individual will be more effective using a wheelchair. The extent to which this model remains operative is reflected

TABLE 4.1 Ethical Models for Medical Decision Making

Model	Roles	Goal	Guiding Principle
Paternalistic	provider-patient	provider determined	beneficence
Contractual	provider-consumer	negotiated	autonomy
Educational	provider-patient	provider determined	
			beneficence→autonomy
	provider-consumer	negotiated	
Deliberative	members of the rehabilitation community	co-determined	empathy

in a recent study by Farnsworth (1991) who found that over two thirds of the requests for competency were initiated by staff due to patient disagreement on treatment or disposition. While this observation may be explained by a number of potential causes, it is likely that providers who believe that they are in the best position to make these treatment decisions may question the competency of those patients who disagree. This model is inappropriate in the rehabilitation setting for a number of reasons: (1) the growing recognition of individual autonomy for persons with disability; (2) the need to foster active participation by the patient in the rehabilitation treatment; and (3) the difficulty of determining the impact of rehabilitation interventions across physical, psychological, environmental, family, work place, and community systems without the patient's active involvement.

The Contractual Model

The contractual model is based on the notion of increased patient autonomy and participation through the use of informed consent. The provider informs the patient of the potential treatment plan, risks and benefits. The patient becomes an informed consumer who may question various treatment plans and outcomes. Providers are still obligated to provide appropriate medical care; however, the care provided is that which is agreed to by the patient/consumer. The patient/consumer is a more active participant in the treatment planning and implementation process. This active role encompasses the ability, and the option, of refusal of treatment. The primary ethical principle guiding this model is one of autonomy.

The Hastings Center has noted several limitations of this model when applied in the rehabilitation setting (Caplan, Callahan, & Haas, 1987). The application is limited by (1) the multiple providers involved who determine various aspects of treatment, each with different goals, agendas, and moral codes; (2) difficulty in obtaining informed consent for all the components of the treatment plan due to components that are often in flux; (3) limitations on the providers' ability to describe likely outcomes of a rehabilitation program as the patient plays a critical role in determining outcome; (4) the increasing role played by third parties who are not formally included in the contractual model of the patient-provider, relationship; (5) questions as to whether patients can make informed choices early in rehabilitation based on an inability to appreciate risks and benefits of choices; and (6) the presumption of autonomous functioning in someone who is coping with significant loss.

The use of this model in medical decision making is reflected in the common practice of the inpatient rehabilitation team meeting with patients and their family to explain the course of rehabilitation and desirable outcomes. In this meeting the benefits of the program, the patient's role, and expected outcomes are commonly addressed. While formal written informed consent is usually not obtained, agreement to participate serves as implied informed consent. At this stage of medical care the patient's ability to question the course of action is likely to be limited, although it is assumed the patient has made an informed choice.

As stated in the Hastings Center Report, "The challenge facing medical professionals in rehabilitation is frequently not how to respect autonomy, or whether to obtain informed consent at every stage of the rehabilitation process but, rather, what steps and activities, and with what degree of persuasion or even coercion, are morally permissible in the hope of restoring autonomy" (Caplan et al., 1987, p. 11). The nature of the interaction has a propensity to be marked by negotiation between provider and patient/consumer, where the patient is sold on the advisability of accepting certain goals (subacute placement, independence, autonomy, physical activity) reflecting prevailing societal and/or staff values.

The Educational Model

This decision model proposed by Caplan and colleagues (1987) is characterized by initial decisions guided by beneficence with the goal of restoring long-term autonomy. Early in rehabilitation, providers assume greater leeway in making decisions, assuming that the sudden illness or injury make it difficult for patients to make fully informed decisions. As time, education, and therapy progress, the patient becomes a fully participating partner in the treatment process. While the model suggests early limitations in autonomy and need for paternalistic attitudes, patients retain certain rights—right to counsel, informed consent in life-threatening situations, and involvement in the decision-making process.

The educational model of medical decision making is reflected in the rehabilitation of the individual with traumatic brain injury. Early in the rehabilitation process physical, occupational or cognitive therapy may be initiated without the individual understanding the rationale, goal, or even need for treatment. As the individual progresses and there is a return in cognitive functioning or an increase in awareness of impairments, the individual's ability to influence treatment goals increases and the patient's decisions regarding discharge and placement options are respected.

While the movement to contractual and educational models reflects the developments in society discussed earlier, the means for achieving these goals are unclear and there remains a strong spirit of beneficence. Note that in the educational model the emphasis is on unidirectional education, where we, as professionals, strive to educate patients in our perspective and approach which is infused with our values. While this may not be the intent or spirit of the model, the language and context may serve to support an emphasis on patients adapting to our environment rather than mutual accommodation. This unintended role assignment may underlie the current adversarial, legalistic approach to resolving treatment decision dilemmas, even if an individual decision never reaches a formal judicial forum. The solution to resolving ethical dilemmas is not to invoke rights—the patient's right to refuse treatment, the right to equal access, staff's right to terminate medical care—but rather to reframe or reconfigure the situation. Specifically, the values and environment that inform the discussion on ethics must be reconfigured. This option is reflected in the deliberative model presented in Table 1.

The Deliberative Model

This model is characterized by the assumption that both parties are members of the rehabilitation community. The interaction between patient and provider is marked by deliberation. The notion of deliberation has been most completely articulated by Emanuel (1991) who suggests we need to broaden our understanding of what informs our discussion of ethical issues in health care settings. Rehabilitation patients are thrust into a medical setting and culture they did not choose. Emanuel posits that this culture, like others, has a political process that patients must enter into if they are to become active members. We become members of this rehabilitation health care culture through participation in a deliberative process. This deliberative process is one where, through reflection, choice and discussion, an individual comes to join in a common interest, thereby entailing responsibility in the culture. Those who do not engage in this process and do not join the culture entail no responsibility for their behavior or participation, leading to patient and staff dissatisfaction. Persons who have the opportunity to participate in community through deliberation achieve autonomy and realize the capacity for responsibility. They come to see, through their participation, that they are members of the community bound together by a common interest.

Mourer (1991) observes that refusal of treatment or reluctance to participate in rehabilitation raises a crisis that the patient as well as the provider must master. There is significant potential for a defensive response by the patient engendering anger, anticipation of retribution, guilt, or avoidance. As more control is ceded to the patient it raises for providers a sense of helplessness and loss of control in "our own" environment. The concept of rehabilitation, as an environment or a process, which is "ours," is seriously challenged by adopting a deliberative model for addressing ethical issues. Redefining this community as one that is owned mutually by provider and patient begins to provide us with a potential means of solving the ethical problems that arise. The deliberative process serves to balance the patients' initial lack of choice which defines their original entrance into the rehabilitation community. Individuals do not choose to participate in the rehabilitation culture, they are selected. In most cases both patients and staff arrive at the rehabilitation setting after a background, training, and socialization in acute medicine. This acute medical setting is likely to reinforce roles, attitudes and behavior that are inconsistent with equality and autonomy. A model that draws our attention to the need for a deliberation process is desirable.

What tools exist to facilitate this deliberative process? Technological advances or legal developments are often thought to be the source of ethical problems in health care settings. Thus, each of these areas are in turn considered as potential solutions to the ethical dilemmas. Rather, it may be that in rehabilitation and chronic disease, ethical problems grow not out of technological or legal factors but out of the difficulties incumbent in determining and achieving enhanced quality of life. We may rediscover tools to better manage potential ethical dilemmas by moving from a focus on technical and legal aspects in the practice of medicine and embracing the human dimension of healing and rehabilitation. Psychology can make an important contribution. The nature and intricacies of the provider-patient relationship are often the source of ethical dilemmas. Psychology has well established principles for developing and maintaining constructive therapeutic relationships. Psychology may make an important contribution by bringing these skills and knowledge to bear in the prevention and resolution of ethical predicaments.

THE ROLE OF EMPATHY IN RESOLVING ETHICAL ISSUES

It is often conflicts of values or perceptions in the context of emotionally laden relationships that bring ethical dilemma to the fore. We have seen how this predicament is more likely to arise in the rehabilitation setting, given the duration and nature of the treatment process. The fact that these dilemmas are characterized by emotions, competing perceptions and values makes empathy a critical tool in resolving these situations. Psychologists seldom have formal training in ethics or legal issues. Psychology does have special expertise to offer the rehabilitation patient and treatment team in the area of understanding conflicts in values, perceptions, and the emotional context of the communication. Empathy is a one key tool whereby the psychologist can facilitate the patient's entrance into deliberative participation in the rehabilitation process.

Empathy is the fundamental mode of human relatedness, wherein emotional connection allows one person to understand the inner experience of another (Kohut, 1971). Empathy requires the individual to engage in two simultaneous processes—perceiving the emotional cues aroused in oneself by the other individual and maintaining the cognitive capacity to understand and reflect these events. This empathetic interaction occurs as an interpersonal process where the accuracy of the empathetic response is checked and clarified with the other. This ongoing process of empathetic understanding of the other and clarification of the perceived feelings, values, and wishes is the hallmark of therapeutic interaction. Diamond (1988) contends that many ethical dilemmas are a result of failure in empathy. Empathetic attunement requires that the parties be able, and willing, to express and receive emotional messages. Rehabilitation patients' ability to communicate their experience may be limited due to closed head injury, cardiovascular accident, respiratory difficulty, language impairment or pseudobulbar palsy. These individuals are exposed to a medical environment which initially encourages passivity, fostering limited autonomous communication. The stress of extended hospitalization may also bring to the surface interpersonal, characterological and premorbid psychopathology that interferes with the communication of inner experience. In the case of personality disorders, the patients' inability to empathize with others may be so severe that they are unable to enter as an equal partner into the rehabilitation community. With these individuals, empathetic understanding of their predicament may require a decision that the most ethical treatment is the establishment of a therapeutic environment characterized by firm boundaries and consistent expectations of appropriate behavior. Firm limits and boundaries are necessary to promote ethical use of rehabilitation resources by the society and affords individuals with severe personality disorders an opportunity to avail themselves of the rehabilitation experience. Rehabilitation staff and psychologists may experience empathetic barriers with patients in the form of differences in life experience, social class, cultural background or expectations. Hostility arising from patient passivity or rejection of the rehabilitation ethic, defensiveness about the value of our work, and strong emotional responses both in and out of awareness also limit our ability to empathize. It is not uncommon to hear, even from rehabilitation staff, "if I were him, I would want to be dead." Such comments indicate the extent of empathetic failure by rehabilitation staff. Effective empathy allows us to know from the patients' perspective why they wish to pursue a particular course of rehabilitation or refuse treatment or are unable to fully participate in a rehabilitation community.

Recent observations in developmental psychology and the psychology of women have reemphasized the importance of empathy and communal interests in facilitating human development (Jordan, Kaplan, Miller, Stiver, & Surrey, 1991). A central focus of this work is a reexamination of developmental theory and its relevance for understanding the nature of empathetic relationships. The most recent work reflects data indicating a growing appreciation of the interdependence of children and parents. These theorists maintain that there has been an overemphasis on increasing need for separation, autonomy and personal independence. This school has noted in "David Bakan's terms how society emphasizes the 'agenetic ethic' (self-protective, assertive, individualistic, pushing toward achievement) at the expense of the 'communal ethic' (being at one with other organisms, characterized by contact or union)." Progress in rehabilitation is often conceptualized in this same manner with a strong emphasis on moving people toward autonomy and independence. While this may be an integral and important goal for rehabilitation, it is possible we may overemphasize these goals at the expense of interdependence, deliberation and empathetic understanding. The deliberative model calls for the therapist or team to expand and enhance the empathetic understanding of the patient for alternative feelings, values, experiences. The model for relationships described by Jordan and colleagues (1991), where the rehabilitation milieu is based on empathic attunement, interdependence and deliberation may facilitate the rehabilitation process.

TRAINING REHABILITATION PSYCHOLOGISTS FOR ETHICAL DILEMMAS

Pedagogic issues related to ethics in rehabilitation psychology have emphasized the need to educate students and providers regarding the underlying principles of ethics and legal decisions relating to these situations. However useful training in these principles or legal decisions may be, it does not replace essential principles of psychological practice. Emphasizing the principles underlying therapeutic relationships may prove instrumental in resolving ethical dilemmas that arise in rehabilitation. The following recommendations are offered to aid in training psychologists for practice in the rehabilitation setting and to address the incumbent ethical dilemmas.

First, avoid premature specialization in the training of psychologists. There is considerable debate regarding the training necessary for psychologists who will practice in the rehabilitation settings. A number of authors (Belar, 1988; Elliott & Gramling, 1990) have described the disadvantages associated with early specialization. Faculty and mentors have the responsibility of training psychologists during the predoctoral phase in the core psychological principles and techniques of clinical practice. Students and practitioners need to be firmly rooted in their therapeutic skills, clinical practice and professional identity in order to work effectively in the rehabilitation setting with the multiple disciplines and their varying roles and models of patient care.

Second, training received by psychologists to prevent and address situations giving rise to ethical dilemmas should emphasize those principles, skills and qualities that are fundamental to psychology and the therapeutic relationship. This training reinforces the basic therapeutic principles that our primary alliance is with the patient rather than the referring physician, institution or rehabilitation team. The therapeutic skills and qualities that have been identified in psychotherapy outcome research, including empathy (see Bergin & Garfield, 1986), need to be recognized and taught as potential tools for preventing and resolving ethical dilemmas.

Third, mechanisms that lead psychologists to question the fundamental assumptions of the systems within which we operate need to be established. In our desire to be an integral part of the rehabilitation team and medical community we may easily lose our objectivity regarding the practices of the system in which we are working. Supervisors, mentors and colleagues in peer supervision have the responsibility to bring to students' and each other's attention the need for questioning basic assumptions that exist in rehabilitation settings. For example, questioning staff decisions to discontinue treatment as well as avoiding the labeling of patients who refuse treatment grow out of this vigilance.

Fourth, didactic education on ethical principles should be an integral part of each level of training. Training in the Code of Ethics for psychologists and general instruction in the broad ethical principles that guide medical decision making should be the focus at the predoctoral level. Rather than emphasizing medical or rehabilitation ethical decisions, predoctoral students may benefit by applying this information to more traditional therapeutic relationships in order to master the application of therapeutic and ethical principles in more familiar situations. In the postdoctoral phase, didactic training in ethical principles and legal issues relevant to health care and rehabilitation settings is warranted. While the APA requires training in ethical and professional issues as part of an APA-approved doctoral training program, this requirement does not exist at the postdoctoral level. Consideration should be given to including required training on ethical models and issues as part of postdoctoral programs nationally and continuing education requirements at the state level. Similarly, those seeking certification at the diplomate level should demonstrate proficiency in handling ethical issues in their area of specialization.

Fifth, those practicing health care and rehabilitation settings should seek practicum experience on ethical consultation services. Most major medical centers have ethical consultation services to provide support to health care practitioners in difficult cases. Psychologists working in rehabilitation settings will benefit by obtaining practicum experience or supervision on this consultation service. Preferably the experience could take place with the guidance of another psychologist whose professional role is firmly established.

Training in ethical principles, while necessary, is not sufficient. A greater emphasis on, and practice of, empathy and deliberative interaction and other principles of therapeutic relationship may provide assistance in preventing and resolving potential ethical dilemmas in health and rehabilitation settings.

REFERENCES

American Health Consultants Inc. (1991). *Medical Ethics Advisor,* 7(1), 1–4.

American Psychological Association. (1992). Ethical principles of psychologists and code of conduct. *American Psychologist, 47,* 1597–1611.

Bakan, D. (1966). *The duality of human existence: An essay on psychology and religion.* Boston: Beacon Press.

Batavia, A. I. (1991). A disability rights-independent living perspective on euthanasia. *Western Journal of Medicine, 154,* 616–617.

Belar, C. D. (1988). Education in behavioral medicine: Perspectives from psychology. *Annals of Behavioral Medicine, 10,* 11–14.

Bergin, A. E., & Garfield, S. L. (1986). *Handbook of psychotherapy and behavior change.* New York: Wiley.

Caplan, A. L., Callahan, D., & Haas, J. (1987). *Ethical and policy issues in rehabilitation medicine.* Briarcliff Manor, NY: A Hastings Center Report.

Cushman, L. A., & Dijkers, M. P. (1990). Depressed mood in spinal cord injured patients: Staff perceptions and patient realities. *Archives of Physical Medicine Rehabilitation, 71,* 191–197.

DeJong, G. (1979). Independent living from social movement to analytic paradigm. *Archives of Physical Medicine and Rehabilitation, 60,* 435–446.

Diamond, D. B. (1988). Psychologic conflict underlying bioethical dilemmas in a chronic disease hospital. *General Hospital Psychiatry, 10,* 250–254.

Emanuel, E. J. (1991). *The ends of human life.* Cambridge, MA: Harvard University Press.

Elliott, T., & Gramling, S. (1990). Psychologists and rehabilitation: New roles and old training models. *American Psychologist, 45,* 762–765.

Farnsworth, M. G. (1990). Competency evaluations in a general hospital. *Psychosomatics, 31,* 60–66.

Frank, R. G., Elliott, T. R., Corcoran, J. R., & Wonderlich, S. A. (1987). Depression after spinal cord injury: Is it necessary? *Clinical Psychology Review, 7,* 1–20.

Gunther, M. S. (1987). Catastrophic illness and the care givers: Real burdens and solutions with respect to the role of the behavioral sciences. In B. Caplan (Ed.), *Rehabilitation psychology desk reference* (pp. 219–243). Rockville, MD: Aspen Publishers.

Hartke, R. J. (1991). *Psychological aspects of geriatric rehabilitation.* Gaithersburg, MD: Aspen Publishing.

Jordan, J. V., Kaplan, A. G., Miller, J. B., Stiver, I. P., & Surrey, J. L. (1991). *Women's growth in connection.* New York: Guilford Press.

Kohut, H. (1971). *The analysis of the self.* New York: International Universities Press.

Longmore, P. K. (1991). The strange death of David Rivlin. *Western Journal of Medicine, 154,* 615–616.

Mourer, S. (1991). The refusal of treatment: Staff reaction and recommendations. *SCI Psychosocial Process, 4(3),* 72–76.

Parsons, T. (1951). *The social system.* New York: Free Press.

Reidy, K., Crozier, K. S., Caplan, B., Kutys, M., & Sinnott, M. C. (1992). Treatment refusals during rehabilitation: Ethical concerns of the interdisciplinary rehabilitation team. *SCI Psychosocial Process, 5(10),* 44–51.

Smith, D. H., & Veatch, R. M. (1987). *Guidelines on the termination of life-sustaining treatment and care of the dying.* A Report by the Hastings Center. Bloomington, IN: Indiana University Press.

Tucker, S. J. (1980). The psychology of spinal cord injury: Patient-staff interactions. *Rehabilitation Literature, 41(5-6),* 114–121.

Wright, B. A. (1988). Attitudes and the fundamental negative bias. In H. E. Yuker (Ed.), *Attitudes towards persons with disabilities* (pp. 3–21). New York: Springer Publishing.

Wright, B. A. (1993). Division of Rehabilitation Psychology: Roots, guiding principle, and a persistent concern. *Rehabilitation Psychology, 36,* 63–65.

5

Coping with A Journey Toward Recovery: From the Inside Out

Dale Walsh

I have worked in the field of mental health for about 20 years. I can talk about this part of my life easily. I have also been a survivor of a long-term psychiatric disability for most of my childhood and adult life, and I am a survivor of the mental health system, both public and private. This is the harder part of my life to talk about. I have walked on both sides of the fence, so to speak. I want to share with you my own personal path toward recovery and what I see as a consumer practitioner to be necessary to support the recovery process of people who use the mental health system.

First, a word about language. There is no clear consensus within either the professional mental health community or among the people who have actually experienced psychiatric treatment as to what we are to be called. In the 1970s, when people who were former "patients" started to come together and share their experiences, they called themselves just that—ex-patients or former patients. Later, as the movement developed and grew and people collectively began to express their anger, some people used the name "psychiatric inmate" to make clear their dissatisfaction with the prevailing power inequities of the medical model and with the way they were treated. In California, the term "client" came to be used, because it met the dual goals of neutrality and descriptiveness. And in the 1980s the term "consumer" began to be used, mostly by the mental health system and by family groups (usually groups of parents who had an adult child with a severe psychiatric disability) in an attempt to find a label which was non-stigmatizing, yet acceptable to them. Other people who have been through the mental health system and consider themselves in recovery may use the phrase

This chapter is based on a presentation at the Alliance for the Mentally Ill/Department of Mental Health Curriculum and Training Committee Annual Conference in Boston, MA April 19, 1996

From *Psychiatric Rehabilitation Journal, 20*(2) (Fall 1996), 85–89. Reprinted with permission.

"psychiatric survivors." This debate over language is more than semantics. What people choose to call themselves is a key element in forming a group identity. It is also an indication of people's felt sense of empowerment and the place they feel they occupy within the hierarchy of the system of mental health care or services. It is important for the mental health system to be respectful and to take careful note of the names or phrases used to describe the people who use their services. Since I knew I was one, I have called myself a "survivor" or "person with a psychiatric disability." Recently I have been with some colleagues who prefer the phrase "person with a psychiatric label." I like that because the phrase speaks to the stigma carried and experienced by those of us who have been through psychiatric "treatment."

I have been dealing with the aftereffects, the stigma, and the shame of having a psychiatric disability for most of my life. As a child I was overly good. I was very anxious. I had multiple physical problems, nightmares, and trouble sleeping. As an adult, I have always been restricted in performing many of life's everyday functions—going to a shopping mall or to the bank, taking vacations or doing other leisure activities, going to social events like weddings, and working full time. Many times just leaving my house has been too anxiety provoking for me to handle. I have had many episodes of depression so severe that basic functioning has been difficult. Most of the time I live with some level of anxiety and a sense of terror and foreboding that come not from the present but from my past history of abuse. Feeling safe in the world is something I work on a daily basis.

For many years I believed in a traditional medical model. I had a disease. I was sick. I was told I was mentally ill, that I should learn to cope with my anxiety, my depression, my pain, and my panic. I never told anyone about the voices, but they were there, too. I was told I should change my expectations of myself and realize I would always have to live a very restricted life.

After I was diagnosed, I was put in a box up on a shelf. Occasionally I was taken down and my medication was changed. But no one really talked to me. No one helped me figure out why I should be content to take my medication and be grateful things were not worse. After all, at least I did not have to live my life in the back wards of a state hospital.

Because of my history and because of the society in which I lived, I easily turned the notion of illness into thinking there was something wrong with me. I was the problem. I felt deformed, everything I did was wrong. I had no place in the world. I was a freak. I was deeply ashamed of who I was and I tried my best to cover up my abnormality. I learned from those around me that psychiatric disability and its aftereffects were something to hide. As a result I lived marginally. I worked in a constant state of terror and tried to look normal. For the most part I succeeded—but at a tremendous cost to myself in terms of my energy, my self-image, my fear, and my inferiority. There were times when the stresses got to be too much and I ended up hospitalized, defeated, and feeling a failure because I couldn't tolerate even the day-to-day problems of what seemed to be a fairly simple life.

I worked in the field of mental health and I was very careful not to let anyone know my shameful secret. I was constantly terrified someone would find me out. I kept myself in entry-level positions because I was having a hard enough time without the added stresses of climbing up the ladder in my field. I went to therapy. I took my medication and waited to feel better. I waited and waited. . . .

I sometimes felt angry at my caregivers, but mostly I felt angry at myself. At times my symptoms were better but I wasn't. I felt powerless. I felt empty. I looked outside myself to the doctors and professionals to cure me, or at least take away some of my pain. But they didn't. Maybe I was one of those hopeless cases. I felt despair and deep loneliness.

This old patriarchal system of treatment and culture of disease is characterized by a hierarchical arrangement of power, a mechanistic view of the mind, causality due to organic forces outside the person's self, an emphasis on a person's deficits, and treatment administered by an expert—always at a professional distance. Did they think they might catch it? Why were they all so careful to maintain that professional distance? For years I felt trapped because I knew no other way to look at myself and my process.

Then about 8 years ago I read *The Courage to Heal.* I started talking to people—professionals and survivors who knew about the effects of trauma and psychiatric disability. I was lucky enough to stumble on 12 Step and other self-help groups. Finally my symptoms, my dreams, and my fears started making sense. I discovered the principles and the practices of recovery. I discovered hope. I had lived for years in despair because the pills and the therapy did not make me better. I began to see that if my life was to become better, I would have to do it myself. I saw that other people with histories similar to mine had been able to move beyond their symptoms. I started working with a therapist who was able to communicate to me that she trusted and believed in my own capacity to grow and move forward. She was willing to assist me but she respected my own pacing. I began to believe I could actually participate in a healing process. As I looked within myself I discovered over the following years, slowly and sometimes painfully, that healing, making positive changes in my life, and feeling better, were all possible. Especially helpful to this process were several self-help groups where I didn't have to hide, where people understood and were engaged in struggles similar to mine. I saw people who were further along in their recovery who served as role models. I also got to know people who were not so far along as I was—whom I could mentor. Giving back and learning how to get out of myself and into someone else's frame of reference has been, and continues to be, an important step in my recovery.

What I found through my own experience is that in order to travel the path of true recovery I could not rely on externals, wait, hope to be rescued, or be made better because of someone or something outside me. Instead, I learned that both the power and the possibility of change reside within me. I could make decisions that would affect my life. But I found I could not do this alone. I needed a supportive community around me. Slowly and gradually I found people who understood. I found friends and support people who could help me hold the hope when I was going through tough times and when I reached what felt like an insurmountable obstacle. These people believed in my capacity to heal. As I learned to take risks, I found that I could actually set and accomplish goals very much like people who were chronically normal.

Recovery is not a return to a former level of functioning. I have heard so many people—professionals and survivors alike—say that mental illness is not curable. I agree that we can never go back to our "premorbid" selves. The experience of the disability, and the stigma attached to it, changes us forever. Instead, recovery is a deeply personal and unique process of changing one's attitudes, values, self concept, and goals. It is finding ways to live a hopeful, satisfying, active, and contributing life. Everyone is changed by major happenings in their lives. We cannot return to the past. Recovery involves the development of a new meaning and purpose in one's life. It is looking realistically at both the limitations and the possibilities. It is much more than mere symptom relief.

As I continued on my path of recovery, I found I could handle responsible jobs. I am now slowly expanding my social network as I feel safer in the world and more comfortable with who I am. And, very importantly, I have come out of the closet and announced publicly, as a representative of those with psychiatric labels, who I am, where I have been, and where we as a community of oppressed people can go if we can find our voices, recapture our power, and exercise it to take charge of our lives and our journey toward wholeness. I am still in recovery, for it is a process—not a sudden landing.

Discovering and participating in this culture of healing has given me the hope and courage to travel the path of recovery. This is a culture of inclusion, hope, caring, and cooperation; of empowerment, equality, and humor; of dignity, respect, and trust. Forming relationships and creating systems of mental health care based on these principles are vital to supporting the growth of people who are users of the system. Traditionally, people who have been labeled as mentally ill have been considered to have poor judgment. They need to be taken care of. They do not know what is best for them. They are told what is wrong with them, what they need, what their future is to be like, and what is in their best interest. The stigma and discrimination that those of us who are labeled as mentally ill have suffered steals our hope, isolates us, and is a barrier to our healing.

Part of healing and recovery is the ability to participate as full citizens in the life of the community. As psychiatric survivors begin to break their silence and advocate for their humanity, the call and demand for basic civil rights becomes increasingly stronger. People want to be able to make their own choices about their own lives. They want to be seen, heard, and taken seriously. They want to be part of the decision making which so deeply affects their everyday experiences. This taking back of power and being taken seriously are both necessary components of recovery.

The notion that there is a recovery process that goes on internally within each person with a psychiatric label, often very separate from the treatment the person receives, is a new and somewhat threatening concept of the psychiatric treatment community. As recovery begins to be talked about and recognized by psychiatric survivors, it offers a way of taking back dignity, self-responsibility, and a sense of hope for the future.

By taking back power from the system of care, a consumer/survivor acknowledges that the ability to cope and heal comes from within. No one else, including the best of service providers, can do anything but facilitate the healing process. However, this facilitation—if it takes the form of good attention, respect, validation, and genuine connection—is an essential part of recovery.

Empowerment is a vital component of our recovery. Allowing and supporting a change within a program, agency, or system requires trust among administrators, staff members, and the people served. This change requires a shift, from power being retained exclusively by administrators to it being shared among all constituencies. It requires a willingness to take risks in not only allowing—but actively encouraging—people to work toward their own goals. It means that choice and self-determination are to be considered foremost when consumer/survivors and staff members are developing treatment and rehabilitation plans. When treatment or rehabilitation is seen as more than prescribing the right formula, and when the emphasis is placed on maintaining the functioning and identity of the person, an atmosphere that promotes recovery is created. We who use the mental health system need to play a significant role in the shaping of the services, policies, and research that affect us. We need to have a place at the table and become participants in a shared dialogue.

When people assert control over their own lives and make their own decisions, they also take on responsibility for the consequences of their decisions. Often, as service providers, we want to protect people from failure. We know, or at least think we know, what is best. We do not like to see people fail—both because of the pain it may cause to the person, but also because of the pain and feelings of failure we may experience. Sometimes when psychiatric survivors decide to make changes in their lives, they may not succeed. And, like other people, they may or may not learn from their failures. Like other people, they have a right to take risks. And sometimes they succeed, surpassing all expectations.

How many of you have tried something new and found it did not work? An investment perhaps? Or maybe a new relationship, or a marriage? You were allowed to take these risks even if the money you put into the investment was money you could not afford to lose, even if the relationship was the same kind of destructive relationship you had been through in the past. Maybe you learned from these situations, but maybe you didn't. People with psychiatric labels have these same rights. Part of sharing power is nurturing, encouraging, and fostering these rights.

Decision making in an environment that fosters recovery involves more people and more time. It is much easier for an administrator to make a decision alone than to bring it to the community for discussion and input. Often, decision making has to be taught to people who have grown accustomed to having their decisions made for them, who have been told so many times that, because of their "illness," they are unable to make responsible choices, and that any preferences they do express should be discounted because they are sick and unstable.

It takes time, patience, and a lot of listening to teach people to take the major risk of making their own choices again. But this type of power sharing through conversation can provide for a climate of equality, which can insure that all people can be free to express and reach for their own hopes and aspirations. Power sharing allows both staff members and clients alike to become much more involved in, and invested in, their own growth. In an environment that fosters recovery, the barriers of discrimination and stigma, which destroy self esteem, perpetuate learned helplessness, and convince people they are incapable of self-determination, are broken down.

Many people who have been diagnosed as mentally ill hate labels and object strongly when people are called schizophrenic, bipolar, or borderline. After people are diagnosed, everything that happens to them is seen through the filter of their labels. A couple of years ago I was admitted to a hospital on an emergency basis. The next morning I called my office to say I wouldn't be in because I was in the hospital. At the time I worked in a very progressive agency with several people who themselves had psychiatric disabilities. My colleagues assumed I was in a psychiatric unit. These same colleagues called every psychiatric unit in the Boston area trying to find me. In reality, I had been admitted to the hospital because of a respiratory infection. They had assumed that if I was in the hospital on an emergency basis of course I was having a psychiatric emergency.

An environment that fosters recovery must be one in which hope is an essential component of each activity. Often people with psychiatric labels have lost hope. They see their disability as a death sentence. They think they can never get any better. When you are in the midst of despair it is almost impossible to see the other side. Too often providers echo these feelings and cement them into reality for those with whom they work. Have you ever found yourself angry at a person who has given up hope? I have.

During difficult times it can be easier to give up. Do we blame ourselves? Sometimes. This can serve to fuel our own despair. More often, though, I think professionals blame the people who are in despair. Despairing clients are seen as lazy, non-compliant, and manipulative, and they don't want to get better. They don't want help. They should be discharged from the program so they can hit bottom—then maybe they will appreciate how good they had it.

In a system where this continually happens, people within the system and the system itself can get caught up in the despair and become rigid, distancing, and lifeless. As an administrator, I try to use these times to take an honest look at the services my agency is providing: are they relevant to what people need and want? Are staff members burning out and in need of support from me or from each other?

In these days of more work and fewer resources I often find that the issues, the traumas, and the life experiences of the people who use the mental health center trigger myself and my staff. We can only be with people in their pain to the extent we are willing to be with our own pain within our own life experiences. I model this with my staff by talking about the feelings the work evokes in me. And I invite others to share also. I have found that creating an environment of safety for staff members as well as for clients is necessary for this open sharing to go on. Safety to reveal one's own vulnerabilities without fear of sanctions is vital for an environment that fosters recovery. Confidentiality, respect, and sincere attempts to empathize and demonstrate understanding to others are components of such an environment. Well developed interpersonal skills, on the part of both staff members and administrators, can serve to support the atmosphere of safety and compassion.

When I decided to return to school to get my doctorate, I did so for several reasons. First of all I wanted to learn more. Second, I thought that the title "doctor" before my name would help me feel validated, and that I had a place in the world. And third, because I wanted to give back some of what had been given to me by those who supported my recovery. As I looked at various programs I was disappointed at the values and the sterility of the various programs. Then I talked to someone at Boston University, where I had gotten my master's many years before. I liked the idea of rehabilitation with its emphasis on functioning rather than illness and limitations. It was suggested to me that I read some of Bill Anthony's work to see if the principles expressed resonated with my own. As I did, I found that both the principles and practices gave a context and a structure as well as a guide for helpers to foster recovery instead of encouraging passivity and compliance. In psychiatric rehabilitation the person and his or her preferences and thoughts are essential to the process. When I learned of the values of involvement, choice, comprehensiveness, support, and growth potential, I saw these were the same values that helped free me from feeling trapped in traditional treatment. I was excited at the possibility of learning how to put these values into practice with other survivors of the psychiatric system. I learned in the very best way possible—by teaching. I taught courses in rehabilitation counseling for 4 years. Over the past several years I have been using these principles to help mental health systems put a recovery paradigm into practice. I have seen, in myself and in the people with whom I work, that when these values form the basis of the structure and programming within a system, people learn to take responsibility for themselves and their actions. These principles provide the soil for people to choose to grow and change. I have come to think of psychiatric rehabilitation as providing an eternal structure, while recovery is the internal process.

Through recovery I have found myself capable of making changes toward more satisfaction and success in my life. The quality of my life has greatly improved. I still have my limitations—I am not a finished product. And from an acceptance of my limitations has become a belief in my own unique possibilities. I have the power to move toward wholeness.

Part I: *Study Questions and Disability Awareness Exercise*

1. Discuss the role of autonomy in the rehabilitation process. Is this role similar for all people coping with disability?
2. Identify the barriers to rehabilitation candidates' autonomy and discuss how they can be reduced.
3. Discuss the "common ground" between psychiatric and physical rehabilitation.
4. Compare the benefits/deficits for persons who have disabilities when they are viewed from the perspective of the "minority group" versus the "functional limits" model.
5. Identify and discuss the similarities and differences between women and men living the disability experience. Discuss the same topic considering persons who are members of ethnic and racial minorities.
6. Should women with severe disabilities be encouraged or forced by law not to have children? What about men?
7. Are the goals of recovery, as related to psychiatric disability, compatible with the goals of rehabilitation for people experiencing a physical disability?
8. Why is the minority group model challenging the functional limitations model?
9. What are the limitations of the medical model, and the minority group model?
10. What are the differences between a sociopolitical perspective and the medical and/or economic definition of disability?
11. Discuss the distinction between existential anxiety and aesthetic anxiety from Hahn's perspective.
12. How has the sociopolitical perspective of disability been empowering to people with disabilities?
13. How does ADA relate to the broad issues raised by genetic testing?
14. Is the eugenics movement an historic or futuristic force in society?
15. How are stereotypes, incorrect assumptions and disability related?
16. Why is the medical model limited from Treischman's perspective?
17. Discuss the assets and limitations of alternative medicine as it relates to the disability experience.
18. Do the energy model principles relate equally to emotional and physical disabilities?
19. Are the ethical principles of health care compromised or enhanced in a managed care/managed cost environment?
20. Who should manage health and rehabilitation care? Why?

21. What role should consumers have on a rehabilitation team? What issues should they not be allowed to decide, if any?
22. What are the strengths and weaknesses of the deliberative model?
23. How can labels be empowering? Disempowering?
24. In what ways has or can the ADA be disempowering to people with disabilities?
25. Is the process of recovery similar for people with physical and/or emotional disabilities?

WELCOME BACK

The following exercise is designed to sensitize participants to the impact of a disabling condition.

Goals

1. To raise the awareness of participants to the qualitative dimensions of disability.
2. To enable participants to evaluate the differential impact of a disabling condition on their interpersonal relationships.
3. To explore with participants the most helpful approaches in dealing with disability.
4. To list the most devastating disabilities that could occur in participants' lives.

Procedure

1. Participants are asked to list the three most important people in their lives.
2. Each member is asked to list three specific disabilities that he or she would least want to experience personally.
3. Participants write a brief statement about each disability focusing on why they would not want it.
4. The leader then asks the group members to take the most undesirable disability and list five specific ways in which it would affect their relationship with each person listed if they were hospitalized and away from that person for one year.
5. The group leader asks the participants to verbalize their feelings and discuss what they have written.
6. The leader asks which of the three persons would be most supportive and why.
7. The leader asks group members what would be most helpful to facilitate their integration back into the community.

8. Group members are asked to select the age they would prefer the disability to occur and explain why.
9. Consider how participants' lives would be altered if a traumatic disability occurred early or later in life, that is age 5, 10, 15, 20, 30, 40, 50, 60, 70.
10. Leader stresses the point that disability can occur any time during the lifespan.

Part II

Family and Developmental Issues in Disability

Disabilities may be present congenitally, or they may be acquired at any time during the lifespan. Part II focuses on the role of the family in promoting healthy development in children and other family members with disabilities or chronic illness. Both physical and mental disabilities are explored.

There is obviously an interactive relationship between children with disabilities and their family, school, and peer social systems. In chapter 6, Miller provides a developmental, biopsychosocial framework for understanding this interaction to promote the child's development and health functioning. Specific intervention strategies are presented. The importance of balance between quality of life and disability management is emphasized.

The relationship between chronic physical disorders in children and their subsequent risk of psychopathology is the focus of chapter 7 by Huebner and Thomas. Three aspects of attachment (neurobiological, interpersonal and intrapersonal, and societal) are reviewed. The authors suggest that these processes are interactive and may be potentially related to the development of emotional maladjustment. The importance of a securely attached child and the development of strong bonds between the child and his parents and caregivers is emphasized. Implications of altered attachment in adults with disabilities and the need for further research regarding the role of attachment are presented.

Helping families treat severe mental illness is the purpose of chapter 8 by Mueser. The evolution and description of family intervention programs and the ingredients of effective family intervention are discussed. Behavioral family therapy for psychiatric disorders, a widely applicable family treatment model, is described as a strategy to minimize relapse and optimize outcome. Future directions for this area are suggested.

In chapter 9, Weingarten and Weingarten Worthen (mother and daughter) each describes her own illness in personal statements and her responses to the other's illness to facilitate the understanding of differences in how well their illnesses are understood. Three narrative concepts—coherence, closure, and independence—are presented as a basis of understanding differences, facilitating coping, and empowering family members.

6

Promoting Healthy Function and Development in Chronically Ill Children: A Primary Care Approach

Bruce D. Miller

The task of childhood is to achieve healthy functioning and development. This process occurs not only in the physical domain, but also in cognitive, emotional, and psychosocial realms. It is a biopsychosocial process, one that is nourished by the family and the child's psychosocial surround. Unfortunately, childhood chronic illness can severely impair psychosocial functions and impede growth (3, 13). In treating a child with chronic illness, the maintenance of physical well-being is necessary but, in itself, not sufficient. Good medical care necessitates a biopsychosocial approach because biological, psychological, and social factors influence one another, and mutually influence the child's ability to grow and thrive. Furthermore, a developmental perspective is essential in understanding and treating children and adolescents with chronic illness.

The purpose of this article is to introduce a developmental, biopsychosocial model for the primary care of childhood chronic illness. We have shaped this integrative treatment model as an approach to the following goals: *to minimize the impact of the disease on the physical and emotional development and functioning of the child; to achieve optimum balance between disease management and quality of life for the patient and family; and to facilitate the adaptive functioning of the psychosocial surround of the chronically ill child.*

This developmental, biopsychosocial approach to the treatment of childhood chronic illness is admittedly complex. Many primary health care providers may determine that they themselves do not have the necessary time, skill, training, or

I thank Beatrice Wood, Ph.D., for helping me to recognize the systemic nature of the work I have been doing with chronically ill children and their families, and for encouraging me to set down these ideas conceptually so that they may be shared with students and colleagues.

From *Family Systems Medicine, 13*(2) (1995), 187–200. Reprinted with permission.

inclination to provide this comprehensive treatment for their patients. Nor should they be expected or feel obligated to provide this multilevel primary care by themselves. However, we do believe that many of the practical suggestions presented herein are easily incorporated into regular medical management. Furthermore, we propose simple preventive, systemic interventions that may avert the development of later psychosocial problems requiring complicated and time-consuming intervention.

If the primary health care provider does not wish to extend treatment beyond basic medical intervention and education, someone else may collaborate in managing the psychosocial and family aspects of this illness. Specially trained nurse clinicians or other psychosocial or family specialists may provide some of the more psychosocially related functions. We have found that the best arrangement is to have available a psychosocial consultant who is an ongoing member of the health care team, and who is trained in the assessment and treatment of both individual and family dysfunction. This consultant may be a social worker, family therapist, psychiatrist, or psychologist who has special training in working with chronically ill children and their families. The key to effective intervention involving a psychosocial-medical collaboration is the maintenance of a fluent, well-coordinated and mutually supportive effort by all of the participating health care providers. Each health care team will develop its own division of labor and coordination of functions according to the needs and logistics of its particular practice. Many medical-psychosocial, collaborative health care approaches are possible (see upcoming special issue of *Family Systems Medicine*). When I use the term "health care provider" (HCP) throughout this article, we are referring to some member of the "health care team" whose training and assigned role would be determined by the individual practice setting. The choice of which health care team member will carry out the specific tasks detailed herein will be determined according to what works best for that particular health care team, depending on the expertise of each team member.

CHILDHOOD CHRONIC ILLNESSES

The most common and disruptive chronic illnesses that have their onset in childhood or adolescence are respiratory allergies (9%), asthma (4%), eczema and skin allergies (3%), heart disease (2%), epilepsy (.2%), and diabetes (.1%) (13). Each of these specific illnesses has its own particular psychosocial and developmental challenges and sequelae, depending on the age of onset, whether it is episodic or chronic, progressive, life-threatening or not. Several excellent publications address the psychosocial aspects and treatment of specific childhood chronic illnesses (see 19 for a selected list). There is tremendous complexity involved in the interactions among factors influencing the well-being of a chronically ill child or adolescent: the type and severity of illness, resources of the family and community, and sophistication and capacity of the health care provider team. However, there are a few developmental and biopsychosocial dimensions that childhood chronic illnesses have in common, thus providing the basis for a general, but simple, treatment model that is manageable for primary care.

THE PSYCHOSOCIAL SURROUND

Adaptive functioning of the psychosocial surround promotes healthy growth and development in the chronically ill child. The chronically ill child and adolescent must negotiate issues of self-image and presentation, adaptation to chronic illness with its physical and emotional sequelae, and compliance with medical treatment. All this is required in addition to fulfilling the normative tasks of individual growth and development. Difficulties in meeting the challenges of chronic illness and in fulfilling normative developmental tasks can result in significant emotional disorder, psychosocial impairment, and developmental delay (3). Healthy growth and development depends heavily upon the successful adaptation of the critical contexts in the child's psychosocial surround: the family, the school, the peer group, and the health care system (see Figure 6.1). The chronic illness of the child influences the interaction of these systems with the child, and the interaction of the systems with one another. In turn, the way in which family, school, and peer groups respond to the chronically ill child either enhances the child's physical and psychosocial functioning and normal development, or undermines it. I will discuss how childhood chronic illness impacts upon each of these psychosocial domains and how these domains influence one another and the child's physical and psychosocial well-being. I will illustrate how health care providers (HCP) can play a key role in establishing healthy versus maladaptive processes among these domains.

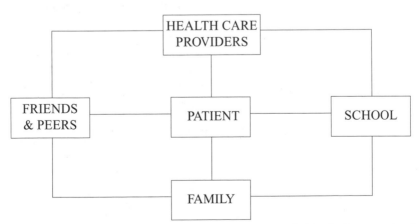

FIGURE 6.1 The chronically ill child/adolescent: Critical elements in the psychosocial surround.

THE FAMILY CONTEXT

The family is the developing child's most important source of support and developmental impetus and direction (see Figure 6.2). As such, the family can be a powerful ally to the health care provider in assisting the child to respond to illness in adaptive and creative ways. Or, the family can be a hindrance if it functions maladaptively. It is important to appreciate the reciprocal, interactive nature of chronic illness and family functioning, with the potential for either adaptive or maladaptive influence (2, 4, 8, 11, 12, 14, 15, 18–21). Families in which the child and the disease are the primary focus for life are at risk for developing maladaptive, interlocking patterns of functioning, which in turn may influence the disease process, psychosocial function, and development. In such cases, one parent may become intensely involved and protective of the sick child, shielding him or her from appropriate discipline from the other parent. This dysfunction can cause marital discord, which in turn may stress the sick child and siblings. If the family believes that stress can affect the sick child's illness (many families do), family members may adopt a strategy of conflict avoidance, which can prevent resolution of normal and illness-related disagreements. Such nonresolution of conflict is not only detrimental to marital and family relations; it can also undermine adequate management of the illness and its psychosocial sequelae. Health care providers can discuss early in treatment the importance of balance in these areas, and thus assist families in finding a happy medium that will adequately protect the child's physical well-being, while promoting healthy development.

Occasionally, families are so threatened by the chronic illness or are so preoccupied by other severe physical or psychiatric illnesses, or by overwhelming life events or situations, that they have difficulty acknowledging and managing the illness. The patient's medical and psychosocial well-being may then be neglected through missed appointments and failure to monitor the child's symptoms and medication. When families operate in this manner, they require inten-

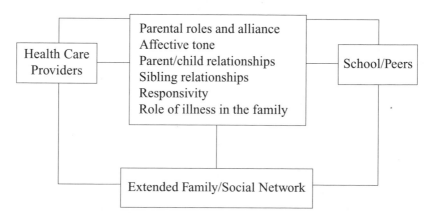

FIGURE 6.2 The chronically ill child/adolescent: Family context.

sive and persistent psychosocial outreach and intervention (2). It may be necessary for the health care provider to access resources and involvement of social service agencies, such as child protective services, if the family is unable to provide adequate medical and psychosocial care for the patient.

A perspective on the economic issues for a family with a chronically ill child must be maintained by the health care provider. The financial drain of health care for a chronically ill child may produce severe stress, which can disrupt the well-being of the responsible adults and the family as a whole. It can raise the general level of anxiety and depression, which tends to exaggerate maladaptive family patterns of functioning. Extended family members can be a source of financial and emotional support and guidance for the nuclear family, or they can be a hindrance. Usually, adequate information regarding the disease and the issue of balance between medical management and psychosocial development will organize the extended family as important resources for the child and family. The health care provider can facilitate this process by encouraging the family to inform involved extended family members directly as to these issues, or these extended family members can be included in relevant family meetings with a health care provider.

Treating patients with separated, divorced, or remarried parents is a common experience and one that requires special attention with respect to the level of involvement of the noncustodial parent in the child's life. Both parents, and their respective families, should be informed and educated as much as possible with regard to the medical and psychosocial aspects of their child's illness. It is not always prudent to rely on the custodial parent to transmit this information to the other parent. The health care provider should consider requesting permission to inform the noncustodial parent as to the child's illness and progress. This is becoming increasingly important as joint custody becomes more prevalent. The noncustodial or joint custodial parent and stepparents should be involved in the medical, school, and peer contextual interactions as appropriate, depending upon the level of this parent's involvement with the child. If conflict between the divorced parents is having an impact on the patient, the health care provider must intervene vigorously, and probably repeatedly, with both parents and the child (not necessarily together) to minimize the negative effect on the child and his or her illness. Assistance from psychosocial specialists experienced in helping separated, divorced, and stepfamilies may be beneficial to the primary health care provider in resolving these difficulties.

The family is the child's gateway to the school and peer worlds. Healthy patient and family adaptation to the child's illness, and integrated interaction and sharing of information with persons outside of the family, can promote adaptive interaction of the child in these other contexts. Given the pivotal position of the family in the adaptation of the child to his or her psychosocial surround, it is critical that the health care provider assess family functioning and provide intervention as necessary. There are several levels at which the primary health care provider can become involved in this process, from simply providing educational information to conducting intensive individual and/or family therapeutic intervention (5). The level at which the primary care provider decides to be involved is a matter of personal choice and type and degree of training. However, at minimum, someone on the health care team should be proficient in recognizing individual psychological disorder or maladaptive family patterns when they occur, and provide or arrange for psychosocial intervention when indicated. One successful arrangement is an ongoing collaboration with a psychosocial specialist as a member of the health care provider team (see 10 for inpatient application and 18 for outpatient application).

THE SCHOOL CONTEXT

In addition to being the center for intellectual and academic development, the school is a tremendously influential psychosocial context for children and adolescents. The way in which the school responds to the child's or adolescent's illness will affect the quality of medical management. It will also affect the child's academic achievement, and color the psychosocial experience by influencing daily functioning, self-esteem, emotional status, and social development (see Figure 6.3).

Most problems in managing issues relating to chronic illness in the school context come from lack of knowledge or from an imbalance in degree of focus upon the disease. The child's illness may be either completely ignored, which impairs adequate medical management, or it may be overly focused upon, which brings serious psychosocial consequences. Some schools overreact to the illness, unduly restricting the child and treating him or her as an invalid. In other cases, the potential for episodes of illness is ignored, with no plans for care should the need arise (many times the school is not even informed of the child's illness). Occasionally schools even reject a child by refusing admission or by trying to

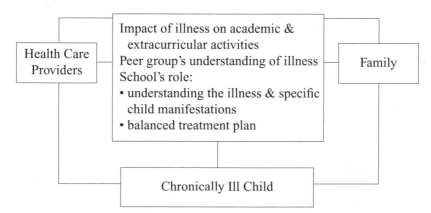

FIGURE 6.3 The chronically ill child/adolescent: School context.

transfer him or her to another school. Alternatively, schools may encourage homebound teaching if they are not provided with adequate guidance and technical support to help the child manage his or her illness. While homebound teaching may suffice academically, it can seriously impede psychosocial development and should be avoided.

The key to healthy adaptation of the school to the child's illness is knowledge with regard to the illness, a communication link with the health care team and family, and a balance between overprotection and neglect. The information provided to the school should include a general understanding of the illness, and the meaning of the illness for the child's participation in academic and in formal and informal extracurricular activities. It is important that all appropriate school personnel be included in the educative process, including the child's teachers, school doctor and nurse, gym teachers and coaches, bus driver, and, perhaps most importantly, the school office staff, which is often responsible for making decisions about steps to take in the event of illness.

The best way for this information to be provided to the school is through a joint meeting of a member of the health care team, the family, and the appropriate school personnel. The health care provider's presence is important in order to convey the relevant medical information, and to convey a balanced concern for medical, educational, and psychosocial issues. The health care provider can also answer medical questions and dispel myths and fears, emphasize that a given chronic illness is different for each afflicted child, and describe the manifestations of the illness that are specific for the child in question. The parents' presence is important so that their preferences regarding the child's activities at school can be taken into account and they can establish an open communication channel and a collaborative relationship with the school around their child's illness. It is important for both father and mother be present so that each of their perspectives and opinions can be considered. The child's presence is also critical so that he or she can help develop the plan for medical management and activities, and comment on whether particular aspects of the plan will work for him or her. The health care provider can facilitate balance if the parents, child, or school propose a plan that leans too far in either a protective or neglectful direction. The goal of the meeting should be a coherent, mutually agreed upon plan that everyone can endorse. The plan should include a written course of action to be taken in the event of an illness episode occurring in the school.

From time to time a child's illness may cause discomfort among classmates or teachers. This can cause rejection or ignoring of the child, or an undue fascination and overfocus on the disease. A project in the context of a science or health class can dispel myths and fears and provide a more comfortable social context for the whole class. Since many children are afflicted with chronic illnesses that are widely misunderstood, these illnesses can be good topics for a health or science project. Ideally, children should be involved directly in the project by having them take an active role in gathering factual information from chronically ill children and from written sources. This can be particularly effective in creating an atmosphere of balanced acceptance with regard to their chronically ill classmates and friends. The health care provider may suggest such a class project to the school counselor.

THE PEER SOCIAL SYSTEM

The social system of peers is underappreciated as an essential context for psychosocial and emotional development. This is the primary domain in which social problem solving evolves and relationship building occurs. There are structured social contexts such as sports, scouting, music, and dance lessons, and unstructured contexts such as informal play and social gatherings. It is important that some of these activities take place in an informal social setting, since absence of structure promotes the child's individual mastery of the social domain.

Chronic illness can compromise this process because the chronically ill child may have difficulty "fitting in" and being accepted (see Figure 6.4). Problems may occur if the child acts differently from the other children because of fearfulness about becoming ill. Additionally, the child may have become accustomed to more than his or her share of attention by virtue of being so attended to because of the illness. This skewed expectation may create a feeling of rejection in the chronically ill child when he or she is in a context of normal, social give and take. To make matters worse, peers may ignore or reject the child out of fear or repulsion based upon ignorance or myths they have acquired regarding the child's particular illness. Attempts on the part of the child to rectify this experiential deficit of attention will not endear the child to peers. Alternatively, peers may "treat the child with kid gloves" and be overly protective and overly fascinated by the illness. Although apparently stimulated by caring motives, this focus on the illness of the child may actually isolate the child and thus impede normal socio-emotional and identity development. Parents may discourage their children from inviting a chronically ill child into their home or may otherwise restrict

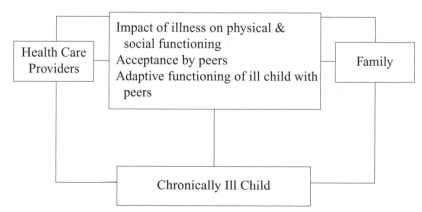

FIGURE 6.4 The chronically ill child/adolescent: Peer/social context.

healthy interaction between their children and the ill child. This often comes about through fear of that child's becoming ill and frightening their own children. Alternatively, parents may have concerns that they, as the responsible adult, may not be able to respond safely in the event of an illness episode.

Education and balance are, once again, key ingredients in constructing an adaptive social context for the chronically ill child. And, naturally, the best approach to this situation is proactive. The health care provider can encourage the child and family to find ways to inform peers and their parents about general aspects of the child's illness, and specifically about how it affects this particular child. Questions can be answered regarding concerns parents have about the illness, and the potential emotional hazards to their own children. Parents (and peers, depending on their age) should be given instructions about how to respond in the event of an illness episode.

It should be readily apparent that the capacity to build these bridges to the peer system depends upon the extent to which the chronically ill child and family members have their own thoughts, feelings, and plans worked out with regard to the child's illness. The health care provider can facilitate this process by educating the family as to the importance of the peer social context for their child's socioemotional development, by encouraging the family to help the child build social bridges, and by providing guidance and support to the family in these endeavors.

DEVELOPMENTAL ISSUES

The necessary developmental trend in the medical management of chronic illness and its psychosocial concomitants is a gradual shift toward the child's self-management of the medical and socioemotional aspects of the illness.

Pre-School Children

Some childhood chronic illnesses are diagnosed before age two. These young children are normatively quite dependent and may require more extensive and frequent medical management both at home and in the doctor's office. Families make significant adaptive changes in their daily living patterns to help their young child manage his or her illness. At the same time, it is important that even young children become active participants in managing their chronic illness. For example, young children with asthma can be taught to notice when breathing is easy and when it is strained, and medicine or respiratory treatments can be self-administered with close parental observation and supervision. Active participation will help these children begin to achieve mastery over their illness and develop a sense of effectiveness and control of their bodies—both essential elements of healthy physical and psychosocial development. In addition, the child's sense of efficacy through actual mastery of the illness assists the child and the family to accept the disease and its limitations within the family's social surround. Thus, a balance must be struck, even at an early age, between family management and self-care of chronic illness. The health care provider can build essential groundwork for a developmentally synchronized increase in the child's active responsibility in the management of and adaptation to chronic illness.

Elementary School Children

As chronically ill children make the transition from home into school, important adjustments must be made in order to facilitate the adaptive process of managing the illness and its associated features. With entry into school, these children must assume a more active and responsible role in the assessment and management of their illness. They must be able to recognize symptom states, express their needs in this regard, and effect treatment. To do so, they will need to interact and negotiate directly with school personnel without the assistance and protection of their parents. As discussed above, this key transition necessitates increasing the autonomy of the chronically ill child as well as the education of those with whom the child will interact outside the home—that is, school personnel, caretakers, and peers (see Figures 6.3 and 6.4).

In order for chronically ill children to progress toward autonomy, they must acquire both the information to manage the illness and the confidence to assert themselves in the administration of medical management, and the adults with whom they interact must be willing and able to facilitate this process. This process of shifting from dependence toward independence (in self-care) requires the maintenance of a delicate balance between adults and child both at home and away from home, and must be actively monitored and facilitated by the health care providers throughout the pre-teen and teenage years.

Adolescence

The shift toward self-management of chronic illnesses picks up momentum during adolescence. However, the transition to full responsibility for the management of medical and psychosocial aspects of their illness will be smoother if it is a continuation of a gradual shift toward independent self-care that has been taking place all along at a developmentally appropriate rate. Again, balance is key in this process. Sometimes families and health care providers retain too much responsibility for the disease. Alternatively, they may abdicate responsibility to the adolescent prematurely. Not infrequently, adolescents will demand this control as part of their general attempt to take charge of their destiny. This is not in itself inappropriate. However, a common error is to hand over responsibility to adolescents because of their chronological age or in response to the intensity of their demands for control. This is not wise. Adolescents must demonstrate through their behavior, not through argument, that they can manage their illness responsibly. But to do so, adolescents need to have some aspects of self-care given over to them in order to demonstrate their mastery. The primary health care provider can guide and assist patients and their families in achieving appropriate balance in this process. Quite often, both the family and the chronically ill adolescent will neglect to take this important developmental step. This delay may be due to fear, or from not wanting to rock the boat, or even simply because of inertia. The primary health care provider can serve as a developmental stimulus by initiating the shift toward more self-care if the family is not naturally evolving in this direction.

At times, disease management can become the focus around which adolescents attempt to rebel during the process of individuation. Parents and adolescents can become locked in counterproductive and potentially dangerous power struggles around disease issues. The danger comes from a polarization whereby parental concern leads to increased attempts to control the adolescent, which can push the adolescent farther in the direction of self-neglect or impulsive acting out around the disease. Usually this problem can be averted if the process of increasing self-care has been part of the ongoing treatment in keeping with developmental milestones. However, once a family is engaged in this highly maladaptive pattern of struggle, the health care provider must take an active leadership role in reorganizing and redirecting the struggle toward more normatively appropriate and safe issues. If the patient or family do not respond to simple redirection, their struggle may be part of other dysfunction in the family and/or may be indicative of emotional disorder in the adolescent or other family members. If this is the case, then family and individual therapeutic intervention is indicated, and a designated psychosocial specialist on the health care team should become more intensively involved with the patient and family.

Special caution must be exercised if a caretaker or health care provider has reason to believe that a child or adolescent may be depressed, because anxiety and depression have been associated with asthma, inflammatory bowel disease, diabetes, epilepsy, cystic fibrosis, and other childhood chronic illness (1, 17). In addition, there is evidence that in some disease, such as asthma, depression is associated with morbidity and mortality (6, 7, 9, 11, 16). (It should be noted that symptoms of depression in children can present in various forms and may be easily missed.) If depression or severe anxiety is suspected, prompt and consistent individual and family assessment treatment is required in order to evaluate and remedy this problem. Again, this is best accomplished by a psychosocial professional who is part of the health care team.

Adolescence carries with it special challenges for chronically ill children. Puberty itself brings psychological and emotional changes that may inherently destabilize and further complicate disease management. In addition to developing an identity, learning about love and sex, achieving a new balance of autonomy and belonging, chronically ill adolescents have special challenges that interact with these developmental tasks. For example, adolescents with chronic illness must develop an identity which does *not* revolve around their being "an asthmatic," "a diabetic," "an epileptic," and so on. In addition, adolescents must engage in the highly competitive set of social, academic, and extracurricular activities while, at times, having to contend with direct and indirect consequences of their illness. For example, issues of physical self-image may be confounded by the cosmetically displeasing side effects of some medications. In addition, the ever-present problem of mood lability in adolescents may be complicated and intensified by problems of irritability and/or affective dysregulation caused by particular medications.

Preparing to leave home is an especially trying time for chronically ill adolescents and their families; for example, the stress of junior year of high school for college-bound adolescents may be met with increased disease activity and emotional turmoil. For adolescents not bound for college, there may be exacerbations of their illness as they contemplate or seek employment or expect to move out of the home. This difficult transition should be prepared for by encouraging the child's gradual assumption of self-care and self-reliance in dealing with the emotional and psychosocial sequelae of the illness. The health care provider can assist the adolescent patient's transition to functional independence by facilitating this process well ahead of its actual time phase.

The enormous complexity and challenge surrounding the interaction of the medical, psychosocial, and developmental factors in adolescent chronic illness require an allied, informed, firm, but flexible coordination on the part of those in the medical and psychosocial surround. It must be appreciated that adolescence is a time of shaping, reshaping, and forging one's way toward the adult (that is, responsible) position. Errors will undoubtedly be made and disease activity will be expressed at times, despite efforts to insure proper management. Parents, health care providers, and school personnel must strike a balance between firm limit setting and nurturance, while maintaining a nonpunitive, supportive, and understanding stance toward the chronically ill adolescent.

TASKS FOR THE HEALTH CARE TEAM

The health care team must maintain an active and interactive role in addressing the biopsychosocial aspects of treatment for chronically ill children, adolescents, and their families. This developmentally oriented model for pediatric care identifies three levels of primary care responsibility:

   physiological and pharmacological intervention and management (biological level)
   consideration of and provision for the specific developmental, psychosocial, and emotional needs of the child throughout treatment and followup (psychological level)
   integrated treatment plan and implementation, including the interactive effects of the child's chronic illness within the family, school, and peer contexts (social level)

This biopsychosocial approach is essential for adequate treatment of childhood chronic illness because biological, psychological, and social factors (see

Figure 6.5) all interact to determine the child's physical and psychosocial well-being and development (10, 19).

Anticipatory guidance and proactive intervention can avert future problems in these realms of function and development. For example, early establishment of open communication channels, education regarding the illness, emphasis on a balance of medical management and quality of life and developmental demands, and promoting age-appropriate self-care, can lay the foundation for adaptive functioning of the child-patient, the family, school, and peer systems (see Appendix).

Assessment and Intervention for Medical or Psychosocial Management Problems

Despite the best efforts of the health care team and the child's family, it's likely that medical, psychological, or psychosocial problems will arise during the course of the child's illness, disrupting biopsychosocial balance and development. Such problems may be anticipated at times of developmental transition (leaving home) or environmental/family distress (for example, loss through death or divorce, economic hardship, birth of a sibling). Becoming aware of these transitions and intervening at the psychosocial level can avert potential problems in disease management. It should be noted that many active and potential psychosocial problems will not be discovered except by explicit inquiry by the health care provider who must, therefore, keep track of important changes in the child and family's life. Many health care providers feel that it is an invasion of privacy to inquire into the psychosocial lives of their patients and their families. However, families are quite appreciative of this attentiveness, particularly when it is explained to them that any important change could influence the child's illness or its management. Some frequent indicators of problems in biopsychosocial function are described below. The presence of these indicators signals the primary care provider that an increase in attention to the psychological and/or social aspects of the child's functioning are indicated.

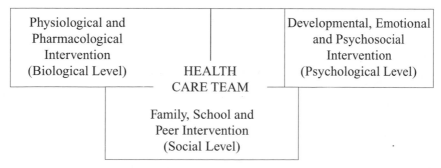

FIGURE 6.5 Biopsychosocial health care model.

Increased or Uncontrolled Disease Activity

When difficulties arise in controlling the chronic illness, it is necessary to attend to developmental and psychosocial dimensions as well as to the biological aspects of the patient-family system. Stress in these aspects of psychosocial functioning can sometimes have an impact on the child's disease. It is essential to inquire into the physiological circumstances, medical management, and patient self-care (or family care of patient). However, in some cases, despite careful attention to the specifics of medical management and self-care, chronically ill children remain unresponsive to medical intervention (12, 16). It is precisely in such cases that inquiry should extend to the developmental, psychological, and psychosocial aspects of the child's functioning. Issues involving family, friends, school, and other relevant developmental concerns for the child must be explored—both directly with the child and indirectly with relevant family members and/or other key persons in the child's life.

Noncompliance

Noncompliance with medical regimen may reflect a lack of knowledge, but if proper education has been provided and the difficulty persists, then the child or adolescent may be suffering from depression. Poor self-care, disregard of symptoms, manipulative use of illness, patient-staff conflict, and patient-parent conflict over medical regimens have been associated with depression and psychological dysfunction in children with refractory illness. It is likely that these symptoms of depression will interfere with compliance. Noncompliance has also been associated with family dysfunction.

Academic or Social Difficulties at School

A drop in grade-point average, loss of motivation for school work, complaining about being "picked on" or "ignored," or dropping out of extracurricular activities may signal emotional disturbance (most often depression or anxiety disorder). These problems at school also may reflect a child's preoccupation with family problems at home, or they may be the result of a worsening in the child's disease process. It is likely that that biological, psychological, and family domains of dysfunction influence and worsen one another. For example, a child's behavioral expression of depression may elicit conflictual family patterns, which then stress the child and exacerbate the physical expression of the illness.

Behavior Problems

Oppositional or defiant behavior may mask depression and anxiety. Although cognitive and behavioral interventions may assist these children and their families, such children may also benefit from the opportunity to reflect upon and express their disappointment, demoralization, or despair about struggling with chronic illness. Family members or even whole families can become demoralized or depressed at times. Guided family discussion of their struggles around these issues serve a valuable role in the patient's and family's regaining a sense of well-being.

Denial of Illness

Clinicians may become unnecessarily concerned with what appears to be denial of illness in children or families. A reluctance to talk about the illness and its effects may represent an adaptive response to the illness. Furthermore, some cultural groups orient and talk less about physical illness. This reluctance should be seen as benign as long as the medical regimen is followed, and as long as the patient and family are functioning and developing adequately in the emotional and psychosocial realms. In these cases, the child and family should not be labeled "in denial," nor is psychological or family intervention indicated.

Refractory Illness

Refractory illness takes an emotional toll on children and families. It can lead to anxiety and depression, which may, in turn, exacerbate the physical condition. Furthermore, anxiety and depression engendered by the refractory nature of the illness can become "functionally autonomous." For these reasons, signs of chronic anxiety or depression require individual and family intervention regardless of whether they "make sense" in the context of unremitting physical illness.

When these indicators of child distress are present, the importance of explicit inquiry into psychosocial factors cannot be overemphasized. Relatively subtle but potent impediments to proper self-care can be discovered. For example, a new teacher who is intolerant or misinformed about the child's chronic illness, a rejection by a misinformed peer (or parents thereof), or an untoward or unexpected parent/sibling issue may cause an imbalance in the child's self-care management. In such an instance, a rather straightforward and direct nonmedical intervention may be the key to getting the child and family back on track.

When straightforward interventions are not sufficient to bring about the needed improvement in biopsychosocial functioning, more intensive psychosocial or physiatric assessment and intervention may be needed. The psychosocial members of the health care team can assist in deciding what combinations of individual and family psychotherapeutic and/or psychopharmacological interventions are best suited to the problems at hand.

SUMMARY

The developmental/biopsychosocial treatment approach to childhood chronic illness offered herein emphasizes five interlocking features:

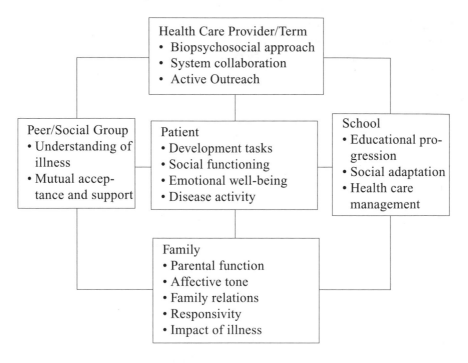

FIGURE 6.6 The chronically ill child/adolescent in psychosocial context.

1. consideration of the biological, psychological, and social aspects of chronic illness that interact with one another and influence disease management and psychosocial functioning and development of the ill child (see Figure 6.6)

2. the importance of balance between disease management and quality of life and developmental needs of the patients and their families

3. appreciation and facilitation of a developmentally synchronized shift toward self-care of the illness and its social and emotional aspects

4. the central role played by the health care team in integrating the developmental/biopsychosocial aspects of comprehensive treatment for childhood chronic illness (see Figure 6.5)

5. the importance of anticipatory guidance and proactive biopsychosocial intervention

REFERENCES

Ader, R., Felton, D.A., & Cohen, N. (eds.). *Psychoneuroimmunology* (2nd ed.). San Diego, CA: Academic Press, 1991.

Boxer, G.H., Carson, J., & Miller, B.D. Neglect contributing to tertiary hospitalization in childhood asthma. *Child Abuse and Neglect 12:* 491–501, 1988.

Cadman, D., Boyle, M., Szatmari, P., & Offord, D.R. Chronic illness, disability and mental and social well-being: Findings of the Ontario child health study. *Pediatrics 79:* 805–813, 1987.

Campbell, T.L. Family's impact on health: A critical review. *Family Systems Medicine* 4(2/3): 135–328, 1986.

Doherty, W.J., & Baird, M.A. Developmental levels in family-centered medical care. *Family Medicine 18:* 153–156, 1986.

Friedman, M.S. Psychological factors associated with pediatric asthma death: A review. *Journal of Asthma 21:* 97–117, 1984.

Fritz, G.K., Rubinstein, S., & Lewiston, N.J. Psychological factors in fatal childhood asthma. *American Journal of Orthopsychiatry 57:* 253–257, 1987.

Gustafsson, P.A., Kjellman, N-IM, Ludvigsson, J., & Cederblad, M. Asthma and family interaction. *Archives of Diseases of Childhood 62:* 258–263, 1987.

Miller, B.D. Depression and asthma: A potentially lethal mixture. *Journal of Allergy and Clinical Immunology 80:* 481–486, 1987.

———. Treatment of the refractory asthmatic child. *American Journal of Asthma and Allergy for Pediatricians 4:* 241–247, 1988.

———, & Strunk, R.C. Circumstances surrounding the deaths of children due to asthma: A case-control study. *American Journal of Disease of Children, 143:* 1294–1299, 1989.

Minuchin, S., Baker, L., Rosman, B.L., Liebman, R., Milman, L., & Todd, T.C. A conceptual model of psychosomatic illness in children: Family organization and family therapy. *Archives of General Psychiatry 32:* 1031–1038, 1975.

Newacheck, P.W., & Taylor, W.R. Childhood chronic illness: Prevalence, severity, and impact. *American Journal of Public health 82:* 364–371, 1992.

Reiss, D., Gonzalez, S., & Kramer, N. Family process, chronic illness, and death: On the weakness of strong bonds. *Archives of General Psychiatry 43:* 795–804, 1986.

Rolland, J.S. Toward a psychosocial typology of chronic and life-threatening illness. *Family Systems Medicine 2:* 2 45–262, 1984.

Strunk, R.C., Mrazek, D.A., Wolfson Fuhrmann, G.S., & LaBrecque, J. Physiological and psychological characteristics associated with deaths from asthma in childhood: A case-controlled study. *Journal of American Medical Association 254:* 1193–1198, 1985.

Weiner, H. *Perturbing the organism: The biology of stressful experience.* Chicago: University of Chicago Press, 1992.

Wood, B. (1991). Biopsychosocial care. In W.A. Walker, P.R. Durie, J.R. Hamilton, J.A. Walker-Smith, & J.B. Watkins (eds.), *Pediatric gastrointestinal disease: Pathophysiology, diagnosis, management.* Philadelphia & Toronto: B.C. Decker, Inc., 1991.

———. A developmental biopsychosocial approach to the treatment of chronic illness in children and adolescents. In R.H. Mikesell, D.-D. Lusterman, & S.H. McDaniel (eds.), *Integrating family therapy: Handbook of family psychology and systems theory.* Washington DC: American Psychological Association, 1995.

———, Watkins, J.B., Boyle, J.T., Nogueirra, J., Zimand, E., & Carroll, L. The "psychosomatic family model: An empirical and theoretical analysis. *Family Process 28:* 399–417, 1989.

Zimand, E., & Wood, B. Implications of contrasting patterns of divorce in families of children with gastrointestinal disorders. *Family Systems Medicine 4:* 385–397, 1986.

APPENDIX

Establishing Adaptive Interactions Among Family, School, Peer Group, and Health Care System

Step 1. Open Channels of Communication:

Family: Encourage both parents to come to appointments; if divorced, obtain permission to keep noncustodial parent involved if possible.
School: Identify one school person to coordinate communication with family and health care provider.
Peers: Have parents communicate with parents of patient's friends, and have patient or parents (depending on age of patient) communicate with peers regarding the illness.

Step 2. Provide Education Regarding the Illness:

Family: Provide information about the illness to all parental figures and to siblings; assist and encourage family to share information with extended family members.
School: Have meeting at school with parents, patient, and relevant school personnel (nurse, homeroom teacher, gym teacher, bus driver). Outline the characteristics of the illness, specific for that child. Devise a written plan for medical treatment and for what do to in the event of an illness episode.
Peers: Have family educate peers and their parents as to the nature of the patient's illness.

Step 3. Emphasize Balance Between Medical Management of the Disease and Quality of Life and Developmental Demands:

Family: Help the family not to neglect psychosocial and developmental needs in favor of the child's physical well-being and growth.
School: Assist the school in achieving balanced expectations of the child with regard to disease management and participation in academics and extracurricular activities.
Peers: Encourage patient to be involved with informal neighborhood peer activities. Emphasize to parents the critical nature of peer relationships for psychosocial development.

Step 4. Initiate Age-appropriate Self-care and Facilitate Increases in Self-care in Accordance with the Child's Development:

Family: Guide the family in home care routines that maximize the patient's active participation in management of the illness and its psychosocial concomitants.

School: Prepare the child for self-care activities at school and obtain the school's coordination.

Peers: Encourage the family to inform peers and their parents as to the care the patient will need to provide for himself or herself, and what assistance might be needed from adults.

7

The Relationship Between Attachment, Psychopathology, and Childhood Disability

Ruth A. Huebner and Kenneth R. Thomas

Historically, the study of childhood psychological dysfunction has been complicated by inadequate diagnostic criteria for children and an insufficient understanding of psychological development between infancy and adulthood (Kazdin, 1988, 1993). Determining the relationship between chronic-physical disorders in children and the subsequent risk for psychopathology is additionally hampered by multiple methodological problems in defining and measuring these two constructs (Breslau, 1985; Pless & Nolan, 1991). Pless and Nolan (1991) summarized the literature in this area and concluded that nearly 10% of children have some form of chronic physical illness with twice the risk of psychopathology. Other authors (Breslau, 19985; Cadman, Boyle, Szatmari, & Offord, 1987; Rutter, 1981; Seidel, Chadwick, & Rutter, 1975) concluded that the risk of psychopathology increases threefold for children with a physical disability, and fourfold in children who have a brain injury. An overall elevation in emotional or behavioral difficulties is typically described in studies on children with chronic disease and disabilities, without delineation or specific diagnostic criteria (Breslau, 1985). In one attempt to delineate emotional disorders, Cadman and his colleagues (1987) randomly sampled 1,869 families, including the children and their teachers, and found an overall increase in neurotic disorders, attentional disorders, conduct disorders, social maladjustment, and multiple psychiatric disorders among children with chronic diseases or disabilities; however, there was no preponderance of any specific emotional disorder.

Julia McGivern, Ph.D., Gary W. Kramer, Ph.D., Jack C. Westman, M.D., and two anonymous reviewers who provided thoughtful comments on earlier versions of this manuscript.

From *Rehabilitation Psychology, 40*(2) (1995), 111–125. Reprinted with permission.

Finding evidence of increased psychopathology is, of course, an easier task than explaining why that pathology may exist. Kazdin (1993) noted that psychological research has neglected children with chronic diseases and physical handicaps; he argued for exploring both risk and protective factors to understand childhood psychological dysfunction and treatment. Attachment processes may be such a risk or protective factor. Securely attached children are more likely to achieve social competence, trust, a strong sense of self, and resilience against stress; in contrast, insecurely attached children are more likely to develop psychopathology (e.g., see Ainsworth, 1978; Cox & Lambrenos, 1992).

Attachment is variously defined by authors from different perspectives as mother-infant interaction patterns (Ainsworth, Blehar, Waters, & Wall, 1978), as mother-infant interaction patterns with related neurobiological system development (Bowlby, 1969), and/or as a socialization process (Kraemer, 1992). The purpose of this paper is to elucidate the relationships among these three components of attachment: (a) neurobiological influences and consequences, (b) interpersonal and intrapersonal factors, and (c) social forces affecting the child and caregiver. The literature search and review included publications on attachment in typical and atypical development, and publications on childhood chronic illness or congenital disability. Disorders such as asthma, cleft palate, cerebral palsy, and congenital anomalies are typically mentioned in the literature, usually without differentiation. Other authors (e.g., see Kraemer, 1992; Wasserman & Allen, 1985) have elaborated on the relationship between neurological development and attachment, but no author has specifically integrated the literature on attachment as described in this paper.

ATTACHMENT THEORY

Classic attachment theory emphasizes the intrapersonal drive for social relatedness and the interpersonal relationships necessary to satisfy that drive. Attachment and loss theory grew out of a psychoanalytic framework with an emphasis on object relations; it is based on the work of John Bowlby (1973, 1979, 1982), who argued that the mother-infant relationship was fundamental to emotional stability rather than mere physical survival. Ainsworth and her associates (Ainsworth, 1978, 1985; Ainsworth & Bell, 1970; Ainsworth et al., 1978) developed a widely used system of classifying attachment behavior into three groups: avoidant/insecurely attached (Group A), securely attached (Group B), and ambivalent/insecurely attached (Group C). Although the names of Bowlby and Ainsworth are often considered synonymous with attachment theory, other psychoanalytic scholars have also contributed significantly to an understanding of attachment (e.g., Eagle, 1984; Fairbairn, 1952; Greenberg & Mitchell, 1983; Mahler, 1968; Mahler, Pine, & Bergman, 1975; Sullivan, 1953; Winnicott, 1960) with the common belief that attachment is fundamental to emotional health and social relationships.

Recently, authors such as Baldwin (1992), Liotti (1984), Safran and Segal (1990), and Westen (1991) have formalized a link between attachment and interpersonal theory and cognitive therapy. According to these authors, fundamental interpersonal schema with expectations and rules for maintaining interpersonal relatedness are formed in early attachment relationships. For example, complex social schema with a hierarchy of representations are found in children at age three (Bretherton, 1985).

NEUROBIOLOGICAL INFLUENCES AND CONSEQUENCES

The strong link between brain injury and psychopathology suggests that one component in the development of psychopathology is altered brain function. However, the literature indicates that neurobiological mechanisms are reciprocally interactive. That is, failures in infant and child attachment may compromise neurobiological development and consequently psychological well-being. Moreover, neurobiological differences may exist as a direct result of brain dysfunction, which may affect relatedness directly with subsequent secondary social deficits. Although it is not clear which specific neurobiological deficits result from inadequate attachment or interfere with normal attachment and social interaction, research is beginning to illuminate these relationships. For example, deficits in neurotransmission processes and neurochemicals, abnormalities in neural responses, and site-specific neurological lesions are being identified in people with severe developmental disorders such as autistic disorder and mental retardation (e.g., see Hooper, Boyd, Hynd, & Rubin, 1993; Huebner, 1992, for reviews of this literature), but neither the etiology nor the developmental implications of these neurological alterations has been established.

Several neurochemical substances which relate to issues of attachment have also been studied in human and nonhuman primate research. These substances are cortisol and the brain biogenic amine systems, including the norepinephrine (NE) system, dopamine (DA) system, and serotonin (5HT) system.

Cortisol

Stress has been shown to be associated with alterations in the immune system, sleep cycle, circadian rhythms, and possibly some aspects of learning (Reite, 1990). Consequently, children with disabilities who are subjected to increased stress due to medical procedures, separation from mothers, and other complications such as cardiopulmonary insufficiency are more likely to suffer stress-related secondary disabilities.

Cortisol is the primary hormone produced by the adrenocortical system in humans; it increases the level of energy available to respond to stress, suppresses inflammation, and facilitates learning (Gunnar, 1989). Too much cortisol secretion may be associated with being overwhelmed by stress, especially novel stress.

Since cortisol levels can be measured by tests on saliva, the research in this area is growing, but the findings are preliminary. Gunnar, in several studies, discovered that both behavioral distress and sleeping were associated with excessive elevation of cortisol levels during medical procedures such as circumcision, suggesting that observation alone is insufficient to measure stress in an infant. According to Gunnar, experience with a stressful event tended to attenuate cortisol secretion, but infants showed substantial variability in their responses to stress. Similarly, Fox (1989) found that infants' and young children's responses to stress fell on two continua of reactivity or arousal and the ability to regulate autonomic nervous system responses. For example, children with high reactivity and high regulation were expressive and social, but those with high reactivity and low regulation were more hyperactive and uncontrollable. These highly reactive infants with low regulation of autonomic nervous system responses were more vulnerable to stress.

From another perspective, Coe, Lubach, and Ershler (1989) found in numerous related studies that psychological distress (in on-human primates) can alter the immune system with potentially long-lasting effects on susceptibility to illness. Conversely, touch, when given by an individual with an attached relationship to the child, may reduce the biological disorders that occur secondary to stress and separation (Reite, 1990). Although preliminary, these research findings may facilitate more precise identification of children who manifest signs of being overwhelmed by stress.

Biogenic Amine Systems

A great deal of research on the neurobiological aspects of attachment has grown from the work of Harry Harlow with non-human primates. Kraemer, Ebert, Schmidt, and McKinney (1989) reared infant monkeys from birth in several attachment conditions (i.e., without any objects; with cloth, stationary wire, or moving wire surrogate mothers; with peers; or with their mothers). They measured the levels of NE over 21 months. Although monkeys raised with peers had higher levels of NE than those raised without objects or with inanimate surrogate mothers, the monkeys raised by their mothers had nearly twice the levels of NE. Low levels of NE are thought to be associated with poor overall adaptation, attention disorders, increased vulnerability to stress, and decreased problem-solving ability. In addition, primates raised in social isolation were noted to have eating disorders; lack aggression-impulse control, and demonstrate hypervigilance, body rocking, self-injurious behavior, and a variety of cognitive deficits. Kraemer (1992) integrated the results of many studies on brain biogenic amine systems and concluded that deficits produced by isolation include disregulation of all three biogenic amine systems (NE, DA, and 5HT), changes in brain cytoarchitecture such as reduction in dendritic branching, and failure to organize an emotional response to stressors.

NEUROBIOLOGICAL CONSEQUENCES

Perhaps in no other disorder is the link between neurobiology and attachment as intriguing as in autistic disorder. Sigman and Mundy (1989) defined a continuum of attachment behaviors in children with autistic disorder and found that these children were attached to their parents, but were more vulnerable to separation from parents than other children. The autistic children's social deficits were related to difficulty with comprehending and sharing emotional reactions rather than to lack of responsiveness. One possible explanation for these findings may be that the neuromechanisms for attachment are altered prior to birth in children with autistic disorder; consequently, the social contacts of parents may be ineffective in developing social responsiveness, with a resulting cascade of impairment in many systems as described in the work of Kraemer et al. (1989) and Kraemer (1992).

The evidence linking increased physical or cognitive disability as secondary to disruption of attachment is sparse, but this potential relationship is an important consideration when examining the effects of interrupted attachment. Magid and McKelvey (1987) described the worst-case scenario for children with attachment disorders as including some sensory abnormalities with decreased ability to feel pain or affectionate touch, phoniness, learning disabilities, abnormalities in eye contact, speech pathology, and many other severe psychopathic behaviors. Similarly, Steinhauer (1991) discussed children with disorganized and disoriented attachment (Group D Attachment response) as exhibiting whining, petulant behavior, huddling, rocking, and wetting in response to stress. Some of these insecure attachment-related behaviors could be perceived as intensifying existing symptoms of physical disabilities or in some cases mimicking a physical disorder.

Attachment may also influence intellectual and motor development. Wasserman and Allen (1985) studied 12 children with disabilities compared to 14 "at-risk" premature children and 9 normal children at 9, 12, 18, and 24 months; they found that children who were ignored at 12 months (50% of those with a disability; none of the normal sample) showed a 30-point drop in IQ by 24 months as measured on a variety of developmental scales. Sorting out the cause of this diminished IQ is difficult since IQ tends to be unstable in young children, and lower cognitive levels could be associated with diminished social reciprocity and maternal fatigue over time. However, Egeland and Farber (1984) studied over 200 mother/infant dyads and also found that those children with more anxious resistant attachment had significantly lower scores on both the mental and motor sections of the Bayley Scales of Infant Development at 9 months.

Psychopathology, possibly stemming from insecure attachment, may also be associated with increased vulnerability to the onset of physical disabilities. Rutter (1981), for example, found in a follow-up study after head trauma that children with mild head injuries ($n = 29$) were more impulsive, disturbed, and overactive before their head injury than a control group, suggesting that behavioral disturbances may increase vulnerability to head trauma.

INTERPERSONAL AND INTRAPERSONAL FACTORS

To understand the context of attachment for children with disabilities, it is necessary to examine both infant characteristics and caregiver responses because it is within this context that interpersonal and intrapersonal characteristics interact in the process of attachment. When considering the influence of infant and child characteristics, researchers view the child as an active participant in the social relationship with caregivers; that is, the child both influences and is influenced by the interaction (e.g., see Rogers, 1988).

Temperamental Characteristics of Children

Overall, children with disabilities are more likely to be born prematurely with low birthweight (Cox & Lambrenos, 1992), and they may require long-term hospitalization. Plunkeet, Meisels, Stiefel, Pasick, and Roloff (1986) compared 33 premature infants, at ages 12 and 18 months, who required hospitalization for more than one month to preterm infants who were hospitalized for less than one month. Although 55% of the long-term hospitalized infants were judged to be securely attached, 36% (compared to 9% of infants with shorter hospital stays) were found to exhibit patterns of insecurity with anxious and resistant behaviors. This study was particularly significant since the authors excluded infants who showed signs of central nervous system disorders, or whose mothers were addicted to drugs or alcohol, were less than 17 at the time of birth, or who had severe mental disorders. Thus, the sample of premature infants was likely to be showing the effects of long-term separation after birth rather than increased biological vulnerability to attachment disorders.

Premature babies are also likely to be more irritable and immature (Cox & Lamgrenos, 1992). Crockenberg (1981) found that irritable and unresponsive babies, those with motor immaturity, or babies with poor physiological regulation were more stressful to mothers and more vulnerable to other maternal or family stressors; conversely, easy temperament babies were more likely to develop secure attachments even in discordant homes.

By three weeks of age, mothers and infants have established a cycle of rhythmic interaction in which the mother and child match levels of vocalization and cuddling (Brooks-Gunn & Luciano, 1985); responsive infants who vocalize and cuddle elicit the same level of interaction from their caregivers. Between 9 and 12 weeks, a typical child develops the ability to change head position and visual gaze, smile, and vocalize (van Wulfften Palthe & Hopkins, 1993). Van Wulfften Palthe and Hopkins theorized that these typical abilities enable a child's first control of and competence in social interactions. Premature or disabled children may have poor ability to interact and focus attention, with decreased visual tracking and reaching, and impaired sensory responses and ability to cuddle (Bendell, 1984). Infants (2-7 months) with a physical disability made less eye contact and fewer protests toward the mother when compared with typical infants

(Barrera & Vella, 1987). Consequently, children with disabilities may be less able to steady their head, focus their gaze, smile, and vocalize in response to others; these limited social abilities may elicit less reciprocal interaction by the mother (Rogers, 1988), and afford a diminished experience of social competence and control for the child.

Disability Characteristics

Although the evidence is not conclusive, severity of disability tends to have a concave, curvilinear relationship with psychological adjustment (Breslan, 1985). That is, individuals with mild or severe disabilities tend to present more psychopathology (Pless & Nolan, 1991). However, the reasons for psychopathology may be different in the mild and severe groups. Children with severe disabilities are more likely to have brain injury and difficulties with cognition and mentation that may mimic psychopathology (Breslau, 1985). Children who have hidden or mild handicaps, on the other hand, may have an ambiguous identity or difficulty in acknowledgment of limitations with subsequent maladjustment (Pless & Nolan, 1991).

The type of disability also seems to make a difference in both security of attachment and overall psychological well being. Children with facial deformities (Wasserman & Allen, 1985), abnormal genitalia, or sensory abnormalities (Collins-Moore, 1984) are more likely to be ignored by their mothers.

Although infants' interactions have been studied extensively, the process of lifespan adaptation to disability has received less attention (Eisner, 1990). However, Breslau (1985) studied 304 children (ages 3-18 years) grouped into four congenital conditions and found that chronicity, with or without neurological injury, was consistently associated with increased amounts of social isolation, conflicts with parents, and repressive anxiety.

Within Family Influences on Attachment

For parents who have a child with a disability, the celebration of birth may be replaced with shock, disbelief, and grief. The family is faced with the high cost of treatment, questions regarding the future, separations from the infant, and sometimes even decisions about rights to life and death (Bendell, 1984). Some parents disengage from their infant in anticipation of a death (Plunkett et al., 1986). Although little is actually known about parent-coping processes, some parental responses may include shock and protective denial, hope for a cure, grieving for the child with vastly different mourning reactions, grieving for themselves and their other existing or planned children, feelings of inadequacy, anger towards many others, and depression (Eisner, 1990). These emotions may divert energy from the attachment process and require professional intervention. Adjustment to having a child with a disability is a dynamic process which changes over time. Barrera and Vella (1987) found that mothers of infants (2-7 months) with disabilities were very similar to controls in responsiveness to their infants; however, these mothers were significantly more commanding and controlling during social interactions with their infants. Over time, the interactional differences may increase; Wasserman and Allen (1985), for example, found low rates of maternal ignoring before 18 months, but by two years of age 50% of mothers with handicapped toddlers ignored their child, even when being watched by research teams. Long-term ignoring may be associated with differences in perception, with mothers being less able to judge and respond to the stress experienced by their children. Tackett, Kerr, and Helmstadter (1990) found in their study of 20 mother/child dyads (8-15-year-old children with physical disabilities and average intelligence) that mothers and their children differed in perceptions of stress and acceptance of the disability. Although the children were keenly aware of stressors such as school, medical procedures, family strife, and peer reactions, the mothers were more stressed about the physical limitations and their own feelings of being different and inadequate. Similarly, Gilbride (1993) found that parents who perceived their child's disability as more severe, whether this was objectively true, held lower expectations and gave less encouragement to their child with a disability. As children move into late adolescence and adulthood, Crittenden (1990) proposed, but did not investigate, the hypothesis that autonomy will be facilitated by family cohesion and adaptability, which are marked by open communication, support, and the emerging of adult attachment styles.

Several authors (Eisner, 1990; Pless & Nolan, 1991; Rutter, 1981; Seidel et al., 1975) have postulated that a physical disability may create increased vulnerability to psychopathology, but that vulnerability is exacerbated and manifested when paired with family dysfunction. Although a causal or directional relationship was not implied, Rutter (1981) found that the rate of psychiatric disorder in children was 20–25% in families with adversity, such as marital discord or prenatal psychopathology, but less than 7% in families without such adversity.
Lastly, families and their children with chronic disease or physical disabilities are often separated for medical procedures. Steinhauer (1991) reviewed the effects of separation and found that children were most susceptible if separation occurred between the ages of 6 months and 4 years; the longer the separation the greater the negative impact. Separation anxiety and suffering was attenuated in those children who were securely attached prior to separation, in those with some prior experience with separation, and when the post-separation environment supported a process of mourning and provided tender support.

SOCIAL FACTORS

Social forces may present both additional risks for psychopathology and/or provide a buffer and support for children with disabilities and their families. The act of labeling a disability is itself fraught with problems since accurate diagnosis and identification or risks and problems are necessary for intervention, but the labels may become part of a self-fulfilling prophecy (Pless & Nolan, 1991).

People with chronic diseases or disabilities may be perceived as "damaged goods" (Phillips, 1990) or categorized as devalued people (Wolfensberger & Tullman, 1991). Regrettably, professionals may unwittingly reinforce or act upon limited or stereotyped expectations and facilitate the process of stigmatization (Rubenfeld, 1988; Sigelman, 1991). Parents are sometimes characterized as over-protective, shopping for treatments, depressed, hostile, overcompensating, and poorly adjusted to their child's disability (MacKinnon & Marlett, 1984).

Both parents and their children with disabilities are vulnerable to prejudice secondary to these stereotypical beliefs. These social pressures are likely to create parental stress and diminish parental resources necessary for nurturance and attachment (Westman, 1991).

Although mothers may feel the most pressure, Tavecchio and van IJzendoorn (1987) challenged the belief that mothers must bear the burden and guilt. These authors proposed that a stable network of caregivers may be optimal to reduce maternal stress and minimize the effects of neglect or overprotection of a child. In support of this proposal, they studied 166 families and found that 70% of the children with working mothers (as compared to nonworking mothers) exhibited equal attachment intensity with both the mother and father.

IMPLICATIONS

When considering this literature on attachment, it is evident that the three fundamental components of attachment processes are powerful and interrelated forces in child development, with potential to modify social competence, neurological development, and psychological adjustment. An appreciation of the dynamics of attachment has important implications for treatment and research.

When assessing a child and his or her family, psychologists must recognize that neurological disorders, developmental delays, or psychopathology have potential to be exacerbated by inadequate attachment to caregivers. Furthermore, a developmental or emotional disorder may be a secondary problem that is founded in inadequate attachment. Although such disorders or delays will alter the interpersonal interaction between the child and the caregivers, a securely attached child will have an innate buffer against psychopathology. In view of these findings, psychologists and other professionals must consider the impact on attachment when intervening within a family. For example, parents are often asked to provide medical, educational, or therapeutic interventions for their child at home. These interventions, although potentially beneficial, may create guilt and stress for the caregivers and ultimately interfere with the benefits of the attachment process. It may be more important, in some cases, to facilitate the bond between child and caregivers than to treat the child. Rogers (1988), for instance, suggested helping caregivers to recognize and interpret the altered or subtle social behavior of the infant and Westman (1991) recommended assessing and facilitating a family's capability to form a parent-professional alliance.

Adults with lifelong chronic diseases or congenital disabilities are likely to have experienced alterations in attachment interactions with their caregivers and continue to have an increased risk of psychopathology. For example, Turner and McLean (1989) found that rates of depression and anxiety were two and half to four times higher in adults with disabilities (*n* = 967). Although Turner and McLean attributed this psychopathology to chronic stress, another variable might be alterations in interpersonal expectations and images stemming from alterations in interpersonal relatedness. Safran and Segal (1990) suggested that interpersonal expectations often become self-fulfilling prophecies in which the individual both construes reality and constructs reality to validate the expectations. While finding employment and securing social support are important for combating depression in adults, examining interpersonal schema and the meaning of ambiguous attachment may enhance social competence and mastery for the adult with a disability. Safran and Segal (1990) provided a guide for such intervention which included using interpersonal processes to activate and explore implicit interpersonal schema and cognitive therapy to alter these schema.

Finally, there is a critical need for research to clarify (a) the coping processes of families and ways to identify families who are most in need of intervention, and (b) the dynamics of adjustment to disability across childhood and into adulthood. A pertinent question is: If attachment processes are fundamental to mental health, then how are attachment deficits manifested in adults and adolescents with physical disabilities?

REFERENCES

Ainsworth, M. D. S. (1978). Toward a general theory of infantile attachment: A comparative review of aspects of the social bond. *Behavioral and Brain Sciences, 1,* 436–2438.

Ainsworth, M. D. S. (1985). Attachment across the life span. *Bulletin of the New York Academy of Medicine, 61,* 792–813.

Ainsworth, M. D. S. & Bell, S. (1970). Attachment, exploration and separation: Illustrated by the behavior of one-year olds in a strange situation. *Child Development, 41,* 49–67.

Ainsworth, M. D. S., Blehar, M. C., Waters, E., & Wall, S. (1978). *Patterns of attachment: A psychological study of the strange situation.* Hillsdale, NJ: Erlbaum.

Baldwin, M. W. (1992). Relational schemas and the processing of social information. *Psychological Bulletin, 112,* 461–484.

Barrera, M. E., & Vella, D. M. (1987). Disabled and nondisabled infants;' interactions with their mothers. *American Journal of Occupational Therapy, 41,* 168–172.

Bendell, R. D. (1984). Psychological problems of infancy. In M. G. Eisenberg, L. C. Sutkin, & M. A. Jansen (Ed.), *Chronic illness and disability through the life span: Effects on self and family* (pp. 23–38). New York: Springer.

Bowlby, J. (1969). *Attachment and loss: Vol. 2: Attachment.* London: Hogarth Press.

Bowlby, J. (1973). *Attachment and loss: Vol. 2: Separation.* New York: Basic Books.

Bowlby, J. (1979). *The making and breaking of affectual bonds.* London: Tavistock.

Bowlby, J. (1980). *Loss: Sadness and depression.* London: Hogarth Press.

Bowlby, J. (1982). *Attachment and loss: Vol. 1: Attachment* (2nd ed.). New York: Basic Books.

Breslau, N. (1985). Psychiatric disorder in children with physical disabilities. *Journal of the American Academy of Child Psychiatry, 24,* 87–94.

Bretherton, I. (1985). Attachment theory: Retrospect and prospect. In I. Bretherton & E. Waters (Eds.), *Growing points of attachment theory and research* (pp. 3–35). Chicago: The University of Chicago Press.

Brooks-Gunn, J., & Luciano, L. (1985). Social competence in young handicapped children: A developmental perspective. In M. Sigman (Ed.), *Children with emotional disorders and developmental disabilities: Assessment and treatment* (pp. 3–22). New York: Grune and Stratton.

Cadman, D., Boyle, M., Szatmari, P., & Offord, D. R. (1987). Chronic illness, disability, and mental and social well-being: Findings of the Ontario child health study. *Pediatrics, 79,* 805–813.

Coe, C. L., Lubach, G., & Ershler, W. B. (1989). Immunological consequences of maternal separation in infant primates. In M. Lewis & J. Worobey (Eds.), *Infant stress and coping* (pp. 65–91). San Francisco: Jossey-Bass Inc.

Collins-Moore, M. S. (1984). Birth and diagnosis: A family crisis. In M. G. Eisenberg, L. C. Sutkin, & M. A. Jansen (Eds.), *Chronic illness and disability through the life span: Effects on self and family* (pp. 39–66). New York: Springer.

Cox, A. D., & Lambrenos, K. (1992). Childhood physical disability and attachment. *Developmental Medicine and Child Neurology, 34,* 1037–1046.

Crittenden, P. M. (1990). Toward a concept of autonomy in adolescents with a disability. *Child Health Care, 19,* 162–168.

Crockenberg, S. B. (1981). Infant irritability, mother responsiveness, and social support influences on the security of infant-mother attachment. *Child Development, 52,* 857–865.

Eagle, M. N. (1984). *Recent developments in psychoanalysis: A critical evaluation.* New York: McGraw-Hill.

Eisner, C. (1990). Psychological effects of chronic disease. *Journal of Child Psychology and Psychiatry, 31,* 85–98.

Egeland, B., & Farber, E. A. (1984). Infant-mother attachment: Factors related to its development and change over time. *Child Development, 55,* 753–771.

Fairbairn, W. R. D. (1952). *An object-relations theory of the personality.* New York: Basic Books.

Fox, N. A. (1989). Infant response to frustrating and mildly stressful events: A positive look at anger in the first year. In M. Lewis & J. Worobey (Eds.), *Infant stress and coping* (pp. 47–64). San Francisco: Jossey-Bass Inc.

Gilbride, D. D. (1993). Parental attitudes toward their child with a disability: Implications for rehabilitation counselors. *Rehabilitation Counseling Bulletin, 36,* 139–150.

Greenberg, J. R., & Mitchell, S. A. (1983). *Object relations in psychoanalytic theory.* Cambridge, MA: Harvard University Press.

Gunnar, M. R. (1989). Studies of the human infant's adrenocortical response to potentially stressful events. In M. Lewis and J. Worobey (Eds.), *Infant stress and coping* (pp. 3–18). San Francisco: Jossey-Bass Inc.

Hooper, S. R., Boyd, T. A., Hynd, G. W., & Rubin, J. (1993). Definitional issues and neurobiological foundations of selected severe neurodevelopmental disorders. *Archives of Clinical Neuropsychology, 8,* 279–307.

Huebner, R. A. (1992). Autistic disorder: A neuropsychological enigma. *American Journal of Occupational Therapy, 46,* 487–501.

Kazdin, A. E. (1988). *Child psychotherapy: Developing and identifying effective treatments.* Boston: Allyn and Bacon.

Kazdin, A. E. (1993). Psychotherapy for children and adolescents: Current progress and future research direction. *American Psychologist, 48,* 644–657.

Kraemer, G. W. (1992). A psychobiological theory of attachment. *Behavioral and Brain Sciences, 15,* 493–541.

Kraemer, G. W., Ebert, M. H., Schmidt, D. E., & McKinney, W. T. (1989). A longitudinal study of the effects of different rearing environments on cerebrospinal fluid norepinephrine and biogenic amine metabolites in rhesus monkeys. *Neuropsychopharmacology, 2,* 175–189.

Liotti, G. (1984). Cognitive therapy, attachment theory, and psychiatric nosology: A clinical and theoretical inquiry into their interdependence. In M. A. Reda & M. J. Mahoney (Eds.), *Cognitive psychotherapies recent development in theory, research, and practice* (pp. 211–232). Cambridge, MA: Ballinger.

MacKinnon, L., & Marlett, N. (1984). A social action perspective: The disabled and their families in context. In J. C. Hansen (Ed.), *Families with handicapped members* (pp. 111–137). Rockville, MD: Aspen.

Mahler, M. S. (1968). *On human symbiosis and the vicissitudes of individuation: Vol. 1: Infantile psychosis.* New York: International Universities Press.

Mahler, M. A., Pine, F., & Bergman, A. (1975). *The psychological birth of the human infant: Symbiosis and individuation.* New York: Basic Books.

Magid, K., & McKelvey, C. A. (1987). *High-risk: Children without a conscience.* New York: Bantam.

Phillips, M. (1990). Damaged goods: Oral narratives of the experience of disability in American culture. *Social Sciences in Medicine, 30,* 849–857.

Pless, B., & Nolan, T. (1991). Revision, replication and neglect: Research on maladjustment in chronic illness. *Journal of Child Psychology and Psychiatry, 32,* 347–365.

Plunkeet, J. W., Meisels, S. J., Stiefel, G. S., Pasick, P. L., & Roloff, D. W. (1986). Patterns of attachment among preterm infants of varying biological risk. *Journal of the American Academy of Child Psychiatry, 25,* 794–800.

Reite, M. (1990). Effects of touch on the immune system. In *Advances in touch: New implications in human development* (pp. 22–31). New Brunswick, NJ: Johnson and Johnson Products.

Rogers, S. J. (1988). Characteristics of social interactions between mothers and their disabled infants: A review. *Child: Care, Health, and Development, 14,* 301–317.

Rubenfeld, P. (1988). The counselor and the disabled client: Is a partnership of equals possible? In S. E. Rubin & N. M. Rubin (Eds.), *Contemporary challenges to the rehabilitation counseling professional* (pp. 31–44). Baltimore: Brooks.

Rutter, M. (1981). Psychological sequelae of brain damage in children. *The American Journal of Psychiatry, 138,* 1533–1544.

Safran, J. D., & Segal, Z. V. (1990). *Interpersonal processes in cognitive therapy.* New York: Basic.

Seidel, U. P., Chadwick, O. F. D., & Rutter, M. (1975). Psychological disorders in crippled children: A comparative study of children with and without brain damage. *Developmental Medicine and Child Neurology, 17,* 563–575.

Sigelman, C. K. (1991). Social distance from stigmatized groups: False consensus and false uniqueness effects on responding. *Rehabilitation Psychology, 36,* 139–151.

Sigman, M., & Mundy, P. (1989). Social attachments in autistic children. *Journal of the American Academy of Child and Adolescent Psychiatry, 28,* 74–81.

Steinhauer, P. D. (1991). Issues of attachment and separation: Mourning and loss in children. In P. D. Steinhauer (Ed.), *The least detrimental alternative* (pp. 13–241). Toronto: University of Toronto Press.

Sullivan, H. S. (1953). *The interpersonal theory of psychiatry.* New York: Norton.

Tackett, P., Kerr, N., & Helmstadter, G. (1990). Stresses as perceived by children with physical disabilities and their mothers. *Journal of Rehabilitation, 3,* 30–34.

Tavecchio, L. W. C., & van IJzendoorn, M. H. (1987). Perceived security and extension of the child's rearing context: A parent-report approach. In L. W. C. Tavecchio & M. H. van IJzendoorn (Eds.), *Attachment in social networks: Contributions to the Bowly-Ainsworth attachment theory* (pp. 35–92). New York: North-Holland.

Turner, J. R., & McLean, P. D. (1989). Physical disability and psychological distress. *Rehabilitation Psychology, 34,* 225–242.

van Wulfften Palthe, T., & Hopkins, B. (1993). A longitudinal study of neural maturation and early mother-infant interaction: A research note. *Journal of Child Psychology and Psychiatry, 34,* 1031–1041.

Wasserman, G. A., & Allen, R. (1985). Maternal withdrawal from handicapped toddlers. *Journal of Child Psychology and Psychiatry, 26,* 381–387.

Westen, D. (1991). Social cognition and object relations. *Psychological Bulletin, 109,* 429–455.

Westman, J. C. (1991). *Who speaks for the children?* Sarasota, FL: Professional Resources Exchange.

Winnicott, D. W. (1960). *The theory of the parent-infant relationship.* New York: International Universities Press.

Wolfensberger, W., & Tullman, S. (1991). A brief outline of the principle of normalization. In M. G. Eisenberg & R. L. Glueckauf (Eds.), *Empirical approaches to the psychosocial aspects of disability* (pp. 202–215). New York: Springer.

8

Helping Families Manage Severe Mental Illness

Kim T. Mueser

The field of psychiatric rehabilitation has made tremendous gains over the past several decades, and nowhere has progress been more evident than in the area of family intervention for severe psychiatric illnesses. Until the 1960s and 1970s, mental health professionals commonly viewed families of mental health consumers as either irrelevant to the process of rehabilitation, or as pathological agents in the etiology of the disorder. Indeed, theories such as the double-bind hypothesis of schizophrenia (Bateson, Jackson, Haley and Weakland, 1958) and the schizophrenogenic mother (Fromm-Reichman, 1949), often served as barriers to establishing a good working alliance between families and professionals. In some cases, these theories have lead to the mistreatment of family members at the hands of professionals (Appleton, 1974). Fortunately, there has been a paradigm shift in recent years and families are now viewed as important allies in the rehabilitation process (Mueser & Glynn, 1995).

Several factors can be identified that contributed to a shift in attitudes of mental health professionals towards the families of mental health consumers. First, the accumulating evidence that genetic factors may play a role in the etiology of major psychiatric illnesses such as schizophrenia (Gottesman, 1990) and major affective disorders (Goodwin & Jamison, 1990), coupled with overwhelming evidence regarding the beneficial effects of psychotropic medications for these disorders (Meltzer, 1987), made psychogenic theories of etiology less tenable. Second, early efforts at family therapy based on psychogenic models met with dismal success raising questions about the utility of these models (Terkelsen, 1983). Third, a growing number of studies found that family factors, such as excessive criticism or hostility, were related to higher relapse and rehospitalization rates (Bebbington & Kuipers, 1994); findings suggested that some families could benefit from learning about how to cope more effectively with a

From *Psychiatric Rehabilitation Skills, 1*(2) (1996), 21–42. Reprinted with permission.

relative's psychiatric illness. Fourth, and last, the family advocacy and consumer movement developed partly because their needs were not being adequately met by mental health professionals, including involvement in the decision making process (Lefley & Johnson, 1990).

As mental health professionals began to recognize the potential value of working and collaborating with families of the mentally ill, a variety of different models of family intervention were developed and empirically evaluated. For example, Anderson, Reiss and Hogarty (1986) developed a model of family intervention which combines techniques from family systems therapy and psychoeducation. Leff and colleagues (1985) developed an approach primarily based on providing education about psychiatric illnesses, both in a group and an individual family format. McFarlane and colleagues (1993) developed a model in which families meet in multiple family groups, provide mutual family support, and problem solve about common difficulties.

Although each of these family models employs some behavioral techniques, none of them are explicitly behavioral in their overall approach to assessment and intervention. Two other models have a strong behavioral orientation. Barrowclough and Tarrier's (1992) model combines education about psychiatric disorder with training in stress management, relapse prevention, and goal attainment. Falloon, Boyd, and McGill (1984) developed a model, described in more detail later in this article, which combines education with communication skills training and problem solving training. Table 9.1 summarizes different validated family treatment programs and provides references for treatment manuals and research supporting each model.

Until recently, most research on family intervention for severe psychiatric illness has been conducted with individuals who have either schizophrenia or schizoaffective disorder. The results of these investigations have been very promising. A total of 16 controlled studies have been conducted which have monitored clients' relapse rates for at least one to two years and which compare either family intervention to no family intervention or evaluate the effects of different models of family intervention (Penn & Mueser, 1996; see also review by Dixon & Lehman, 1995). The findings from the controlled research on family intervention for schizophrenia have been very encouraging. In general, studies that provided family treatment, either to individual families or in a multiple family group format, reported two-year cumulative relapse rates between 20 and 40 percent. In contrast, clients who received no family intervention had two-year relapse rates that were usually in the range of 60 to 80 percent. The differences in relapse rates between family intervention and no family treatment were present, despite the fact that clients in all studies were maintained on antipsychotic medication, provided case management and had access to other psychiatric services. Other areas of functioning, such as the social adjustment of the client and burden on family members, were infrequently measured, but when assessed, improved with family intervention as well.

TABLE 8.1 Summary of Different Empirically Validated Models of Family Treatment for Schizophrenia

Originators	Model Components	Treatment Format	Treatment Manuals	Support Research
Falloon (1984)	• Assessment • Education • Communication Skills Training • Problem Solving Training • Special Problems	Single Family	Falloon et al. (1984) Mueser & Glynn (1995)	Falloon et al. (1985) Randolph et al. (1994)
Anderson et al. (1986)	• Joining with the Family • Education • Re-entry of Client into Family • Enhancing Work and Social Adjustment • Maintenance	Single Family	Anderson et al. (1986)	Hogarty et al. (1991)
Barrowclough & Tarrier (1992)	• Assessment • Education • Stress Management Training • Planning for a Relapse • Goal Setting and Attainment	Single Family	Barrowclough & Tarrier (1992)	Tarrier et al. (1989, in press)
Leff et al. (1985)	• Assessment • Education • Relatives' Group • Individual Family Sessions to Reduce Expressed Emotion or Client-Relative Contact	Single/Multiple Family	Kuipers et al. (1992)	Leff et al. (1985, 1990)
McFarlane et al. (1991)	• Joining with the Family • Education • Relapse Prevention • Problem Solving to Improve Psychosocial Functioning • Creating a Social Network	Multiple Family	McFarlane et al. (1991)	McFarlane et al. (1995)

INGREDIENTS OF EFFECTIVE
FAMILY INTERVENTION

Despite the many different models of family therapy which have been studied, effective family intervention programs share a number of common features. Table 9.2 contains a list of common features of family intervention programs for psychiatric disorders, which are discussed below.

Educate Families About Psychiatric
Illnesses and Their Management

Education is at the core of all successful family interventions for psychiatric disorders. Education can span a broader array of different topics, including symptoms of the illness, how diagnosis is established, prevalence, long-term course, medications and their side effects, the role of stress in precipitating relapses, and strategies for coping with common problems. In recent years, a number of useful self-help books have been published for families about coping with disorders such as schizophrenia (Mueser & Gingerich, 1994; Torrey, 1995), bipolar disorder (Berger & Berger, 1991), depression (Papolos & Papolos, 1988), post-traumatic stress disorder (Matsakis, 1992), and obsessive compulsive disorder (Foa & Wilson, 1991). Clinicians may find it useful to consult an educational needs survey conducted by Mueser and colleagues (1992) to identify possible topics for educating families. Information on self-help books for different psychiatric disorders can be found in reviews by Reavis and colleagues (1995) and Santrock and colleagues (1994).

TABLE 9.2 Common Features of Effective Family Intervention Programs

- Educate families about psychiatric illnesses and their management
- Show concern, sympathy, and empathy to family members who are coping with mental illness
- Avoid blaming the family or pathologizing their efforts to cope
- Foster the development of all family members
- Enhance adherence to medication and decrease substance abuse and stress
- Improve communication and problem solving skills in family members
- Provide treatment that is flexible and tailored to the individual needs of families
- Encourage family members to develop social supports outside their family network
- Instill hope for the future
- Take a long-term perspective

Show Concern, Sympathy, and Empathy to Family Members Who Are Coping

Family members often experience high levels of stress and personal suffering in their efforts to cope with a mental illness in a relative (Vine, 1982). It is important to recognize difficulties the family members face and to show genuine concern and empathy for the trials they have faced. Empathic understanding is perhaps the first and most important quality mental health professionals can bring to establishing a working relationship with the family members of a person with severe mental illness. Feeling understood, and the validation of coping with the stressful experiences of living with a mentally ill person, are necessary for relatives to trust mental health professionals and work productively together.

Avoid Blaming the Family or Pathologizing Their Efforts to Cope

As evident from the numerous accounts of relatives coping with a major mental illness in a close family member, a wide range of consequences are common, ranging from depression to anxiety, anger, fear, and despair. Not uncommonly, mental illness in the family leads to conflict between family members and high levels of tension. Mental health professionals must be careful to avoid pathologizing the reactions of family members to a mentally ill relative or to blame families for having a negative impact on the course of the illness. Finding fault in family members and over pathologizing their behavior invariably interferes with the ability to form a good working alliance with the family. A fruitful position is to assume that all family members are doing their best to cope effectively with a mental illness at home. While such coping efforts may not be optimal, and may at times even be counterproductive, they truly represent the best coping efforts of family members.

Foster the Development of All Family Members

Relatives, particularly parents, often submerge their personal goals and ideals in efforts to cope with and help a mentally ill family member. By focusing only on the needs of the ill member, professionals may inadvertently support family members in believing that the needs of one person are more important than another. Instead, many family members benefit from the message that everyone in the family is important and deserves to have a decent quality of life. Encouraging the development of all family members has two primary advantages. First, it removes some of the burden on the ill family member by not making him or her the sole focus of all family work. Clients often appreciate not always being the center of attention in family sessions. Second, facilitating the development of all family members can be very effective at reducing stress in the family, since tension can result from family members not actively pursuing their own goals.

Attending to the special needs of siblings is important (Mueser & Gingerich, 1994), especially in parental households in which siblings may assume greater caregiving roles over time as parents age and die. Siblings of persons with severe mental illness often experience a range of different emotions, including guilt, sadness, and fear about their own or their children's susceptibility to mental illness. Furthermore, siblings are often confused about the nature of the psychiatric illness, and desire information about how to relate to their brother or sister, and how to assist them in managing their illness. Several first-person accounts by siblings have been published that describe the impact of mental illness on the family, and illustrate the importance of involving siblings and addressing their unique needs in family work (Moorman, 1992; Swados, 1991). Horowitz, Tesler, Fisher & Gamache, (1992) have reported that siblings with a more positive attitude towards a client are more likely to provide assistance, and suggests that the strengthening of sibling bonds may facilitate the transfer of care giving as parents grow old and are unable to fulfill this responsibility.

The needs of spouses also deserve special consideration. Marriage typically assumes a sharing of decision-making and responsibilities between partners, an expectation that is often shattered following the development of a psychiatric disorder in one person. Indeed, divorce rates following the development of psychiatric illness in one partner are quite high. Helping healthy spouses balance between their needs and their partner's, and dealing with the frustrations inherent in living with a close person who has a psychiatric disability, are important goals of family intervention. Similarly, children of a parent with a psychiatric disorder have unique needs. Even before they have grown up, children must often assume a care giving role for a parent with mental illness, which can result in feelings of resentment, anxiety, and mourning over their loss of childhood. Dealing with these feelings, maintaining a relationship with the ill parent, and encouraging the personal development of offspring are critical elements of successful work with these families.

Enhance Adherence to Medication and Decrease Substance Abuse and Stress

Non-adherence to medication is a common contributing factor to relapse in major psychiatric disorders (Corrigan, Liberman, & Engel, 1990). Effective family interventions promote adherence to medication by helping family members understand the purposes of medication, some common side effects, and strategies for enhancing adherence to medication. In addition, considering the strong relationship between both substance abuse and stress in contributing to relapse in psychiatric disorders (Drake, Mueser, Clark & Wallach, 1996), reducing these influences is an important goal of family intervention. These generic goals of family intervention stem quite naturally from the stress-vulnerability-coping skills model of psychiatric disorders (Mueser & Glynn, 1995).

Improve Communication and Problem Solving Skills in Family Members

Research on family expressed emotion (EE) has pointed to the possible negative effects of certain communication styles. Therefore, effective family interventions help family members develop better strategies for communicating and solving problems together. These strategies can either be explicitly encouraged over the course of family intervention, or alternatively, can be taught through specific skills training techniques.

Provide Treatment That is Flexible and Tailored to the Individual Needs of Families

Although a number of programs have been developed for helping families cope with psychiatric illness, family interventions must be flexible and tailored to the needs of individual families. Individual assessment of the needs of all family members is critical, and assessments should be conducted on a routine basis throughout the course of treatment. There are multiple variations in family needs, which may change over time. Some families may benefit more from a multiple family group, whereas others need individual counseling. Some families gain primarily from learning more about the psychiatric disorder and principles of treatment, whereas other families benefit more from a focus on communication and problem-solving. Effective family interventions are flexible in recognizing that needs of families differ, both across families and over time.

Encourage Family Members to Develop Social Supports Outside Their Family Network

Families often report feeling isolated after the onset of a psychiatric illness (Dearth, Labenski, Mott, & Pellegrini, 1986), and many families have constricted social support networks (Kreisman & Joy, 1974). Sometimes relatives stop seeing old friends and allow close relationships to drift apart as they become overwhelmed by the mental illness of the family member. It is helpful to encourage family members to reestablish old friendships or to expand their social networks by reaching out to others coping with similar experiences. Some relatives find that joining advocacy organizations such as the Alliance for the Mentally Ill provides a good opportunity for social support from other families with similar experiences. Other families get support from old friends, or establish new relationships based on mutual interests.

Instill Hope for the Future

Families often come into contact with mental health professionals after years of strenuous effort dealing with the illness. Not surprisingly, many relatives despair of never being able to cope successfully. Similarly, clients with severe psychiatric disorders often experience a sense of futility related to dealing with their illness, which may be fueled by the social stigma attached to mental illness (Fink & Tasman, 1992). The upshot is that many families do not feel that change is possible, and consequently may not make efforts to improve the status quo. A critical function of family intervention is to instill in family members that it is never too late to change, and that improvement is not only possible, but likely, if the family works together. Improving family members' self-efficacy, and engaging them actively in exploring options for change, tends to decrease the "learned helplessness" phenomenon common in families with a history of unsuccessful coping. Hope is the necessary first ingredient for change in family members, who may have had a history of unsuccessful coping in the past.

Take a Long-Term Perspective

Effective family interventions for psychiatric disorders must take a long-term perspective on improving family functioning, and eschew "quick-fixes" including short-term educational programs. All of the successful family treatments for schizophrenia have provided treatment for at least nine months, and some interventions have been given over a period of several years. In contrast, studies employing short-term family intervention programs (e.g., lasting between several weeks and several months) provide, at best, short-term benefits which rapidly dissipate after treatment stops (Penn & Mueser, 1996). Bellack and Mueser (1993) suggest that it is not more realistic to assume that brief, time-limited psychosocial interventions will produce long-term benefits than it is to expect benefits from a time-limited course of psychotropic medication.

There are several reasons why taking a long-term perspective when working with families is critical to achieving success. First, families require time to absorb and assimilate information about psychiatric disorders and their treatment. Time is needed to reflect on the information, to perceive its relevance in terms of their own situations, and to put it in the broader context of understanding the nature of the psychiatric illness. Second, the needs of family members evolve over time, so that short-term interventions resolve problems only in the short-term. Third, many families appear to benefit from the long-term support inherent in these family intervention programs. This support may come from mental health professionals or, in the case of multiple family support groups, from other families. Fourth, and last, working with families over extended periods of time ensures that not only do they become members of the treatment team, but they continue to work with the team over the course of the illness, including critical transitions (e.g., when the client begins competitive employment, during transitions to more independent living).

Some families appear to benefit from a time-limited course of family intervention, lasting between nine months and two to three years. For example, Tarrier and colleagues (in press) reported that benefits from nine months of behavioral family therapy persisted for over five years. However, other families may require ongoing contact for longer periods of time. Mental health professionals need to be aware of the different needs of families, and titrate the dose of family intervention accordingly.

BEHAVIORAL FAMILY THERAPY

Behavioral Family Therapy (BFT) is one of the most widely studied models of family intervention for psychiatric disorders (Penn & Mueser, 1996). This model was originally developed by Falloon, Boyd, and McGill (1984) for schizophrenia, and has since been adapted to a broad range of psychiatric disorders by Mueser and Glynn (1995). A brief synopsis of BFT is provided below.

BFT is a model of family intervention that is usually provided to families on an individual basis, although the approach has also been used in a multiple family group format. BFT is typically provided on a declining contact basis, starting with weekly sessions for approximately three months, followed by biweekly sessions for another three to six months followed by monthly sessions thereafter for at least three more months. Although BFT was originally developed as a model to be provided directly in the homes of family members, research also indicates that family sessions can be effective when provided in a clinic. Often a combination of home-based and clinic-based sessions is optimal, with home-based sessions offered at the beginning of treatment to facilitate the engagement of the family.

BFT is provided to those family members most involved in caring for the member with the mental illness. This may include parents, siblings, spouses, other relatives, or even close friends. Whenever possible, family sessions include the client. The BFT model is divided into five sequential stages, with a recycling of each stage conducted on an "as needed" basis: *assessment, education, communication skills training, problem solving training, and special problems.*

The purpose of the *assessment* phase is to evaluate the strengths and weaknesses of the family as a unit, as well as for each family member. In addition, family members' understanding of the psychiatric illness and its treatment is evaluated. Assessments are conducted through a combination of individual interviews with each family member, a family-based interview, and engaging the family in problem solving discussions. The assessment stage enables the clinician to arrive at case formulation of the goals of BFT for a specific family. Goals include both family-oriented goals as well as individual goals identified by each member.

Following assessment, several sessions are devoted to providing *education* to family members about psychiatric illness an the principles of its management. During these educational sessions, the mentally ill family member is cast as the "expert", and his or her experience with specific psychiatric symptoms is elicited and discussed. The educational curriculum covers three broad areas: the psychiatric illness (symptoms, how a diagnosis is established, long-term course and outcome), medication (effects on acute symptoms and relapse prevention, side effects, interactions with drugs and alcohol, adherence issues), and the stress-vulnerability model (the role of stress in precipitating relapses, how coping skills can mediate noxious stress). Education is often provided to family members through the use of handouts, posters, and/or audiovisual aids. Mueser and Glynn (1995) have developed educational handouts on a variety of severe psychiatric disorders (schizophrenia, schizoaffective disorder, bipolar disorder, major depression, obsessive-compulsive disorder, posttraumatic stress disorder), different classes of psychotropic medication (antipsychotics, antidepressants, mood stabilizers, sedative hypnotics), and the stress-vulnerability model. These handouts can be reproduced from this book and distributed to family members to facilitate the educational process. Usually between two and four educational sessions are conducted, although the material is often reviewed again in later sessions.

Communication skills training involves teaching family members specific skills to facilitate nonstressful communication and problem solving. Skills are taught using the principles of social skills training (Liberman, DeRisi, & Mueser, 1989). Targeted communication skills, such as expressing positive feelings, making positive requests, and expressing negative feelings, emphasize making communications brief, to the point, behaviorally specific, and when appropriate, making specific feeling statements (e.g., "I felt mad when . . ."). Typically, between four and eight sessions are devoted to communication skills training.

After family members have developed sufficient communication skills, attention shifts to improving the ability of the family to *problem solve.* The underlying philosophy of problem solving training is that if families can solve problems on their own, they will be empowered to attain their own personal goals without the assistance of mental health professionals. Problem solving training focuses on helping family members learn a structured approach to discussing and resolving individual or family problems. Families are encouraged to establish a weekly problem solving meeting, during which time they get together and work on problems. Each problem solving meeting is chaired by one family member, with another family member playing the role of secretary. Some families prefer to elect a new chairperson or secretary for each problem, whereas others elect a chairperson and secretary who serves these functions during all problem solving efforts. The chairperson leads the family through a sequence of steps designed to minimize conflict and maximize successful resolution of the problem or attainment of a specified goal: define the problem to everyone's satisfaction, brainstorm possible solutions, evaluate the advantages and disadvantages of each solution, select the best solution or combination of solutions, plan how to implement the solution, and meet again at a later time to review progress towards resolving the problem.

When family members have improved their collective ability to solve problems together, the clinician works with family members to address any other problems that are still outstanding.

Special problems are those areas in need of improvement that families are unable to resolve through problem solving, and may well benefit from the application of a specific clinical strategy. A wide variety of other problem areas may be addressed, which may require the clinician's expertise and use of specific cognitive-behavioral strategies. For example, a token economy program may be set up at home to encourage a client to improve his or her self-care skills, graduated exposure may be taught to address an anxiety problem, or supplementary skills training can be taught to facilitate clients' social interactions. Many families benefit from the education, communication skills training, and problem solving training and do not require special efforts to address additional problems. When additional problems are addressed, the clinician enlists the help of family members in implementing specific strategies to address the target problems.

Although most of the research on BFT thus far has been conducted with clients who have schizophrenia (Penn & Mueser, 1996), several studies are currently underway examining the efficacy of BFT in other disorders. In a symposium at the 1995 meeting of the Association for the Advancement of Behavior Therapy, three research groups presented preliminary data on the effects of BFT on chronic posttraumatic stress disorder (Glynn et al., 1995) and bipolar disorder (Miklowit & Simmoneau, 1995; Clarkin, Carpenter, Wilner & Perlick, 1995). This research stands to fill an important gap in our understanding of the effects of BFT on other severe psychiatric disorders.

TEAMWORK BETWEEN
PROFESSIONALS AND FAMILIES

Family advocacy organizations, such as the National Alliance for the Mentally Ill, have often had an uneasy relationship with professionals who have advocated family intervention, concerned that such treatments may reflect another way of blaming families for the illness. At least part of this concern appears to stem from the research on Expressed Emotion, which has suggested a link between negative or stressful communication styles and increased vulnerability to relapse in clients with psychiatric disorders (Bebbington & Kuipers, 1994). Indeed, it is understandable that some relatives might be concerned that the emphasis of some family treatment programs on teaching specific skills (e.g., communication skills) suggests professionals, at least partly, blame relatives for the psychiatric illness. On the other hand, many family members are interested in improving their ability to communicate with their relative and learning specific problem solving skills (Mueser et al., 1992).

An important goal of family treatment programs is to equip families with information and skills that will be useful in the long-term management of psychiatric disorders. However, an equally critical goal is to foster collaboration and teamwork between family members and professionals. Both parties have significant contributions to make in improving psychiatric outcomes. The strengths of professionals lie in their technical knowledge and access to special resources for the mentally ill (e.g., medication, rehabilitation programs). Relatives' strengths lie in their intimate knowledge of the client, and their love and commitment to the client. Although family intervention programs may initially emphasize teaching of information and skills, their ultimate success is determined by their ability to get families and professionals working together. In some settings, families are invited to become members of the treatment team. In others, teamwork is sought without families being formally recognized as "team members" or even participating in regular team meetings. In either case, mutual respect, communication, and shared goals (while acknowledging differences) are the fundamental elements of a productive relationship between professionals and families.

PUTTING FAMILY WORK INTO PRACTICE

Family work for the severely mentally ill has grown over the past two decades, but most families remain unengaged in treatment and do not receive support from local chapters of the Alliance for the Mentally Ill. Despite the evidence supporting the effects of family intervention programs for persons with severe psychiatric disorders, there are obstacles that need to be overcome in order to make it more widely available to families. For example, what services should be made available to families who are unable to commit to long-term therapy such as BFT? How can family services be provided in a cost-effective way? How can third-party payers be encouraged to reimburse for family intervention?

There are no definitive answers to these questions. Their solutions depend upon the actual needs of families in a particular setting and the creativity of the service providers. Research on family intervention suggests that more intensive or more individualized family programs, such as BFT, are not necessarily more effective. For example, the Treatment Strategies for Schizophrenia study (Schooler et al., 1997), which compared monthly family support groups with support groups plus more intensive BFT, did not find differences in rehospitalization rates over two years, although rates were quite low for both groups. In addition, McFarlane et al. (1995) reported that multiple family groups resulted in *significantly* lower cumulative relapse rates over two years than individual family intervention. These studies suggest that multiple family groups may be a cost-effective alternative to single family treatment for many families, although some families may need more individualized intervention. Furthermore, shorter-term treatment should be available to families who are unable to participate in long-term treatment, or who do not need it. There is need to develop a range of treatment services for families, including individual and multiple family group formats, as well as individual counseling, to meet their diverse needs.

Who is going to pay for family intervention? Fifteen years ago the same questions were posed about a novel case management approach, Assertive Community Treatment (ACT), which had been shown in early studies to have promising effects on reducing hospitalizations and improving functioning in the community (Stein & Test, 1980). In subsequent years, numerous controlled studies confirmed the effects of ACT on reducing hospitalizations (Mueser, Bond, & Drake, 1996), and today this and similar case management models (e.g., intensive case management), are widely practiced for clients with severe mental illness who are high service utilizers. If family therapy is to achieve similar acceptance, its proponents must educate third-party payers about the benefits of family intervention, especially its effects on reducing relapses and rehospitalizations. Two studies which examined the cost-benefit of family programs both concluded that providing family intervention resulted in lower overall costs, including the cost of the family therapy (Cardin, Magill, & Falloon, 1986; Tarrier, Lowson, & Barrowclough, 1991).

FUTURE DIRECTIONS

Family intervention for severe psychiatric disorders can have a range of beneficial effects, including reducing vulnerability to relapse and improving the quality of family relationships. Despite gains in understanding how to work effectively with families, there is much work that still needs to be done.

Although the evidence supporting family intervention is strong, most mental health centers and psychiatric hospitals do not provide family therapy, and those that do usually provide only short-term educational-based interventions. Families are rarely invited to become members of the treatment team, and tension is often high between families and mental health professionals. There is a need for professionals to reach out to family members and recognize them as a valuable resource for the management of severe psychiatric disorders.

It is also important to understand more about which family intervention models are most effective for which families. There are a variety of different treatment models available, but little work has been done examining whether particular client or family characteristics predict response to one or another model of family treatment. For example, is BFT more effective for families with high levels of tension and conflict because of its focus on communication skills training? Is the multiple group family format more suitable for families who are isolated or lack adequate social support? In addition, work is needed to address whether different models of family intervention may be suitable at different stages of the illness for a particular family. For example, some families may benefit from an initial course of BFT, followed by participation in a more extended multiple family support group.

Another area in need of further research is the timing of family intervention. Few guidelines exist to help clinicians determine when, if ever, family intervention can be stopped. Exploratory work is needed to help clinicians evaluate both the appropriate intensity and duration of family intervention. A related issue concerns when during the course of an illness family intervention should be provided. The negative symptoms of schizophrenia typically worsen during the first five years of the illness (McGlashan & Fenton, 1992), yet most family therapy research has been conducted with clients who have had the illness for many years. It is possible that family intervention provided early, after the onset of psychiatric illnesses, may have a beneficial effect on improving the long-term trajectory of the illness.

On the other hand, a strong case can also be made for late family intervention. Many families face new and challenging issues as parents grow older and ask the question of "who will take care of my ill relative when I die?" (Mueser & Gingerich, 1994). Siblings are often turned to as top candidates to be both trustee and substitute decision-maker for treatment decisions. Yet many siblings are not prepared to assume these roles; their knowledge about psychiatric disorders may be limited, they may be ambivalent about taking on such responsibilities, and they may be concerned about their ability to balance their own lives with that of their ill sibling. Family programs may help address these issues and, when mutually desired, facilitate the transfer of the care giving role from the parents to the siblings and their families.

There have been tremendous gains in recent years in understanding how families and professionals can work together to improve the outcome of severe psychiatric disorders. Perhaps the biggest surprise to mental health professionals has been that teaming up with family members has made their work both easier and more rewarding. Professionals, relatives, and mental health consumers can all share in the excitement of knowing that the future of severe mental illness grows brighter each day.

REFERENCES

Anderson, C.M., Reiss, D.J., & Hogarty, G.E. (1986). *Schizophrenia and the Family.* New York: Guilford Press.

Appleton, W.S. (1974). Mistreatment of patients' families by psychiatrists. *American Journal of Psychiatry, 131,* 655–657.

Barrowclough, C., & Tarrier, N. (1992). *Families of schizophrenic patients: Cognitive behavioral intervention.* London, England: Chapman & Hall.

Bateson, G., Jackson, D.D., Haley, J., & Weakland, J. (1958). Toward a theory of schizophrenia. *Behavioral Science, 1,* 251–264.

Bebbington, P., & Kuipers, L. (1994). The predictive utility of expressed emotion in schizophrenia: An aggregate analysis. *Psychological Medicine, 24,* 707–718.

Bellack, A.S., & Mueser, K.T. (1993). Psychosocial treatment for schizophrenia. *Schizophrenia Bulletin, 19,* 317–336.

Berger, D., & Berger, L. (1991). *We heard the angels of madness: A family guide to coping with manic depression.* New York: Quill.

Cardin, V.A., McGill, C.W., & Falloon, I.R.H. (1986). An economic analysis: Costs, benefits and effectiveness. In Falloon, I.R.H. (Ed.), *Family management of schizophrenia.* Johns Hopkins University Press, Baltimore, MD.

Clarkin, J.F., Carpenter, D., Wilner, P., & Perlick, D. (1995). Psychoeducational/behavioral marital intervention with bipolar disorder. Presented at the 29th Annual Convention of the Association for the Advancement of Behavior Therapy, Washington, D.C.

Corrigan, P.W., Liberman, R.P., & Engel, J.D. (1990). From noncompliance to collaboration in the treatment of schizophrenia. *Hospital and Community Psychiatry, 41,* 1203–1211.

Dearth, N., Labenski, B.J., Mott, M.E., & Pellegrini, L.M. (1986). The course, treatment and outcome of substance disorder in persons with severe mental illness. *American*

Journal of Orthopsychiatry, 66, 42–51.

Dixon, L.B., & Lehman, A.F. (1995). Family interventions for schizophrenia. *Schizophrenia Bulletin, 21,* 631–643.

Drake, R.E., Mueser, K.T., Clark, R.E., & Wallach, M.A. (1996). The course, treatment and outcome of substance disorder in persons with severe mental illness. *American Journal of Orthopsychiatry, 66,* 42–51.

Falloon, I.R.H., Boyd, J.L., & McGill, C.W. (1984). *Family care of schizophrenia: A problem-solving approach to the treatment of mental illness.* New York: Guilford.

Falloon, I.R.H., Boyd, J.L., McGill, C.W., Williamson, M., Razani, J., Moss, H.B., Gilderman, A.M., & Sompson, G.M. (1985). Family management in the prevention of morbidity of schizophrenia: Clinical outcome of a two year longitudinal study. *Archives of General Psychiatry, 42,* 887–896.

Fink, P.J., & Tasman, A. (1992). *Stigma and Mental Illness.* Washington, DC: American Psychiatric Press.

Foa, E.B., & Wilson, R. (1991). *Stop obsessing! How to overcome your obsessions and compulsions.* New York: Bantam.

Fromm-Reichman, F. (1949). Notes on the development of treatment of schizophrenics by psychoanalytic psychotherapy. *Psychiatry, 11,* 263–273.

Goodwin, F.K., & Jamison, K.R. (1990). *Manic depressive illness.* New York: Oxford University Press.

Gottesman, I.I. (1990). *Schizophrenia genesis: The origins of madness.* New York: W.II. Freeman.

Glynn, S.M., Randolph, E.T., Eth, S., Boxer, L., Urbaitis, M., & Crothers, J. (1995) Extending behavioral family therapy in the clinic: Moving from schizophrenia to chronic combat-related PTSD. Presented at the 29th Annual Convention of the Association for the Advancement of Behavior Therapy, Washington, D.C.

Hogarty, G.E., Anderson, C., Reiss, D., Kornblith, S., Greenwald, D., Ulrich, R., & Carter, M. (1991). Family psycho education, social skills training, and maintenance chemotherapy in the aftercare treatment of schizophrenia: II. Two year effects of a controlled study on relapse and adjustment. *Archives of General Psychiatry, 48,* 340–347.

Horowitz, A.V., Tesler, R.C., Fisher, G.A., & Gamache, G.M. (1992). The role of adult siblings in providing social support to the severely mentally ill. *Journal of Marriage and the Family, 54,* 233–241.

Kreisman, D.E., & Joy, V.D. (1974). Family response to the mental illness of a relative: A review of the literature. *Schizophrenia Bulletin, 10,* 34–57.

Kuipers, L., Leff, J., & Lam, D. (1992). *Family work for schizophrenia: A practical guide.* London: Gaskell.

Leff, J.P., Berkowitz, R., Shavit, N., Strachan, A., & Vaughn, C. (1990). A trial of family therapy versus a relatives' group for schizophrenia: Two-year follow-up. *British Journal of Psychiatry, 157,* 571–577.

Leff, J., Kuipers, L., Berkowitz, R., & Sturgeon, D. (1985). A control trial of social intervention in the family of schizophrenic patients. Two-year follow-up. *British Journal of Psychiatry, 146,* 594–600.

Leff, J., & Vaughn, C. (1985). *Expressed emotion in families: Its significance for mental illness.* New York: Guilford Press.

Lefley, H.P., & Johnson, D.L. (Eds.) (1990). *Families as allies in treatment of the mentally ill: New directions of mental health professionals.* Washington, DC: American Psychiatric Press.

Liberman, R.P., DeRisi, W.R., & Mueser, K.T. (1989). *Social skills training for psychiatric patients.* Needham Heights, MA: Allyn & Bacon.

Matsakis, A. (1992). *I can't get over it: A handbook for trauma survivors.* Oakland, CA: New Harbinger.

McFarlane, W.R., Deakins, S.M., Gingerich, S.L., Dunne, E., Horan, B., & Newmark, M. (1991). *Multiple-family psychoeducational group treatment manual.* New York: New York State Psychiatric Institute.

McFarlane, W.R., Dunne, E., Lukens, E., Newmark, M., McLaughlin-Toran, J., Deakins, S., & Horen, B. (1993). From research to clinical practice: Dissemination of new York State's family psychoeducation project. *Hospital & Community Psychiatry, 44,* 265–270.

McFarlane, W.R., Lukens, E., Link, B., Dushay, R., Deakins, S.A., Newmark, M., Dunne, E.J., Horen, B., & Toran, J. (1995). Multiple-family groups and psychoeducation in the treatment of schizophrenia. *Archives of General Psychiatry, 52,* 679–687.

McGlashan, T.H., & Fenton, W.S. (1992). The positive-negative distinction in schizophrenia: Review of natural history validators. *Archives of General Psychiatry, 49,* 63–72.

Meltzer, H.Y. (Ed.) (1987). Psychopharmacology: *The third generation of progress.* New York: Raven.

Miklowtiz, D.J., Simoneau, T.L. (1995). Behavioral family therapy for bipolar disorder. Presented at the 29th Annual Convention of the Association for the Advancement of Behavior Therapy. Washington, D.C.

Moorman, M. (1992). *My sister's keeper.* New York: W.W. Norton.

Mueser, K.T., Bellack, A.S., Wade, J.H., Sayers, S.L., & Rosenthal, C.K. (1992). An assessment of the educational needs of chronic psychiatric patients and their relatives. *British Journal of Psychiatry, 160,* 674–680.

Mueser, K.T., Bond, G.R., & Drake, R.E. (1996). Case management of the severely mentally ill: A review of the research. Manuscript under review.

Mueser, K.T., & Gingerich, S. (1994). *Coping with schizophrenia: A guide for families.* Oakland, CA: New Harbinger Publications, Inc.

Mueser, K.T., Gingerich, S.L., Rosenthal, C.K. (1993). Educational family therapy for schizophrenia: A new treatment model for clinical service and research. *Schizophrenia Research, 3,* 99–108.

Mueser, K.T., & Glynn, S.M. (1995). *Behavioral family therapy for psychiatric disorders.* Boston: Allyn & Bacon.

Papolos, D.F., & Papolos, J. (1988). *Overcoming depression.* New York: Harper & Row.

Penn, D.L., & Mueser, K.T. (1996). Research update on the psychosocial treatment of schizophrenia. *American Journal of Psychiatry, 15,* 607–617.

Randolph, E.T., Eth, S., Glynn, S., Paz, G.B., Leong, G.B., Shaner, A.L., Strachan, A., Van Vort, W., Escobar, J., & Liberman, R.P. (1994). Behavioral family management in schizophrenia: Outcome from a clinic-based intervention. *British Journal of Psychiatry, 144,* 501–506.

Reavis, P.A., Epstein, B.A., & Piotrowicz, L.M. (1995). Book reviews: Selected books on mental illness and treatment for patients and their families. *Psychiatric Services, 46,* 1292–1302.

Santrock, J.W., Minnett, A.M., & Campbell, B.D. (1994). T*he authoritative guide to self-help books.* New York: Guilford.

Schooler, N.R., Keith, S.J., Severe, J.B., Matthews, S.M., Bellack, A.S., Glick, I.D., Hargreaves, W.A., Kane, J.M., Ninan, P.T., Frances, A., Jacobs, M., Lieberman, J.A., Mance, R., Simpson, G.M., & Woerner, M.G. (1997). Relapse and rehospitalization during maintenance treatment of schizophrenia: The effects of dose reduction and family treatment. *Archives of General Psychiatry, 54,* 453–463.

Stein, L.I., & Test, M.A. (1980). Alterative to mental hospital treatment: I. Conceptual model, treatment program, and clinical evaluation. *Archives of General Psychiatry, 37,* 392–397.

Swados, E. (1991). *The four of us.* New York: Farar, Straus, and Giroux.

Tarrier, N., Barrowclough, C., Vaughn, C., Bamrah, J., Porceddu, K., Watts, S., & Freeman, H. (1989). Community management of schizophrenia: A two-year follow-up of a behavioral intervention with families. *British Journal of Psychiatry, 154,* 625–628.

Tarrier, N., Barrowclough, C., Porceddu, K., Fitzpatrick, E. (in press). The Salford Family Intervention Project for schizophrenic relapse prevention: Five and eight year accumulating relapses. *British Journal of Psychiatry.*

Tarrier, N., Lowson, K., & Barrowclough, C. (1991). Some aspects of family interventions in schizophrenia: II. Financial considerations. *British Journal of Psychiatry, 159,* 481–484.

Terkelsen, K.G. (1983). Schizophrenia and the family: II. Adverse effects of family therapy *Family process, 22,* 191 200.

Torrey, E.F. (1995). *Surviving schizophrenia* (3rd Ed.) New York: Harper & Row.

Vine, P. (1982). *Families in pain.* New York: Pantheon.

9

A Narrative Approach to Understanding the Illness Experiences of a Mother and Daughter*

Kathy Weingarten and

Miranda Eve Weingarten Worthen

We are a mother and daughter, the female half of a four-person family, and the half that does not live in reliable bodies. One of us, the mother, Kathy, has had breast cancer. The other, the daughter, Miranda, age 16, was born with a rare genetic disorder called Beckwith-Wiedemann Syndrome, about which almost no one—lay or professional person—has ever heard.

Many factors contribute to a family's ability to cope with the illness of a member, including, for example, the member's role, the severity and chronicity of the illness, and the treatment regimen. In this article we would like to address another dimension. We believe that a family's ability to cope with an illness is also profoundly affected by the degree to which the illness is understood by the family's networks. We will discuss the impact of having a condition that is either poorly or well understood in terms of one's own ability to cope with it and one's ability to involve others in coping with the experience of disease.

We will contend that Miranda, by virtue of having a rare genetic disorder that is poorly understood, has more difficulty finding people—professionals nd friends—with whom she can share her experience, and that this produces an isolation quite different from Kathy's experience. An important consequence of this difference is that the members of our family play a vital role in Miranda's devel-

This chapter is based on a paper given at a Harvard Medical School conference on "Intergrated Care: Psychosocial Needs and Medical Crises," May 7, 1995.
From *Families, Systems, & Health, 15*(1) 1997, 41-54. Reprinted with permission.

oping understanding of herself, and that we are centrally involved in her construction of her story about herself.

Our approach to our subject is based on narrative theory, applied within a postmodern paradigm (Bruner, 1990; Griffith & Griffith, 1994; Sampson, 1993; White & Epston, 1990). According to this paradigm, what we know we know with others. Reality isn't fixed, but rather is negotiated within the communities of which we are a part; meaning is primarily socially constructed. From this perspective, the self continually creates itself through narratives that include other people who are reciprocally woven into these narratives (Weingarten, 1991). This weaving together occurs through language, which doesn't represent reality but, rather, is constitutive of it.

A postmodern narrative approach emphasizes meaning-making as a key feature of human experience. As Jerome Bruner writes, "By virtue of participation in culture, meaning is rendered *public* and *shared*. Our culturally adapted way of life depends upon shared meanings and shared concepts" (1990, p. 13). However, as we will make clear, we do not all have equal access to those meaning-making resources that facilitate the sharing of meaning. The difference in access to meaning-making resources profoundly influences the experience we have of our own illnesses and the experience others have of us. That is, differential access to meaning-making resources affects our weaving.

Although we will primarily discuss the way we are each woven into each other's narrative of self in relation to our illnesses, the wider context of our lives is profoundly affected by the love and support we share with our husband/father and son/brother. These two men, in their own ways, make our lives possible. Hilary, my husband and Miranda's father, plays multiple roles with us: physician, interpreter of other physicians, nurturer, inventor, driver, crisis manager, cook, and night duty nurse, among the many roles that could be enumerated. Ben, my son and Miranda's brother, provides constant comfort with his generosity of spirit, fondness for play, willingness to share his friends with his family, and his easy-going approach to almost any of life's contingencies.

ILLNESS IN AN EXTENDED FAMILY CONTEXT

Because we are using our own illness experiences to illustrate the points that we are making, it will be useful to place our illness narratives in an intergenerational perspective (Chilman, Nunnally, & Fox, 1988; Eisenberg, Sutkin, & Jansen, 1984; Koocher & McDonald, 1992; Penn, 1983; Rolland, 1994; Walsh & Anderson, 1988; Walsh & McGoldrick, 1991). The first author will describe this history.

My husband, Hilary Worthen, a primary care physician, and I, a clinical psychologist and family therapist, became parents in the context of my mother's dying from a rare malignant tumor. Our first child, Ben, was born 6 weeks before my mother died. Miranda, our second child, was born 2 years and 9 months after her brother. Her birth occurred 11 months after my father had a heart attack and 9 months after he underwent a complicated triple bypass.

Miranda was diagnosed with Beckwith-Wiedemann Syndrome at 4 hours of age. The pediatrician who had delivered her, by chance, had delivered another baby with Beckwith-Wiedemann Syndrome exactly one year before. (Later, we were to learn that at that time, 1979, there were only eight known children with Beckwith-Wiedemann Syndrome in our region.)

Beckwith-Wiedemann Syndrome, or BWS, is caused by a mutation in chromosome 11, and most cases are thought to be sporadic as opposed to inherited. Infants with BWS usually have an enlarged tongue (macroglossia), linear indentations of the ear lobes, abnormalities of the umbilicus, for instance omphalocele, and are atypically large. Many affected infants have hypoglycemia at birth, and it is speculated that this, if untreated, is responsible for the frequent occurrence of mental retardation. Children with BWS are at greater risk than the normal population of developing malignant tumors; of having enlarged internal organs; and of developing overgrowth of half of their limbs (hemihypertrophy).

During those 4 hours, before we learned that Miranda had BWS, I talked to family and friends, describing our new baby as beautiful and adorable—as any new mother would—and remarking on three features, which later would become the cornerstones of a medical diagnosis. To my maternal eye, it was amazing that she was full-term 4 weeks early; I thought that she had the cutest little creases on her earlobes; and she kept her tongue at an angle outside her mouth, like a kitten about to lick a bowl of milk. I went on and on about these features, never once imagining that my rapturous descriptions of these three observed phenomena would be redescribed by a medical language that would transform these already beloved features from sources of joy to sources of worry (Kleinman, 1988).

I was diagnosed with breast cancer in 1988, and within the next year I had multiple surgeries, chemotherapy, and radiation therapy. By that year, our children had had quite a lot of experience living with people who were being treated for cancer. Hilary's parents, who live in Vermont, were both diagnosed and treated for cancer in Boston. Both parents lived with us for the course of their treatments: a surgical recovery from stomach cancer for the children's grandmother, and a 4-month course of surgery and radiation therapy for their grandfather.

The past 3 years have been the most difficult in Miranda's experience of living with her syndrome, though for us—her father and me—the first 6 years of her life were just as challenging. Additionally, Miranda is deeply disturbed by the knowledge that many of her relatives have had cancer and several have had breast cancer. While she worries about the pervasiveness of cancer in her family, she is aware that it produces a community of shared experience for me. This shared experience is missing for her because there is no one in the extended family who shares her condition.

In this next section, we each recount aspects of our own experience living with, in Kathy's case, breast cancer, and in Miranda's case, Beckwith-Wiedemann Syndrome. For each of us there is a natural separation of the narrative into three phases. We will each respond briefly to the other's story, sharing how we have been affected by the other's condition.

In writing this section of the article, we were amazed by how many ways we could tell any of the anecdotes we do in fact record here, and how complex the process was of selecting the ones we finally chose to create these particular narratives. We were struck that even when we are in control of the telling, rather than, for instance, when we are responding to the queries of healthcare providers, that we ourselves are often uncertain about which points are most important for us to stitch together into the fabric that becomes the story that constitutes our lives.

Living with Breast Cancer

Kathy's Version

I was first diagnosed with breast cancer at age 42, in December of 1988. Ben was 12 and Miranda was nine years old. I learned of my diagnosis over the phone, in the middle of an afternoon that was already packed with carpools and grocery-shopping. In other words, breast cancer was invading my body, but it was interrupting the lives of my children as well as my life and, of course, my husband's.

The visit to my surgeon with Hilary to review the diagnosis, prognosis, and probably treatment was followed by a tearful and then practical conversation about what to tell the children. There was something definitive and discrete to tell them. We knew what I had and we knew what would be done about it. We were in agreement to tell our children that night, but to go slowly, answering only the questions they asked. It was a tactic that worked for Ben and immediately failed for Miranda. She felt cut out of the loop, confident that we knew things we weren't telling her, and this, she told me, made her mad.

The evening was long and painful. Ben was warily optimistic, our parents supportive and devastated, and Miranda was typically laser-like in her probes.

That night, in bed, unable to sleep, Hilary and I talked and cried. I felt awful; I blamed myself for being the cause of our family's upheaval. It took hours before I was able to say that the cancer, not I, had been the agent of our sudden sorrow.

For me, the hardest role to fill as a person with cancer was that of mother. In that role, I was frequently in conflict with myself. A child wanted help with homework when I was desperate for a nap. A child had a school recital when I was scheduled for chemotherapy. I wanted to be alone when a child wanted to be close and cuddly. I rarely gave in to my wishes, and for this I have mixed feelings. No one encouraged me to put my own needs first; I now believe that I was living out the precepts of the dominant cultural discourse about mothers: a "good" mother is selfless and a "bad" mother is selfish (Weingarten, 1994, 1995). The problem was that appropriate self-care didn't fit into the dichotomy, and so it was marginalized as an activity to which I could only aspire.

Fifteen months after treatment ended, in 1990, I made the decision to write about my experiences. The process of turning pain into prose was one of the most exciting times of my life. By placing my story out in the world, by hearing from so many people that my story had resonance with theirs, I created a community of understanding with many people beyond that of my healthcare providers, colleagues, family, and friends.

Miranda's Version

I remember when my mother first told me that she had cancer. We were in the den and I was on a huge brown wicker rocking chair that looked like it had wheels. I remember that my first impulse was to flip the chair over so that it would become like a rocket ship. I wanted to imagine that I was somewhere else. I don't remember anything else about the night.

I went through a metamorphosis that started when my mother was diagnosed and ended a few years later. I changed from being a loud, rambunctious child who was not afraid to ask for anything that I wanted—the typical egocentric little child—to being obsessed with giving my mother all the care she would tolerate, and then some. I became tuned in to all her needs. For instance, I would massage her feet for long periods of time and would constantly pester her with hugs. I unconsciously chose to abandon those years of my childhood in favor of helping her.

Kathy's Version

The second time I was diagnosed with breast cancer was 4-1/2 years later, in 1993. I was terribly disappointed, but not scared. The recurrence was local, my prognosis wouldn't change, I did not need chemotherapy, and I recovered well from surgery.

I felt fine about being without a breast. The aesthetics were even pleasing to me. When else had I had a chance to see a major asymmetry on my body? At 17, Ben was past the age when saying his mother had breast cancer or discussing mastectomies would have been embarrassing, but Miranda and her friends were not. My primary experience of this period followed the course of Miranda's adjustment from fear to rage to worry to uneasy acceptance. In this aspect, I would say that my response to having a breast removed was less typical than Miranda's response. Most of my friends were shocked that I didn't fear "disfigurement," a concept that had no saliency for me.

Miranda's Version

For the first 2 weeks, I was furious at my mother. She had promised that she would tell me about any changes in her medical status because she knew that I felt most comfortable knowing all the facts. But this time, she had held out on me and didn't tell me until after the biopsy came back positive. Being enraged was a much better tactic than the one I had taken earlier, the one of internalizing my fear.

I was going to start high school in the fall, and I was terrified that having a mother with only one breast would scare potential new friends away. I was convinced that my peers would be too insecure to understand rationally what had happened, and that they would not want to be friends with me. I feared that I would be stigmatized as the daughter of a mutant.

My current friends validated my fears in one of the meetings of a mother/daughter group that we had. They too were frightened of what my mother would look like with her breast gone and with a huge scar in its place. She calmed their fears by showing them what it really looked like. They looked at her, ready to submerge their faces in the intact chests of their own mothers. I looked at them and then at her with a mixture of awe and pride.

That was a major turning point for me. Through conversations with my mother, I was able to transmute my fear of her rejection by society into political action. I learned to speak out against the overwhelming oppression of "lookism," an excessive, but culturally determined, concern with appearance (Pipher, 1994).

Kathy's Version

Since my mastectomy in 1993, I have continued to develop appropriate denial and to increase my capacity to manage worry and fear. The most painful times are listening to Miranda's fears, and the hardest is not letting my guilt intrude on us. A few months ago, I asked her to think of a present in the $100 dollar range that she might like for her 17th birthday present. She wasn't joking when she announced to Hilary and me that she wanted a mammogram. I am fortunate that she is so present to her feelings, so articulate and passionate about them, and so willing to share them with us.

Miranda's Version

My life has been hijacked by fear of breast cancer. I think about it almost every day, and often become terrified. I wrote these paragraphs a few months ago after one of these terrified moments:

"This evening one of those fears overtook me again. I was sitting in one of our comfortable living room chairs talking about health issues when the veil came toward me. I wanted to run out of the room, to say something totally non sequitur, anything to avoid talking about cancer. I didn't though. If anything I perpetuated the conversation more by relating my own views and asking questions. In the midst of people who I feel know me the best and nurture me the most, I felt alone and scared.

"A black cloak was hovering over my head about to pounce on me and envelop me in terrifying darkness. Not the beautiful darkness of a starless night, but that darkness that exists when all feeling is taken away and all that exists is the void. I wanted to cry, I was so scared of this impending shroud, but I couldn't. I was anxious that crying would stop the conversation and I would never hear what I wanted to hear, but knew would be harmful for me to hear. It was like a gruesome accident on the highway; you don't want to look, but you can't take your eyes off it."

Living with BWS

Miranda's Version

Though my life from its earliest point has been affected by having Beckwith-Wiedemann Syndrome, it is hard to say how I felt about it before I had my own consciousness of it. Most of my information about the earliest part of my life in relation to BWS comes from my parents.

I was always the kid in my elementary school who had a cast on her foot or her arm, or a bandage around her knee. I was proud to say that I had "broken, sprained, or dislocated over forty bones." I never thought of these as fitting under one umbrella problem, other than my "rambunctiousness," which was the term my orthopedist (or as we joking called him, my primary care doctor) used for me. I now know that all of these were probably related to BWS.

There were other early manifestations of BWS that I wasn't proud of, but rather made me confused and embarrassed. Some of these were noticeable to other people—like the size of my tongue and my jaw—and I was teased about them. Others I could keep hidden, but they still made me feel inadequate.

It was only last year that I asked my mother to tell me about her experience of my birth and first few years of life. Up until then I had been content with knowing simply that I was diagnosed with this syndrome 4 hours after I was born; that they thought I was going to die; that my father fed me all night so I wouldn't die; and that my grandfather talked with my mom about the importance of taking the risk of loving me whole-heartedly.

Kathy's Version

We did learn that Miranda had BWS 4 hours after she was born. We were told a worst case scenario: she might be retarded, have malignancies of the internal organs, and asymmetries of her limbs. hardest of all to hear was that the doctors were uncertain that she would live. This uncertainty lasted for 3 months, when she was seen by a specialist who informed us that Miranda had never been at risk of dying, though some infants with BWS are.

The first few weeks were an overwhelming melange of falling in love and living in terror. Many doctors saw Miranda and seemed to take delight in being the first doctor to tell us something else was "wrong." We soon learned that many doctors were extrapolating from similar but not identical medical conditions, and that these extrapolations were often wrong. Because the BWS narrative has so many gaps, doctors filled in as best as they could, often with unintended consequences. One pediatric fellow told us that Miranda would be unable to integrate stimulation from more than one sensory channel at a time. He advised us never, for instance, to talk to and touch her at the same time. Further, he told us that it would be unwise for her to have contact with her older brother until she herself was older and could handle the stimulation. Though distressed by the possibility that we were harming her, we refused to accept his clinical assessment as valid since the consequences for normal baby care and family life would have been calamitous.

The early years with Miranda were full of contradictions. The story we told her about her birth and early years was an expurgated version. By age 6 or 7, she had a version of her life that emphasized heroic elements. We made her larger than life to compensate, I suppose, for our fear that she would have no life. We made her a heroine, a baby whose life force was so strong that she defied the doctors' predictions that she would die.

The actual story was filled with confusion, pain, hard work, and some courage. Hilary and I tried to get the best help that we could, evaluated the recommendations we received against our own growing knowledge of BWS, and then selected assessments, procedures, and treatments that made sense to us. It was lonely, scary, and isolating most of the time. Friends and family supported us but could not immerse themselves in the level of detail that would have been required to help us. Only our pediatrician, Dr. Patricio Vives, walked the walk with us. His wisdom and compassion have sustained us since Miranda was 6, when we had the good fortune to begin working with him.

Miranda's Version

When I was 9, my parents gave me words to help explain my experience and to help me understand that I was not at fault for some of the problems that I was encountering. The words were "Beckwith-Wiedemann Syndrome", and I had never heard them before. They had the immediate effect of assuaging my feelings of stupidity and inadequacy, but I forgot them almost immediately after they had worked their magic.

It was 3 years later before I actually connected my life to BWS. I was being evaluated for braces and my socially incompetent dentist told me that on a scale of one to ten where ten was the worst possible dental situation, I was an eleven. As a person who dutifully brushed her teeth twice a day and whose older brother had been told that his bite was "perfect," I was aghast. I asked him why and he replied boldly that it was because I had BWS. Later, I found out that it was written all over my chart that I didn't know about BWS and that I was not to be told anything about it. The dentist's speaking upset me profoundly, and it made me conscious of having BWS in a way that I never had been before.

I know I connected with it then because, one month later, at my school picnic, I was unable to participate in my last school race because of Achilles tendonitis. Before I would have just left it at that. But I remember thinking I couldn't run because of my syndrome.

Kathy's Version

Throughout Miranda's life, Hilary and I regularly discussed what we should tell her about the physical problems she was having. In a family in which truth is valued alongside love, and honesty is taken for granted, we never lied to her and never told all there was to tell. Our early strategy was to treat each event singly and give her the best explanation we could for whatever problem she was having. After all, we couldn't tell her anything that would be coherent. If she asked us questions, she too would have to live with the uncertainties that gaps in knowledge—and therefore storying—produced.

By the time Miranda was 9 years old, it became clear that our effort to spare her a "label" was spinning off other problems. She blamed herself for physical difficulties that we knew were not under her control. We felt she needed to know about BWS, but we hoped she wouldn't weave it into her developing sense of personhood. We told her a story of BWS that embellished the birth story she already knew with some additional elements. We explained further that BWS affected many parts of the body, and that BWS, not she, was responsible for most of her injuries and difficulties.

We would never have been able to predict the effect on her. She seemed instantly and immediately relieved to know there was a "reason," and yet the reason itself seemed to disappear from her awareness. She never asked us questions about BWS and never used the term herself.

The episode with her dentist at age 12 was pivotal for me too. I had been unable to protect her although I had been sitting next to her and was signaling wildly to the dentist. She left the dentist distraught. Comforting her as best I could, I realized that my more important task was to help her access her own resources to make herself feel better.

Miranda's Version

The last 3 years have been very difficult for me. First, the symptoms of BWS have been worse than I can ever remember: I suffer pain most of the time, whether from headaches, joint dislocations, or other problems related to abnormal formations of my internal organs. Because I spend my time thinking about matters that are very different from my peers, I am alienated from them. I am occupied with evaluating levels of pain, not spring colors. I'm continually thinking whether I want to share anything of my situation, and with whom. I am constantly trying to figure out what I need to report and what I don't. I am trying to avoid saturating my parents with my medical complaints and yet still be honest about what I feel.

My peers often ask me what is wrong with me. They notice that I have been absent for long periods of time and that I often come to school on crutches, with body braces or with slings. I have to decide whether to tell them the whole truth or not. When I have made the decision to tell people, the outcome has not always been positive for me. Some people have been grossed out by what I have told them, and others have not kept my confidence and, instead, repeated what I've said to people I wouldn't have told myself.

This year, I was hospitalized several times. I used to love going to the hospital because I felt safe there. I felt that the doctors were there for the sole purpose of taking care of me and making me feel better. This year, for the first time, doctors questioned my honesty. In a situation in which there was great uncertainty about the cause of my pain, several doctors accused me of not reporting my symptoms accurately. I realize now that having an unusual condition is going to set me up for disbelief. In the face of their lack of knowledge, they took the easy way out and blamed me, relying on a psychological explanation to fill the gap in the story because they didn't have a satisfactory medical explanation. Fortunately, I had the unconditional trust of my parents and my pediatrician who got me to other doctors who finally diagnosed the problem and prescribed appropriate treatment.

I am struggling not to let BWS take over my identity, but to be only a part of it. At the same time, I am trying to expand the category of what a disabled person looks like. When Gloria Steinem turned 40, reporters were disbelieving that a woman looking so young could be 40. She said, "This is what 40 looks like." I am trying to do what she did when people doubt my having a disability. I say, whether out loud or to myself, "This is what a disabled person looks like." I am trying to identify myself with a group of people—disabled people—who are not the same as I am, but who have had similar experiences. I am not going to lose myself in their experiences, but I am going to use them to build my knowledge of myself and my own experience.

Kathy's Version

The last few years have been as hard in their own way as were the first few years. What makes them different is that Miranda is an active participant and collaborator in the decisions that we must make. We are blessed by the fact that she is such a careful and accurate reporter of her experience.

When she is having a great many symptoms, the family focus narrows to get through the crisis. We are on the phone constantly with family and friends who want updates and want to offer support; we are scheduling and going to see doctors; coordinating with her school; keeping our son Ben, who is in college, in touch with what is happening; and trying to make Miranda more comfortable. Sometimes she requires 24-hour face-to-face care.

All of this usually takes place within a context of uncertainty: we often don't know what's going on and what to do about it. A dramatic example of this occurred in March 1995 when Miranda injured her hip while sitting on a couch, and then dislocated both shoulders the next day from using the crutches she was prescribed. We were pretty sure the BWS was responsible for the shoulder dislocations, but the hip? And, what had happened to the hip? More importantly, could it happen again? None of these questions have ever been resolved.

THE ILLNESS EXPERIENCE

A Narrative Analysis

In the last few years, Miranda and I have tried to understand the differences in our two illness experiences and the impact of these differences on our family. Though much can be explained by virtue of the different roles that we play in the family, the differential resources to which these roles give us access, and the nature of the conditions themselves, we have felt certain that other parameters are at play. We have begun to attend to features of the stories we tell about our conditions, and we notice that there are significant differences in our experience that derive directly from the kind of story we can each tell.

By virtue of having a rare genetic disorder that virtually no one has ever heard of, Miranda is more isolated in her experience than I, because I have a disease that affects one in eight women at some time in their life (Brack & Brack, 1990; Butler & Rosenblum, 1991; Hargrove, 1988; Lorde, 1980; Weingarten, 1994; Whitman, 1993). At my age, it is hard to imagine that I might know or meet someone who does not know a woman who has had breast cancer. By contrast, it is hard to imagine that Miranda will ever find anyone who knows someone with her syndrome.

The disparity shows up in the healthcare community as well. In the 17 years that we have been interacting with the medical profession over concerns related to Miranda's syndrome, and we have easily consulted with or met 100 doctors, only five have ever personally worked with a child with Beckwith-Wiedemann Syndrome. By contrast, all my medical providers have other patients with breast cancer.

The difference translates into very particular experiences that we each have on a daily basis. I never feel alone. I know that there are many women and many families going through what I and my family have gone through, even right on my block! Miranda always feels alone. In her world, she is an N of one.

Many people understand the etiology, pathophysiology, and the course of my illness. If I go to my public library, I can find reference books and first-person narratives, even my own book, about living with breast cancer. No one understands Beckwith-Wiedemann Syndrome. It is a disorder with multiple manifestations that can affect a number of organ systems, and no one can predict what is in store for any one person with the Syndrome. If Miranda goes to our public library, she will probably not be able to find even the name Beckwith-Wiedemann Syndrome in any of the 350,000 books in the library.

The name I use to define my medical situation—breast cancer—is defined as a disease, and this fits with my experience of having had breast cancer. Each time I was diagnosed with breast cancer, the treatment that followed corresponded with my ideas of what having a disease entails. Though I had no pain from the lump itself, the surgery, chemotherapy, and radiation therapy I underwent confirmed my belief that I had a disease.

Miranda, however, carries a diagnosis that has no obvious implications. We know that she has BWS, but nothing inevitably follows from that diagnosis the way surgery, for example, follows from the diagnosis of breast cancer. When I told others I had breast cancer, most people could imagine what I was experiencing. When Miranda says she has Beckwith-Wiedemann Syndrome, few people have any idea what that means for her.

Nor have we been able to find a word that conveys to us, much less to others, what she experiences routinely. Does she have a disease, an illness, a condition, a disability, a chronic disability, a chronic illness, a handicap, a disorder, a genetic disorder? We are baffled. No designation maps the territory. Without language, experience dissolves. Without language, experience cannot be shared and community cannot be formed.

In the last few years, since Miranda's physical condition has worsened, it has become imperative to us to find concepts to express the significance of these phenomenological differences between us, to make sense of certain reliable differences in our illness experiences. Drawing on narrative theory, we have located three concepts that we now use routinely to make sense of our experience. These concepts have provided the stepping-off point for the development of a set of coping strategies that have been invaluable for both of us. First, we will present these concepts. Next, we will describe the coping strategies that have derived from our application of these concepts to our illness experiences.

Narrative Concepts

Three characteristics of narrative have relevance to understanding illness experience. These three characteristics are narrative coherence, narrative closure, and narrative interdependence (Chatman, 1978; Weingarten & Cobb, 1995).

Narrative Coherence

Narrative coherence is established by the interrelationships between plot, character roles, and themes or values. In an illness narrative, the patient, the patient's family, and medical personnel all play parts. With the diagnosis of breast cancer, a plot sequence unfolds according to fixed and known responses to data derived from the analysis of breast tissue. The patient will likely have visits with an oncologist, a radiotherapist, a surgeon, and ongoing relationships with them, depending on how the plot unfolds. Family members can be given a likely set of events to expect. The feelings of everyone involved are likely to include sadness, anxiety, worry, and fear. This was so for me. Though at any moment I may have felt confused, the story I could tell was not particularly confusing. In fact, it was quite coherent.

By contrast, these elements applied within the context of Beckwith-Wiedemann Syndrome have the feeling of a deck of cards thrown into the wind. Having such scanty criteria available to us to guide our selection of cards, it always feels just shy of random that we are proceeding, playing, with one deck of cards and not another. Since the significance of any event is unknown, the plot unfolds chaotically. Nor is it clear who the players—besides Miranda, Hilary, and me—should be. Do we go to a geneticist or a pediatrician? Do we find a specialist for each affected organ? How should we feel about it? Is this a disaster waiting to happen? Has a disaster already happened? Are we on the edge of a cliff, or have we fallen over? We have never known, and on one has ever been able to tell us.

Narrative Closure

The second feature that applies to illness narratives is that of narrative closure. Narrative closure occurs when the story that is told seems to have only one way of understanding it. That is, the story resists alternative interpretation. There are two elements that help create narrative closure: completeness and cultural resonance. With regard to completeness, the more "open" the story, that is, the more the story has gaps, the more vulnerable the story is to others filling in these gaps with material of their own. With regard to cultural resonance, the more familiar people are with the situation described, the higher the cultural resonance will be, and the more likely that others will be able to participate with the person whose narrative it is in a way that supports, endorses, and elaborates the story the person has to tell.

On the one hand, breast cancer narratives have a high degree of narrative closure: they resist alternative interpretation because the course of the disease is so well known. For instance, how commonly do you think a woman who has found a large breast lump would find a friend or physician who says, "Oh, gee, don't worry about that large lump you have." One reason such a response is almost unthinkable these days is precisely because so much is known in both the lay and professional communities about breast cancer. There is high cultural resonance.

On the other hand, Beckwith-Wiedemann Syndrome has a low degree of narrative closure. There are multiple gaps in the story and virtually no cultural resonance. Few people know how to respond when faced with the name of the disorder or even the names of the physical manifestations. For instance, as we mentioned, an enlarged tongue (macroglossia) was an early diagnostic feature. Some people associate an enlarged tongue with children who are mentally retarded, some of whom indeed do have large tongues. Our inability to tell anyone what Miranda's large tongue meant led some people to assume she was retarded! The story—her story, our story—had, has gaps just about everywhere and people fill them in as best they can. This has occurred with medical personnel as well.

Narrative Interdependence

Finally, narrative interdependence refers to the interrelatedness of one person's narrative to another's. In families, one member's narrative is usually interrelated to the narratives told by other family members. For better or worse, my breast cancer narrative is related to the stories other women in my family with breast cancer can and do tell. Miranda has her own story that relates to my breast cancer because, as the daughter of a mother with breast cancer, she worries about her own increased risk of acquiring breast cancer.

Miranda's illness narrative has no connection to the illnesses of anyone else in our extended family. Though Beckwith-Wiedemann Syndrome is genetic, she is the first person in the family to be affected by it. This probably means that in her case BWS is a new mutation that appears for the first time in her. However, along another dimension, neither Miranda nor I could tell an authentic account of our lives without reference to the illness experience of the other. In this sense, our illness narratives are profoundly interdependent.

COPING STRATEGIES

I had been in New York at a professional conference the days that Miranda dislocated her hip and shoulders. Hilary kept me posted by phone, and each time I checked my phone messages, there was a long, detailed, and excruciating message about her situation. I realized how impossible my life would be without Hilary; how fortunate we are that we collaborate about her care, functioning like a precision team. I also realized that I had to glean from my own illness experience those elements that made living with it relatively manageable and find a way to graft these into Miranda's illness experience.

The evening I returned, I was unable to sleep. Miranda was in considerable pain, but only the three of us and Ben knew it. Ben called from college daily, but no one else in our network or hers knew. She was in too much pain to consider talking to others, and we were working so hard at the practical matters of tending to her, taking her to her various appointments, and trying to squeeze in our work, that we were, as we often were, isolated from any support.

Partially, I knew that the difficulty of responding to people's questions each time—Why did it happen?—was exhausting and frustrating. We never had explanations that were satisfying to us or to others. Thinking through the narrative categories that I use in my work, the ones I have described above, I realized that we had to find a way to create legitimacy for the narrative we could tell—coherent or not; that we had to find away to increase the cultural resonance of Miranda's story, to decrease her sense of isolation, even if it were to a small "local" group of people who could share our "cultural" meanings; that her story had to link to those of others, both by creating an audience for hers and by finding a community of like-situated persons; and finally, she had to feel empowered about as many aspects of her situation as possible.

The next evening I proposed to Miranda that we design a ceremony and invite a group of trusted friends and helpers with whom to share the history of her living with Beckwith-Wiedemann Syndrome. I shared with her my reasons for this suggestion, and she immediately accepted it.

Miranda's Version

My mother's suggestion really made me aware of just how isolated I was. The idea of a ceremony was relieving. I had hope that I could feel connected to others.

Kathy's Version

Miranda and I designed the invitation and the ceremony itself. On the invitation we explicitly asked people to join a team for her, one that would "oppose despair and nourish hope." Those were her words. The ceremony, we hoped, would help shift her relationship to Beckwith-Wiedemann Syndrome, from one in which she was isolated from others to one in which others could support her. We hoped that by describing the effects of BWS on her life, "unmasking" these effects (White, 1995; White & Epston, 1990), she would find others willing to help her live with BWS.

Miranda's Version

I designed two rituals that were important to me. The first ritual involved candles. At the beginning of the ceremony, I gave each of the twelve people present a candle and I lit the one in front of me. I began to tell the story of my living with BWS. I asked people to light their candle from mine when they understood the magnitude of my experience. As people lit their candles from mine, at different intervals of time, I felt that each lit candle took some of the burden off me.

The second ritual I designed was intended to show the feelings that BWS makes me have. I listed about 30 different feelings on small cards, some of which were positive and some of which were negative. I had purchased two beautiful boxes and selected one for the negative feelings and one for the positive feelings. This was my way of honoring my negative feelings, but also to have a place for them outside my heart. I asked people to brainstorm with me about other positive feelings that they thought they could help me feel thorough their participation on my team. People suggested many words, like "wise," "humorous," "connected," "loved," and "content." I felt understood, and I felt it was possible that they could help me feel these ways.

Kathy's Version

The effects of the ceremony have been profound and long-lasting. Miranda does have a team. Ten women check in with her regularly, can be counted on in crises, and know her story. The difficulty of explaining has dissolved because they all know how slippery BWS is, and they no longer ask questions that make us feel stupid or ashamed when we can't answer them. Nor do they challenge whether or not Miranda is really in pain. They accept, as we did years ago, that the "rules" of BWS are shifty. While the experience of pain is the "most vibrant example of what it is to 'have certainty,' . . . for the other person it is so elusive that 'hearing about pain' may exist as the primary model of what it is 'to have doubt'" (Scarry, 1985).

Following the ceremony, we created documents that better represent the history of her living with BWS (White, 1995). I sent for her medical records from every hospital and medical office where she had been seen, and together we compiled a chronology of medical events—still with some missing pieces, I'm afraid. We also decided to attack head-on the problem of those routine problem checklists that she finds so frustrating because the categories rarely allow her to make checkmarks on the pages, thus rendering invisible the reality of her particular physical problems. Instead, we designed a problem checklist that counts as categories those that fit her problems. She now takes this form to every first visit with a new doctor.

Finally, she has begun to read first-person accounts of disabled people, and accounts of the history of the disability rights movement in this country (Bow, 1992; Grealey, 1994; Merker, 1992; Panzarino, 1994; Resnick, 1984; Saxton & Howe, 1987; Williams, 1992, 1994; Zola, 1982). Her sense of community has shifted.

Miranda's Version

Reading other persons' accounts of their challenges in life has been both oppressive and liberating. At times, I have felt swamped by sadness, but at other times I have felt astonished that other people could have experiences so similar to mine. It makes me think that I can be walking down the street and the person walking next to me might have had experiences like mine at some point in his or her life. I feel much less isolated than I did before.

CONCLUSION

From a narrative perspective, empowerment is related to one person experiencing another person as accepting and elaborating what she has to say without challenging the basic integrity of her story (Cobb, 1992; Weingarten & Cobb, 1995). In this last year, not only has Miranda experienced other' speaking in a way that has elaborated her story without challenging its basic integrity she has also spoken out to stop medical people from speaking in ways that do not empower her, and she has spoken up for others in ways that empower them. Armed with the knowledge that her condition, unlike mine, will rarely be automatically understood, she knows that she must work harder to gain others' understanding. Also, she has learned that she must be always prepared to stop people from drawing false conclusions about her. Writing this article is one more step in developing a more collaborative relationship with BWS, showing that *she* has expert knowledge about it, and empowering herself.

We believe that the empowerment of all members of a family is fundamental to their coping with medical crises. Healthcare providers have the opportunity at all times to cut short, to interrupt, to contradict, to take over, or, alternatively, to respect and to elaborate the illness narratives that family members and the designated patient tell. We hope that our narrative will strengthen your resolves to act in ways that endorse and elaborate, and ultimately empower the people with whom you work. We hope that our writing will have created possibilities of empowerment for people who may now be better understood because of what you have read.

REFERENCES

Bow, F. (1992). *Equal rights for Americans with disabilities.* New York: Franklin Watts.
Brack, P., with Brack, B. (1990). *Moms don't get sick.* Aberdeen SD: Melius Publishers.
Bruner, J. (1990). *Acts of meaning.* Cambridge: Harvard University Press.
Butler, S., & Rosenblum, B. (1991). *Cancer in two voices.* San Francisco: Spinsters Book Company.
Chatman, S. (1978). *Story and discourse.* Ithaca NY: Cornell University Press.
Chilman, C.S., Nunnally, E.W., & F.M. Cox (eds). (1988). *Chronic illness and disability: Families in trouble series* (Vol. 2). Newbury Park CA: Sage Publications.
Cobb, S. (1992). Empowerment and mediation: A narrative perspective [commissioned by National Institute for Dispute Resolution]. *The Negotiation Journal 9*:2245–2260.
Eisenberg, M.G., Sutkin, L.C., & Jansen, M.A. (eds). (1984). *Chronic illness and disability through the life span: Effects on self and family.* New York: Springer Publishing Co.
Grealey, L. (1994). *Autobiography of a face.* New York: Houghton Mifflin.
Griffith, J., & Griffith, M.E. (1994). *The body speaks.* New York: Basic Books.
Hargrove, A.C. (1988). *Getting better: Conversations with myself and other friends while healing from breast cancer.* Minneapolis MN: CompCare Publishers.
Kleinman, A. (1988). *The illness narratives: Suffering, healing, and the human condition.* New York: Basic Books.
Koocher, G., & McDonald, B. (1992). Preventive intervention and family coping with a child's life-threatening or terminal illness (pp. 67–88). In J. Akamatsu, M.A. Stephens, S. Hobfoll, & J.H. Crowther (eds), *Family health psychology.* Washington DC: Hemisphere Publishing.
Lorde, A. (1980). *The cancer journals.* San Francisco: spinsters/aunt lute.
Merker, H. (1992). *Listening: Ways of hearing in a silent world.* New York: Harper Perennial.
Panzarino, C. (1994). *The me in the mirror.* Seattle WA: Seal Press.
Penn, P. (1983). Coalitions and binding interactions in families with chronic illness. *Family Systems Medicine* 1(2):12–25.
Pipher, M. (1994). *Reviving Ophelia: Saving the selves of adolescent girls.* New York: Ballantine Books.
Resnick, M. (1984). The social construction of disability and handicap in America (pp. 29–46). In R. Blum (ed.), *Chronic illness and disabilities in childhood and adolescence.* Orlando FL: Grune & Stratton.
Rolland, J.S. (1994). *Families, illness, and disability.* New York: Basic Books.
Sampson, E.E. (1993). *Celebrating the other: A dialogic account of human nature.* Boulder CO: Westview Press.

Saxton, M., & Howe, F. (eds.) (1987). *With wings: An anthology of literature by and about women with disabilities.* New York: The Feminist Press.

Scarry, E. (1985). *The body in pain: The making and unmaking of the world.* Oxford: Oxford University Press.

Shapiro, J.P. (1993). *No pity: People with disabilities forging a new civil rights movement.* New York: Times Books.

Sontag, S. (1977). *Illness as metaphor.* New York: Farrar, Straus, & Giroux.

Walsh, F., & Anderson, C.M. (eds.). (1988). *Chronic disorders and the family,.* New York: Haworth Press.

————, & McGoldrick, M. (eds.). (1991). *Living beyond loss: Death in the family.* New York: W.W. Norton.

Weingarten, K. (1991). The discourses of intimacy: Adding a social constructionist and feminist view. *Family Process 30:*285–305.

————, (1994). *The mother's voice: Strengthening intimacy in families.* New York: Harcourt Brace.

————, (ed.). (1995). *Cultural resistance: Challenging beliefs about men, women, and therapy.* Binghamton NY: Haworth Press.

————, & Cobb, S. (1995). Timing disclosure sessions: Adding a narrative perspective to clinical work with adult survivors of childhood sexual abuse. *Family Process 34:*257–269.

Weingarten, V. (1977) *Intimations of mortality.* New York: Alfred A. Knopf.

White, M. (1995). *Re-authoring lives: Interviews and essays.* Adelaide, South Australia: Dulwich Centre Publications.

————, & Epston, D. (1990). *Narrative means to therapeutic ends.* New York: W.W. Norton.

Whitman, J. (1993). *Breast cancer journal: A century of petals.* Golden CO: Fulcrum Publishing.

Williams, D. (1992). *Nobody nowhere: The extraordinary autobiography of an autistic.* New York: Avon Books.

————. (1994). *Somebody somewhere: Breaking free from the world of autism.* New York: Times Books.

Zola, I. (1982). *Missing pieces.* Philadelphia PA: Temple University Press.

Part II: *Study Questions and Disability Awareness Exercise*

1. What are the similarities and differences between the loss associated with the birth of a child with a disability as compared to the loss associated with the onset of a disability during the teenage years?
2. Is the loss experienced by the mother and father of a child with a disability the same? Different? How? Why?
3. In what way are the challenges faced by adolescents with chronic illness and disabilities different from those experienced by adults?
4. Why is the biopsychosocial model complex and difficult to implement?
5. How can the family be an ally or a hindrance in treatment and rehabilitation?
6. What are the major components of attachment theory?
7. How do characteristics of the child born with a disability relate to attachment? Provide examples.
8. Why has there been a paradigm shift regarding the role of families in treatment and rehabilitation?
9. Discuss the features of an effective family intervention program.
10. Can behavioral family therapy be applied to families living a physical disability experience?
11. What are the unique stressors related to coping with a rare genetic disorder?
12. In the Weingarten article, how are Kathy's and Miranda's perspectives similar and how are they different?
13. What suggestions would you make to improve the disability experience of both Kathy and Miranda?

RETURN UNOPENED

The parents of children with disabilities face difficult situations for which they are often not prepared and which they must frequently resolve alone. The process of problem resolution can be stressful, painful, and demanding on the family system as well as on the marital relationship. A child might become a source of conflict between the parents regarding the best approach to the child's future care, or the experience may enrich and solidify the family relationships.

Goals

1. To present the potential impact of a child with a disability on selected aspects of the marital relationship.

2. To involve participants in the exploration of their personal reaction to a specific situation.

Procedure

1. Participants read the following role description: "You are the parent of a 2-week-old hospitalized child who has a severe disability. You have not had the child home from the hospital. One spouse wants to put the child in an institution, while the other wants to bring her home."
2. When this is read, all group members will write their responses concerning which position they would take and what they would do.
3. Having written the response, group members explore their reactions to this situation.
4. Group members are then asked to consider what difference it would make to each of them if the child was a female or a male.
5. Repeat steps 2 and 3.

Part III

The Personal Impact of Disability

The personal response to disability, at any given time, can vary on a continuum from denial of its existence to exaggeration of its consequences. This response is dependent upon a number of variables, including environmental, social, biological, and psychological characteristics of the respondent.

Acceptance of loss theory, as initially presented by Beatrice Wright and her associates, has played a major historical role in the thinking and practice of rehabilitation psychology for over 40 years. In chapter 10, Keany and Glueckauf describe the basic tenets of this theory, review and critique studies relevant to it, and summarize conceptual and methodological problems relevant to its application. Future directions and a reformulation of Wright's value changes are presented.

Nunn (chapter 11) views hope and its relationship to the perceived future as critical in our understanding of physical and mental disorders with significant utility in assisting persons in their recovery from mental and physical illness. Hope is defined in relation to its elements, object, subject, stability, phenomenology and relationship to denial, despair, and reality.

People with disabilities who challenge the barriers to their independence and autonomy in our society are often viewed as "angry." Lane (chapter 12) describes the importance of anger and its role in empowering persons with disabilities to seek justice, as well as the psychology of anger and its potentially destructive nature. Expressing anger at God and forgiving God are presented as important elements of a faith journey and vital to personal wholeness.

The devalued role that people with disabilities, particularly women, have in our culture, combined with the frequent insensitivity of others, including parents, peers, and professionals, is described in the personal statement of Susan Buchanan in chapter 13, as contributing to the battered self esteem of persons with disabilities. The need for a change in the beliefs and behaviors of others in facilitating self-respect and autonomy for people with disabilities is emphasized.

10

Disability and Value Change: An Overview and Reanalysis of Acceptance of Loss Theory

Kelly C. M-H. Keany and Robert L. Glueckauf

D isability, whether congenital or adventitious, traumatic or gradual, can exert a major influence on one's values and world view. It is a commonly held belief that rehabilitation is more successful when clients and their significant others are accepting of the disability and are willing to adapt to the many changes disability entails (Marinelli & Dell Orto, 1984). Although numerous articles have been written on value change processes following disability (e.g., Livneh, 1980; Shontz, 1975), the theorizing of Dembo, Leviton, and Wright (1956/1975), and Wright (1960, 1983)[1] continue to occupy a central position in the rehabilitation literature.

Although the notion of acceptance of disability has become part of the daily parlance of rehabilitation, the psychological conditions underlying value change and acceptance of disability have not been adequately delineated or assessed. For example, the widely used Acceptance of Disability scale (Linkowski, 1971) measures global acceptance of one's functional limitations, but it does not directly assess the value changes proposed by Dembo et al. and Wright.

The primary purpose of this article is to re-examine the basic tenets of the acceptance of loss theory, particularly the four value changes associated with acceptance of disability. After summarizing the major components of acceptance, we will critique research on acceptance of disability, focusing on the measurement of value change. Finally, we will present several methodological and

We gratefully acknowledge the comments and guidance from Beatrice A. Wright in this research.

From *Rehabilitation Psychology, 38*(3) (1993), 199–210. Reprinted with permission.

[1]*For brevity, reference to the work of Dembo, Leviton and Wright (1956/1975) and Wright (1960, 1983) will be noted as Dembo et al. and Wright in the rest of this article.*

conceptual suggestions, including Rokeach's analysis of values (1973) and its implications on acceptance of loss following disability.

BASIC TENETS OF ACCEPTANCE OF DISABILITY

The original research of Dembo et al. emphasized the common perception of disability as a misfortune or "value loss" (Dembo et al., 1975, p. 30). If perceived as a misfortune, disability can lead to underestimation of existing abilities and even devaluation of the whole person. Acceptance of disability, however, is an adjustment of a person's value system such that his or her actual or perceived losses from disability do not negatively affect the value of existing abilities. In effect, Dembo et al. and Wright were *"concerned with the conditions facilitating acceptance of one's disability as nondevaluating"* (Wright, p. 159; italics in original).

Wright, building on the work of Dembo et al., proposed four major changes in a person's value system that preclude or limit devaluation: (a) enlargement of the scope of values, (b) subordination of physique relative to other values, (c) containment of disability effects, and (d) transformation of comparative-status value to asset (intrinsic) values. Although these value changes are hypothesized to be interdependent (Wright, 1983), they will be discussed separately below.

Enlargement of the Scope of Values

During the crisis period (usually following trauma of some kind), the person experiences a period of mourning over the cherished values believed to be lost. The period of mourning refers to a continuum, one extreme being all-inclusive suffering, the other being a narrow focus on specific losses with occasional feelings of dysphoria. When a person's preoccupation with loss is intense, the first value change to emerge is "enlargement of the scope of values." The other three value changes are not posited to follow an orderly progression of stages.

Wright suggests that enlargement of scope is initiated when the person begins to recognize the importance of values other than those presumed lost. Such recognition is stimulated by a variety of experiences, including the need to manage activities of daily living and the need to seek relief from being satiated with grief. When a person can find meaning in events, abilities, and goals, then the person is enlarging his or her scope of values.

Subordination of Physique Relative to Other Values

In our society, there is an emphasis on physical perfection, beauty, and ability. During mourning, this emphasis on physique may be significantly heightened if certain of its attributes are perceived as lost. Focus on physique may lead the person to ignore the importance of other values in life, such as friendship, intelligence, work, and creativity. As the scope of values broadens, the relative emphasis on physique decreases; the "worth" of the person begins to be determined by abilities and characteristics in addition to those related to physique. For example, personality and effort may gain in importance relative to appearance or actual ability.

Containment of Disability Effects

Although a physical disability may have an impact on functioning, it can overreach its actual effects and be viewed as globally debilitating, affecting other physical abilities, emotional and intellectual spheres, and even the overall value of the person. Dembo et al. and Wright have called the "power of single characteristics to evoke inferences about a person," the spread effect (Wright, 1983, p. 32). Containment of spread is dependent on the perceiver. For example, spread can be avoided or decreased if the disability or loss is seen as a "possession" rather than a personal characteristic (Dembo et al., 1975, pp. 32–33). That is, if the disability is seen as a personal characteristic, the person and the characteristic become a closely knit unit: a disabled person. Spread is likely to occur because feelings about the disability, viewed as a central, personal characteristic, can affect other aspects of the person, just as other personal characteristics can. If, however, the disability is seen only as a possession, then the person and the disability are perceived as separate: a person with a disability. When introduced as a "quadriplegic," the person and his or her abilities more generally may be associated with limitations. However, if "quadriplegia" is considered but one among many aspects of a person, such as marital status, occupation, or ethnic origin, it is less likely to dominate the impression of the person.

Transformation of Comparative-Status Values to Asset Values

When a personal quality or ability is compared to a standard, a comparative-status value has been given to it. In contrast, asset (intrinsic) values involve evaluation based on qualities inherent in the thing being evaluated, such as its intrinsic worth, usefulness, or beauty. With an asset value, it is possible to focus on the quality of the object, ability, or person being evaluated rather than on its status compared to something or someone else. A wheelchair may be valued for its usefulness as means of mobility, rather than devalued as inferior to walking or running. The effect of asset values is to make it possible to appreciate the value of something which otherwise would be devalued because it falls short of a higher comparative standard. Whereas comparative evaluations are necessary to show progress in rehabilitation or treatment, when a comparative-status statement reflects a judgment of personal worth, particularly a negative judgment, it becomes detrimental to the acceptance process.

Although not encompassing all types of value changes that may occur with acceptance, the four value changes are hypothesized to be strongly related to acceptance of loss (disability) as nondevaluating. They may facilitate a positive

reframing of disability and "free people to act in ways befitting their own characteristics rather than those of an idolized normal standard" (Wright, 1983, p. 183).
Thus, acceptance of loss paves the way for positive adjustment to disability.

Review and Critique of Acceptance of Loss Studies

Several researchers have examined specific value changes associated with acceptance of loss. Wright presented two studies supporting the value change of subordination of physique and acceptance of disability. English and Oberle (1971)
administered a survey on attitudes toward disability to airline stewardesses (who
were expected to place higher emphasis on physique) and female typists (who
were expected to place lower emphasis on physical appearance). They found that
airline stewardesses showed more negative attitudes toward disability than the
typists. Note, however, that the tendency to emphasize physical appearance as a
value was not directly measured. The investigators ranked airline stewardesses'
and typists' aesthetics preferences based on their intuitive assumptions. Even
though these intuitions may seem plausible considering the physical standards
required to become an airline stewardess at the time of the study, it cannot be
assumed that such global impressions closely match empirically based evaluations of the aesthetic preferences of these two samples. Thus, the relationship
between airline stewardesses' purported tendency to emphasize physique and
have a lowered acceptance of disability remains questionable.

Wright (1983) also cited Balunas' doctoral dissertation which showed that
persons with higher acceptance of their own disability, as measured by the
Attitudes Toward Disabled Persons scale (ATDP; Yuker, Block, & Younng, 1966),
were more likely to focus on the personality characteristics of another person
(with or without a disability) than those subjects with a lower acceptance of their
own disability. Balunas found a significant positive correlation between ATDP
scores and the ratings of importance of personality. No correlation was found
with ATDP scores and either ability or appearance. Wright concluded that
Balunas' findings supported the hypothesized direct relationship between subordination of physique and acceptance of disability. It is equally plausible, however,
that this positive association may have resulted from an enlargement of subjects'
scope of values rather than subordination of physique. This ambiguity in interpretation underscores the need for clear operational definitions and specific measures of Wright's proposed value changes.

Focusing on Wright's concepts of spread and containment of disability
effects, Shontz (1984) conducted an analogue study of spread with 48 college
students (36 women, 12 men). Subjects were instructed to list their most important life goals; frequent goals mentioned were characterized as "vocational and
economic" and "prospective home and family" (p. 82). After subsequently imagining the loss of the highest ranked goal, they rated the importance of the goals,
and "everything else in life" (p. 79). Subjects repeated this process until all their

goals were imagined to be lost. Shontz found that many of the subjects demonstrated spread; that is, with the loss of one goal, others were perceived as less important than when initially ranked. Other subjects, however, did not show a decrease in their ratings, which was interpreted as analogous to containment. Although Shontz's analogue method was highly creative, the lack of a "no-loss comparison" condition obfuscates the interpretation of results. Changers in the rank order of goals, reportedly reflecting "spread," may have resulted from causes unrelated to loss, such as experimenter bias, contrast effects, or by simply "taking stock of one's life goals."

Dion, Berscheid, and Walster (1972) offered further support for the spread effect in their study of the physical attractiveness stereotype and its components. Sixty psychology students (30 men and 30 women) perceived "attractive" persons as having a greater number of "socially desirable" personality traits, and as leading better and more successful lives (p. 288). Although this study was not concerned with disability, it provides support for the spread effect and emphasizes the formidable obstacle physical appearance poses when accepting disability.

In one of the few studies using subjects with disabilities, Butts and Shontz (1962; cited in Wright, 1983) examined the relationship between spread and the use of comparative-status evaluations. Subjects included four groups of 14 men: an institutionalized group of persons with schizophrenia, veterans with physical disabilities living in a VA setting, veterans without social-adjustment problems living in a VA setting, and a group of "self-supporting 'normals'" (Butts & Shontz, 1962, p. 326). The researchers selected these four groups based on the assumption that they formed a rank ordering of coping ability, from low to high ability. Spread was assessed by measuring how confident subjects were that, given a few traits about a person, the person would have other personality traits as well. Comparative-mindedness was assessed by asking subjects to evaluate several written descriptions of "everyday life situations" and rating the relative usage of comparative and asset evaluations (Wright, 1983, p. 185).

Butts and Shontz reported that subjects who were judged a priori to have higher coping abilities (e.g., veterans without social adjustment problems in a VA setting and self-supporting normals) tended to use asset evaluations more often than comparative evaluations. Note, however, that subjects' coping abilities were not directly assessed. The investigators ranked the four groups of subjects based on assumptions about their coping ability. As mentioned previously, it may be erroneous to assume that global impressions closely match empirically based measurements. In addition, subjects' usage of social comparisons when judging the "everyday life situations" of others may not be a valid indicator of their own tendency to engage in comparative evaluations in interpersonal situations. Despite these methodological limitations, the overall findings of the study supported Wright's contention that asset evaluations are associated with more effective coping with disability.

A major landmark in the growth of acceptance of loss research was the development of the Acceptance of Disability scale (AD; Linkowski, 1971). Many studies of the psychosocial aspects of disability have employed Linkowski's AD scale as a measure of acceptance (e.g., Glueckauf & Quittner, 1992; Linkowski & Dunn, 1974; Morgan & Leung, 1980; Nadler, Sheinberg, & Jaffe, 1975; see also Linkowski, 1986). Because the AD has been so widely utilized, a discussion of its development and psychometric characteristics follows.

The Acceptance of Disability Scale

Using Wright's four value changes as a guide, Linkowski generated 50 items for his scale, and administered it to two samples: 46 persons being evaluated at a rehabilitation center, and 55 university students with disabilities. Reliability was determined for the first sample (Cronbach's alpha = .93, using the Spearman-Brown prophesy formula). Linkowski performed factor analysis, with principle components extraction and orthogonal rotation, on each sample, and determined the 50-item scale to be unidimensional, measuring the construct of acceptance of disability.

Several conceptual and methodological concerns need to be addressed in evaluating Linkowski's AD scale. First, a key assumption of Wright's (1960) theorizing was the acceptance of disability results from specific value changes; yet the AD scale does not systematically measure Wright's four key value changes. Without direct evidence of the underlying components, it is unclear that the AD actually measures Dembo et al. and Wright's construct of acceptance. The conceptual fit between studies utilizing the AD and acceptance of loss theory may therefore be called into question.

Second, Linkowski's scale development procedures raise further question about the validity of the AD scale. Linkowski asserted that value changes were interdependent, as Wright suggested, and allowed considerable overlap of the broad value domains in the item development phase of the AD scale. Despite this stated interdependence, Linkowski analyzed the scale with factor analysis using orthogonal rotation, when oblique rotation was more appropriate (Kerlinger, 1986). Even so, his sample sizes (ns = 46 and 55) preclude the use of factor analysis as a feasible method of analysis, which requires a much higher subject to item ratio to be interpretable (Nunnally, 1978). In addition, Linkowski failed to remove items not loading on the primary factor, making his unidimensional scale factorially impure (Kerlinger, 1986).

Although we have addressed two potential limitations of Linkowski's AD scale, research focusing on the assessment of the construct and factorial validity of this measure may prove fruitful in the long term. Linkowski's scale has proved to be an effective measure of broad-based acceptance of disability (Linkowski, 1986).

SUMMARY OF CONCEPTUAL AND METHODOLOGICAL PROBLEMS

Three major methodological inadequacies have limited the validity of research on acceptance of loss and value change. First, the majority of studies (e.g.,

English & Oberle, 1971; Shontz, 1984) have used analogue procedure rather than field methods to test relationships between proposed value changes (e.g., subordination of physique) and acceptance of disability.

Second, there has been an underreliance on samples of persons with disabilities. Although the costs of collecting data on individuals with chronic disabilities are high, the increased generalizability and utility of such studies warrants the sacrifice. Note, also, that despite the broad applicability of the overlying acceptance of loss theory, only one study (Butts & Shontz, 1962) included persons with disabilities that were not physical (i.e., schizophrenia). The theory contends that persons without disabilities also go through the process of acceptance of disability; this component has not been adequately studied.

Last, the methodological limitations of Linkowski's (1971) AD scale may influence the validity of the studies utilizing it, insofar as the research is used to garner support for the acceptance of loss theory. Consideration of the problems cited above leads us to offer changes in acceptance of loss theory and research.

Our review of acceptance loss research revealed several conceptual difficulties. There have been few studies focusing on the value change components of acceptance and the process of value change. Many studies of disability rely on a measure of acceptance or adjustment (the AD scale or the ATDP scale) to demonstrate the effects of treatments or education without focusing on an underlying theory of acceptance.

A major component of Dembo et al. and Wright's theory focuses on value change as critical to the process of acceptance, yet the four value changes are not well defined or operationalized. Value changes have been inferred rather than quantitatively measured (e.g., Balunas, cited in Wright, 1983; Shontz, 1984). Linkowski (1971) maintained that he had operationalized the four value changes associated with Dembo et al. and Wright's theory, but his AD scale does not specifically measure them.

Research on acceptance of loss has also been limited by incomplete testing of the major components of Wright's theoretical model. None of the studies reviewed above assessed more than two value dimensions of the model. In addition, when a value change has been studied, there has not been a concomitant measure of acceptance of disability based on the acceptance of loss theory as a check for validity. Acceptance of disability as a combination of all four value changes has yet to be empirically examined.

FUTURE DIRECTIONS FOR RESEARCH

Methodological Suggestions

Measurement of Acceptance of Loss.

Linkowski has developed an easily administered instrument to measure a general construct of the acceptance of disability. Further factor analysis with large numbers of subjects (at least 500 for a good subject-to-item ratio; Nunnally, 1978) might provide evidence of specific underlying components (i.e, value changes), as well as remove extraneous items that do not fit well into any factor. It is possible, however, that this type of static measure of acceptance is inadequate to support the value changes delineated by the theory (Keany, 1993). Although steps were taken in her procedure to differentiate the value changes (stated as items for an acceptance of disability scale), Keany was unable in her masters' research to divide the value changes into distinct clusters. If the results of factor analysis with appropriately large numbers of subjects are inconclusive (i.e., without the hypothesized factor loadings), or provide evidence supporting acceptance as a unidimensional construct, then other methods of measuring value change must be developed. The interdependence of the acceptance of loss components, however, may not be dissected through the use of static measures.

It is crucial to acknowledge that acceptance of loss occurs over time and is subject to multiple influences both within and outside the individual. Longitudinal field studies may help to capture the process of acceptance of loss, and provide evidenced for the theory, as well as suggestions for modification. We strongly urge the use of intensive interviewing procedures in which volunteers with recent disabilities are asked to describe their ongoing and long-term experiences in adapting to the uncertainties of their medical condition. Unobtrusive probes regarding changes in the scope and quality of values can be introduced during the interview process. Qualitative data on value changes following disability are needed to enhance our understanding of how and under what conditions the acceptance process occurs.

Increasing Generalizability Across Subject.

Acceptance of loss theory includes both visible and covert disabilities; Dembo et al. and Wright originally focused on visible physical disability as a loss. Covert physical disabilities, such as diabetes, hearing impairment, and chronic pain, and nonphysical disabilities, such as mental and emotional disabilities, also involve value losses, and thus may elicit devaluation. Because of the specific characteristics of various disabilities, measuring value changes in samples of persons with different disabilities may help in developing acceptance-enhancing interventions tailored to target populations.

Acceptance of loss theory, therefore, recognizes a wide range of disabling conditions, with consideration given to any loss attributable to disability (e.g., losses in intellectual functions, physical ability, or social skills). Enlargement of the scope of values and containment of disability effects focus on the values persons hold, how disability (physical or nonphysical) affects them. The fourth value change, transformation of comparative-status values into asset values, is also largely unaffected by the addition of other disability populations. Subordination of physique, however, originally specified values concerning a person's appearance and ability, which may or may not change with a covert disability. This value change might now be called "subordination of affected values," in which the importance of values related to losses in function is decreased relative to the importance of values unaffected by disability.

Conceptual Suggestions

Operationalization of Key Constructs.

One of the major obstacles to research on acceptance of loss theory has been the difficulty in operationalizing key constructs. Although value changes, such as subordinating physique, have high intuitive appeal, the absence of clear operational definitions for these constructs has led to substantial measurement problems.

We propose that Rokeach's (1973) hierarchical value analysis may enhance our understanding of the structure of value systems and how values change as a result of disability. Furthermore, Rokeach's approach includes a measure of value ranking which can be adapted for acceptance of loss research.

Dembo et al. and Wright depicted disability as a misfortune or "value loss," the loss of something valuable. Value change is described as a restructuring of a person's value system to accommodate changes related to disability. How are value systems restructured following onset of disability? The value changes proposed by Dembo et al. and Wright do not sufficiently explain the changes that take place in a person's value system. An alternative framework, Rokeach's hierarchical analysis of values, may help to illuminate the process of value change associated with acceptance of disability.

Rokeach (1973) defines a value as "an enduring belief that a specific mode of conduct or end-state of existence is personally or socially preferable to an opposite or converse mode of conduct or end-state of existence" (p. 5). For example, honesty is a preferable mode of conduct over dishonesty. Accomplishment is a preferable end-state of existence rather than failure.

Rokeach categorizes values as either terminal or instrumental. Terminal values are idealized or desirable end-states of existence. Examples of terminal values include wisdom, a comfortable life, or a world at peace. Instrumental values are idealized or desirable modes of conduct that are instrumental to the attainment of terminal values. Instrumental values include cheerfulness, logic, responsibility, competence, and so forth. Instrumental values determine how a person behaves in order to reach his or her terminal values. Rokeach (1973) proposed the existence of a relatively small number of terminal values (about 18), and a somewhat larger number of instrumental values (about 60 to 70).

The Value Survey (Rokeach, 1973) is a scale in which a person ranks the terminal values and 18 typical instrumental values proposed by Rokeach (1973). The survey lists terminal and instrumental values on separate pages in alphabetical order, and directs the subject to rank the values of each list "in order of importance to YOU, as guiding principles in YOUR life" (Rokeach, 1973, p. 27). Rokeach reported test-retest reliabilities of .74 for terminal values, and .65 for instrumental values in studies involving college students (Rokeach, 1973).

A value system is an organization of hierarchies; terminal values are arranged in a hierarchy according to importance, and each terminal value has its own hierarchy of instrumental values perceived to be useful in its attainment. There is no absolute minimum or maximum importance a value may possess, but a value's importance determines its position relative to other values in the hierarchy. The value system is "stable enough to reflect the fact of sameness and continuity of a unique personality socialized within a given culture and society, yet unstable enough to permit rearrangements of value priorities" (Rokeach, 1973, p. 11).

Dembo et al. and Wright define misfortune as a value loss; that is, the absence or loss of something valuable. Using Rokeach's (1973) model, misfortune can disrupt a person's value system because pre-disability instrumental and terminal values may no longer be germane or do not mesh with one another. When a person sustains a disability, certain abilities and behavior may no longer be accomplished; that is, certain modes of conduct (instrumental values) are no longer adequate or appropriate for reaching terminal values.

As a person confronts disability and the transition of instrumental value hierarchies occurs, he or she may also find that terminal values, once highly regarded, do not have as much importance as they did before disability. For example, a person might consider a successful life as his or her most important terminal goal. Instrumental values might include ambition, productivity, and job advancement. If this person were to sustain a disabling injury that thwarted instrumental values related to his or her job, changes in his or her value system might include other instrumental values (e.g., honesty or perseverance) becoming more important. In addition, other terminal values might surpass a successful life in importance, such as a healthy life, or family security.

Acceptance, then, is a reorganization of instrumental and terminal values in a person's value system to accommodate life changes brought on by disability. Reorganization occurs through value change.

Reformulation of Wright's Value Changes.

What Wright termed "enlargement of the scope of values" can now be considered a shift within the hierarchies of the value system. In the initial stages of dealing with the implications of disability, instrumental and terminal values perceived to be unattainable because of disability stand out in sharp relief. Because a person may be so preoccupied with affected values, those values that are unaffected may be ignored or considered unimportant. As preoccupation diminishes (Wright, 1983), however, other values in the person's life may gain importance, and he or she can focus on goals and experiences that are not precluded by the disability. The values associated with disability may or may not have lost importance in the person's perception, but the scope of values is enlarged; values unaffected by disability gain enough importance to change position in the value system.

The second domain, "subordination of physique relative to other values," can be reconceptualized as a change in the importance of values associated with physical functioning. Within Rokeach's framework, values associated with physique may include competence, physical ability, and attractiveness. The importance of these values may shift downward in the different hierarchies of instrumental values, whereas other values not so closely related to physical functioning may gain importance (e.g., honesty, imagination, self-control, determination). The relative importance of values associated with physical losses has changed so that their importance or value has been subordinated.

The value change that Wright (1983) called "containment of disability effects" can be characterized as a correction of an inaccurate hierarchical shift During the period of mourning or preoccupation with loss, certain instrumental and terminal values may be judged inappropriate or unattainable because of lost ability. Spread occurs when values other than those directly affected by disability are perceived as similarly inappropriate or unattainable, when in fact they remain viable. Spread may cause the downward shift of values in a hierarchy, or even their complete removal from it. With containment of spread, the importance and appropriateness of these values are recognized and the values regain an important place in the hierarchy.

The fourth value change, "transformation of comparative-status values to asset values," is qualitatively different from Wright's other proposed value changes. It represent a fundamental change in the basis for evaluation of abilities, actions, or traits. That is, instead of a standard of comparison, the intrinsic usefulness or worth of something determines its value. As a result of this fundamental change, the position of affected values in the hierarchies may change. For example, if a person perceives values (e.g., beauty, mobility) only in relation to other persons or to an idealized, unattainable standard, then a shift in values that promotes acceptance may be difficult to achieve. In contrast, if a person perceives an ability or affection as intrinsically important (e.g, a person with AIDS advocating for basic human rights such as equal access to employment), then this evaluation promotes hierarchical shifts that encourage acceptance of disability and self-worth.

Wright (1983) posits several experiences that can occur to overcome mourning and begin the process of value change. One experience could be the onset of disability itself; a traumatic injury may be so shocking that the person recognizes what he or she finds truly important. For example, an attractive, vain person, when seriously burned, may focus on being alive rather than on the permanent scarring that changes his or her appearance. Rokeach (1973), in addition to Wright, discusses the utility of education, observation of others in similar situations (e.g., those with disability), and the realization of contradictions in one's value system, as catalysts of shifts in the value system.

Rokeach's (1973) analysis clarifies the value changes of acceptance and provides a systematic method for recording shifts in value hierarchies (i.e., Rokeach's Value Survey, 1973). Used before, during, and after treatment, Rokeach's Value

Survey may provide evidence for specific shifts of instrumental and terminal values. Knowledge of which values are more likely to be affected in the acceptance of the loss process may be important information about where to most effectively intervene. An upward shift in the "imaginative" instrumental value during the initial stages of rehabilitation might encourage therapists to focus the client on problem-solving and creative use of materials such as adaptive equipment.

SUMMARY AND CONCLUSION

The work of Dembo et al. (1975) and Wright (1983) has guided the thinking and practice of rehabilitation psychologists for almost four decades. Despite its importance, however, the major premises of the acceptance of loss theory remain largely untested. For the field to advance, we must go beyond global evaluations of acceptance of disability during a single point in time to intensive longitudinal analyses of the social psychological process linking onset of disability, value change, and acceptance of loss. We have proposed that Rokeach's (1973) analysis of values may be helpful in clarifying the structure and meaning of value changes following disability. We have also offered specific suggestions for improving the measurement of acceptance of loss and the rigor of research designs.

REFERENCES

Butts, S., & Shontz, F.C. (1962). Comparative evaluation and its relation to coping effectiveness. *American Psychologist, 17,* 326 (Abstract).

Dembo, T., Leviton, G. L., & Wright, B. A. (1975). Adjustment to misfortune: A problem of social-psychological rehabilitation. *Rehabilitation Psychology, 22,* 1-100. (Reprinted from Artificial Limbs, 1956, 3, 4–62.)

Dion, K., Berscheid, E., & Walster, E. (1972). What is beautiful is good. *Journal of Personality and Social Psychology, 24,* 285–290.

English, W. R., & Oberle, J. B. (1971). Toward the development of new methodology for examining attitudes towards disabled persons. *Rehabilitation Counseling Bulletin, 15,* 88–96.

Glueckauf, R. L., & Quittner, A. L. (1992). Assertiveness training for disabled adults in wheelchairs: Self-report, role-play, and activity pattern outcomes. *Journal of Consulting and Clinical Psychology, 60,* 419–425.

Keany K. C. M-H. (1993). *Disability and value change: A review of the adjustment to misfortune theory and the development of the Acceptance of Disability Inventory.* Unpublished masters' thesis, Purdue School of Science, Indiana University-Purdue University at Indianapolis.

Kerlinger, F. N. (1986). *Foundations of behavioral research.* Fort Worth, TX: Holt, Rinehart, & Winston.

Linkowski, D. C. (1986). *The acceptance of disability scale.* (Available from Dr. Linkowski, George Washington University, Washington, DC.)

Linkowski, D. C. (1971). A scale to measure acceptance of disability. *Rehabilitation Counseling Bulletin, 14,* 236–244.

Linkowski, D. C., & Dunn, M. A. (1974). Self-concept and acceptance of disability. *Rehabilitation Counseling Bulletin, 18,* 28–32.

Livneh, H. (1980). The process of adjustment to disability: Feelings, behaviors, and counseling strategies. *Psychosocial Rehabilitation Journal, 4*(2), 26–35.

Marinelli, R. P., & Dell Orto, A. E. (1984). *The psychological and social impact of physical disability.* New York: Springer Publishing Co.

Morgan, B., & Leung, P. (1980). Effects of assertion training on acceptance of disability by physically disabled university students. *Journal of Counseling Psychology, 27,* 209–212.

Nadler, A., Sheinberg, L., & Jaffe, Y. (1975). Coping with stress in male paraplegics through help seeking: The role of acceptance of physical disability in help-seeking and-receiving behaviors. In C. D. Spielberger, I. G. Sarason, and N. A. Milgram (Eds.), *Stress and anxiety* (vol. 8, pp. 375–384). Ramat Aviv, Israel: Tel Aviv University.

Nunnally, J. C. (1978). *Psychometric theory.* New York: McGraw-Hill.

Rokeach, M. (1973). *The nature of values.* New York: Free Press.

Shontz, F. C. (1984). Spread in response to imagined loss: An empirical analogue. *Rehabilitation Psychology, 29,* 77–84.

Shontz, F. C. (1975). *The psychological aspects of physical illness and disability.* New York: Macmillan.

Wright, B. A. (1960). *Physical disability: A psychological approach.* New York: Harper & Row.

Wright, B. A. (1983). *Physical disability: A psychosocial approach* (2nd edition). New York: Harper & Row.

Yuker, H. E., Block, J. R., & Younng, J. H. (1966). *The measurement of attitudes towards disabled persons.* Albertson, NY: Human Resources Center.

11

Personal Hopefulness: A Conceptual Review of the Relevance of the Perceived Future to Psychiatry

Kenneth P. Nunn

T here are good reasons why hope should be considered to a greater degree than it has been in the past. First, the loss of hope has been shown to predict suicide as, or more powerfully, than depressive disorder (Beck, Steer, Kovacs & Garrison, 1985; Dyer & Kreitman, 1984; Wetzel, 1976). Second, the loss of hope and the generalization of hopelessness has been implicated in the mediating pathway between social processes and the personal experience of depression (Brown & Harris, 1978). Third, hope and despair contribute to therapeutic efficacy as a study factor, an outcome factor, an intervening variable and a recovery factor (Brown, Lemyre & Bifulco, 1992; Frank, 1973; Greene, 1989; Snyder, Harris & Anderson, 1991*a*). Fourth, hope and the disorders of hope may be of central importance in mind–body interactions. The role of hope and the loss of hope in the precipitation, perpetuation and emotional burden of physical illness have been considered indirectly and qualitatively (Buehler, 1975; Schmale & Iker, 1971), and more recently directly and quantitatively (Elliott, Witty, Herrick & Hoffmann, 1991; Peterson, Maier & Seligman, 1993; Snyder, Irving & Anderson, 1991*b*). Fifth, our study of post-earthquake morbidity (Nunn, Lewin, Walton & Carr, 1996) demonstrated that personal hopefulness contributed as much to the variance in symptomatology as did earthquake exposure. Sixth, notions such as learned helplessness, which have been influential in

I wish to thank Professor Beverley Raphael for encouraging me to develop my interest in hope and Professor Tony Cox and Professor Vaughan Carr for helping me to rekindle my own hopefulness. I also wish to thank Terry Lewin, Jane Walton and Akin Akinwunme for their contributions to the preparation of this paper and Ms Jocelyne Kenny for preparing the final manuscript.

From *British Journal of Medical Psychology, 69,* (1996), 227–245. Reprinted with permission.

the development of new forms of therapy, are being increasingly reformulated to include the perceived future (Abramson, Alloy & Metalsky, 1989; Seligman, 1992). Finally, a consideration of personal hopefulness will lead to a reevaluation of the significance of concepts such as depression, institutionalism and anxiety. The aims of this paper are to review the definition of, and theoretical issues relating to, hope in the context of psychiatry. The measurement of hope, in particular trait personal hopefulness, has been addressed elsewhere (Nunn *et al.*, 1996).

THE DEFINITION OF HOPE

A definition of hope includes (Murray, 1976):

Temporality—Hope is future oriented and the notion of time is implicit. Experiential time, namely, 'philosophical, social, cultural constructions of the world and their effects on the interpretations of time experience', rather than chronological time, is of most relevance (Ornstein, 1969). The construction of the perceived future has not been elevated to a faculty of brain function in the same way as the construction of the perceived past, namely, memory. Despite this, anticipation, planning, foresight and the executive functions are pivotal to human adaptation (Luria, 1978; McCarthy & Warrington, 1990).

Desirability—Hope includes the 'wished-for' future. Desire impels to the attainment or possession of something. It is a goal oriented, positive emotion directed towards the future and experienced as wanting, striving, longing, yearning, or even craving. Hope is not merely cognitive, but conative and therefore implicit to motivation (Hershberger, 1989). The intensity of desire is a function of the importance or value to the individual of what is hoped for. At a complex level, it is also possible to desire that a feared outcome will not eventuate.

Expectancy—Hope is the belief that the desired future is both possible and probable (Stotland, 1969). Probability here refers to subjectively anticipated likelihoods. Kuvlesky & Bealer (1966) distinguished between aspiration and expectation. Aspiration or desirability without expectancy is more accurately described as wishful thinking. Occasionally, something or someone is so important, so desired, that belief and behavior are contoured to the possible, even when perceived probabilities are low.

Hope, then, is that general tendency to construct and respond to the perceived future *positively. The hopeful* person subjectively assesses what is desired for the future to be *probable or so important* as to constrain belief and behaviour to be grounded upon its *possibility.* This definition conforms to the elements Stotland (1969) identified. His work represents the first scientific overview of hope in psychology. The results of our work and others suggest that

Stotland (1969) was largely correct in his predictions that expectation of outcome was as, or more, critical than control (Hull & Mendolia, 1991) and that hope was as pertinent to anxiety as to depression (see Nunn *et al.*, 1996).

The Object of Hope

There is evidence that hope is directed towards the different domains of human experience in a discriminating fashion. Personal, professional and communal domains of experience may each elicit different expectations for the future (Schmidt, Lamm & Trommsdorff, 1978). Hopefulness in one domain may diminish or enhance hopefulness in another. The overall or global personal hopefulness of an individual, as a pervasive response across all domains of experience, reflects the degree to which these domains correlate with each other. This paper, together with our quantitative research (Nunn *et al.*, 1996), primarily address global personal hopefulness and our instrument (the Hunter Opinions and Personal Expectations Scale), is an example of instruments that measure generalized expectancies (Scheier & Carver, 1987).

The Subject of Hope

Who is desiring, expecting and therefore hoping? Different authors have investigated hopefulness at an individual, family, institutional and cultural level (Obayuwana *et al.*, 1982; Stotland & Kobler, 1965; Tonge, James & Hillam, 1975; Turnbull, 1974). Kellehear (1984) argued that confusion emerges when phenomena at an intrapsychic level are conflated with phenomena at a societal level. It is preferable, therefore, to refer to individual group, family, communal, corporate or collective hope recognizing that different phenomena and principles may emerge at each level. Interestingly, the same distinction has been raised in the helplessness literature (Simkin, Lederer & Seligman, 1983). Further, it is necessary to ask what aspect of functioning is described by the term hopefulness. Some authors see cognitions as primary with affective and behavioural phenomena as secondary (Kovacs & Beck, 1978; Seligman, 1992). This tendency to reduce hope to cognitive events, and then to ascribe causal primacy to cognitions, is inadequate. It fails to explain the hopeful depressive, the despairing person who has suicidal ideation but is not depressed and the person who is neither hopeful nor despairing but is depressed in the context of a cognitive void, lacking positive expectations. It also fails to explain why those with depressive or suicidal ideation are not always affectively impaired. Others see affective and relational phenomena as primary (French, 1958). Averill (1991) uses the term 'intellectual emotions' in which hope, subjectively and behaviourally, is socially and culturally determined. Still others (Luria, 1978) see the components of hope, such as planning, intentionality and expectancy, as fundamental expressions of central nervous system activity. Gray (1990) has emphasized the intimacy of neural hardware for emotions and cognitions despite their seeming separation upon introspection. At this stage, it is probably most helpful to consider hope as a multidimensional responsiveness to the future, without *a priori* statements as to the primacy of one or other aspect of personal functioning in the genesis of personal hopefulness.

The Phenomenology of Hope

Darwin (1890) was perhaps the first to draw detailed attention to the phenomenology of despair. Despair was grouped with low spirits, anxiety, grief and dejection. Behavioural and cognitive theorists have concentrated on describing what people without hope think and do (Beck, 1967). Until recently (Averill, Catlin & Chon, 1990; Seligman, 1992) little has been written about what hopeful people think and do. The activities of hope, both cognitive and behavioural, are distinguished by their implicit investment in the future. However, the interpretation of behaviours is ambiguous. Preparing one's will and testament may reveal personal despair or vicarious hopefulness for one's children. Cognitions are less ambiguous.

Stotland's trilogy of books remains the most comprehensive cognitive psychology of hope (Kobler & Stotland, 1964; Stotland & Kobler, 1965; Stotland, 1969). Stotland's most important contribution has been in his formulation of testable hypotheses of hope, namely: that motivation is proportional to the perceived importance and probability of attaining a goal; that the greater the perceived importance and probability of attaining a goal, the greater the affect experienced; that when perceived importance of attaining a goal is high and perceived probability low, anxiety is experienced; and that motivation to goal attainment is increased by anxiety. He saw the early experiments on learned helplessness as examples of learned hopelessness. Stotland's work, along with Kobler, was essentially descriptive and definitional. They did not measure hope quantitatively or explore its role in non-clinical populations.

Averill *et al.* (1990) have carried out a series of studies on the social construction of hope as an emotion. In their view, optimism is more enduring, more intellectual, more accurate in the assessment of likelihoods and less personal than hope. Optimism is generally used in the psychological literature by those who wish to limit the concept of perception of and responsiveness to the future to a cognitive framework. The subject of optimism will be addressed later in this paper when examining Seligman's work. However, what can be said is that the distinguishing features of hope are cognitive and conative, not cognitive alone. It is, therefore, premature to discriminate between the phenomenology of hope and that of optimism. Further, as Averill *et al.* (1990) argue, there are no discriminating affective or behavioural features of hope, in contrast to despair. This is not to say that there are no affective and behavioural concomitants of hope, but rather that these are not specific. Positive and negative affectivity (Clark, Watson & Mineka, 1994; Watson, Clark & Harkness, 1994) are shaped by the perceived future (Lazarus, 1991). This future-oriented binary shaping of emotional tone is referred to by Lazarus (1991) as primary appraisal and is based on the perceived importance of an event and the perceived likely outcome.

The Stability and Predictiveness of Personal Hopefulness

If the construct of personal hopefulness is salient to the human condition, it ought to be predictive of future experience. If it is worth measuring, it must be relatively enduring. This is not to ignore fluctuations in hope, but to postulate both state and trait aspects which may or may not interact. Eysenck & Eysenck (1970) argued that optimism was a characteristic of stable extroverts with choleric temperaments, whilst pessimism was a feature of unstable introverts with melancholic temperaments. Our final measure (Nunn *et al.*, 1996) is one of trait or dispositional hopefulness rather than state or episodic hopefulness. We attempted to measure state personal hopefulness but were unsuccessful in that our measure was too stable over time. If expectations are probed in any measure it is likely that stability is introduced because of the enduring nature of expectations in comparison with affect or more episodic cognitions. Individual hopes may wax and wane but perceptions of one's global future are very stable.

Hope by Exclusion

There is a danger of defining hope by exclusion of despair or, in more general terms, of defining mental health by exclusion of disorder. There are people who do not fear the worst but do not expect their hope to be fulfilled. They are without hope but not despairing. It is unfortunate that the term hopelessness in the literature designates 'global negative expectations' rather than 'the absence of global positive expectations'. There is no term for the experience of being without positive or negative expectations. It is also possible, as mentioned earlier, that positive expectations might be directed towards feared outcomes not occurring. For this reason the term despair is preferable when referring to negative global expectations and hopelessness should be reserved for the absence of positive expectations. However, the established and popular usage will require ambiguity for some time to come.

It does not follow that hope is the absence of despair, that despair is the absence of hope, or that they cannot coexist (Tonge *et al.*, 1975). The possibility of negative and positive affects and expectations coexisting, subject to different determinants and directed towards different domains of experience must be borne in mind in any research methodology. An analogous situation occurred in the studies on well-being where positive and negative affect were found to be independent dimensions (Bradburn, 1969). The best predictor of well-being was the discrepancy between the scores of positive and negative affect. Diener's (1984) review of subjective well-being elaborated some of the complexities of this finding, highlighting the importance of not confusing the determinants of morbidity and well-being. Surprisingly, the learned optimism literature treats optimism and pessimism as polar opposites (Peterson *et al.,* 1993).

The Reality Basis of Hope

Hope, like Utopia, is associated all too commonly with unrealistic aspirations. It is the stock-in-trade of the politician, the charismatic healer and the charlatan. 'Fraudulent hope is one of the greatest malefactors . . .' (Bloch, 1986, p. 5). It may thus be dismissed as intangibly subjective. However, it may also have been treated adversely by the psychoanalytic tradition in which hope is affiliated with denial. Hope was seen as a denial of vulnerability (Menninger, 1959). There had, until recently, been a neglect of invulnerability and resilience (Rutter, 1985). However, hope does not preclude realism.

The concept of denial requires some clarification. The belief that what is desirable is probable, may or may not be based on the realities of the situation. There are some people who remain hopeful when most others concede that the situation appears hopeless. It is also possible for a person to take cognizance of the constraints of reality, but not to base hopefulness upon them. A person may fail to acknowledge reality constraints and also fail to be hopeful. Lack of realism can characterize despair as well as hope (Moltmann, 1967). Seligman (1992) maintains that pessimists are more realistic. The evidence he cites is largely in relation to mild depression and mostly assesses the comparative accuracy of the perceptions of pessimistic versus optimistic participants descriptively and not predictively. Gollin, Terrell & Johnson (1977) and Alloy & Ahrens (1987) did show that non-depressed people overestimate their chances of success while depressed people estimate accurately. However, Seligman's group suggest that under extreme or boundary conditions depressed participants distort while the non-depressed do not (Peterson *et al.,* 1993). The debate about positive illusions and psychological well-being has not been resolved (Colvin & Block, 1994; Taylor & Brown, 1994). Personal hopefulness and the construct of 'denial' as a coping mechanism are complex notions to do with responding to reality. Personal hopefulness is the response of a person associated with the belief that what is desirable is possible. Denial does not merely interpret reality differently. Rather, it negates that reality (Vaillant, 1977).

Nor must it always be assumed that hope is *ipso facto* adaptive and despair maladaptive. Lazarus' (1981) argument for a cost-benefit analysis of denial is equally applicable to hope. There is the possibility that hope may sometimes function paradoxically or that despair in specific domains may be therapeutic (Bennett & Bennett, 1984; Watzlawick, 1983). Norem & Cantor (1986) have shown how some people use pessimistic cognitive strategies, defensive pessimism, to cope with situations that threaten self-esteem or failure. They were able to demonstrate that interference with this strategy by reassurance and encouragement produced deficits in performance. Seligman (1992) has emphasized the importance of flexible optimism which encourages the choice of optimism in low-risk situations, where there is little to lose by being optimistic, or where pessimism is impairing performance.

COMPONENTS OF PERSONAL HOPEFULNESS

Mastery—the Future

The theme of perceived mastery of the future comprises four main notions: personal agency (or responsibility); personal adequacy (efficacy and or competence); environmental malleability (or responsiveness); and illness responsiveness. Personal responsibility for one's future and perceived adequacy to meet the demands, cope (Luthar & Zigler, 1991) and fulfil one's aspirations and maintain a sense of control recur frequently in the literature (Bandura, 1977; Rotter, 1966; Seligman, 1975). Personal agency and adequacy need to be complemented with that individual's perception of the environment as yielding or not yielding to their desires and coping strategies. Environmental responsiveness and illness response have elements in common when the self is experienced as struggling against the body. Brown & Inouye (1978) have also demonstrated the possibility that helplessness (and, *ergo* hopefulness) may be learned through modelling, again emphasizing possible environmental contributors. Bandura's notion of perceived self-efficacy does not give a central role to external circumstance (a benign or hostile environment, luck, religious faith) in influencing outcome expectancy. Further, Bandura sees outcome expectancy as the subjective probability that a given act produces a given outcome. Scheier & Carver (1985, 1987) and Stotland (1969) take outcome expectancy to mean the subjective probability that a desired outcome will occur, whether or not the individual contributes to it.

In the psychosomatic literature, the positive response of an individual to illness in terms of a 'fighting spirit' or negatively in terms of 'giving up' implies an existential posture of mastery or defeat (Greer, 1983; Schmale, 1972). Similarly, the responsiveness of an individual's illness to personal activities, attitudes and coping strategies has been documented (Meares, 1983; Peterson & Bossio, 1991; Ray & Baum, 1985). Mastery contrasts with the notion of helplessness. Hopelessness and helplessness are frequently linked in clinical description, in both therapist and patient (Adler, 1972). The key issues of control of the future, with its many threats, and the possibility of contributing to a positive outcome, is recurrent. Zimmerman (1990) has linked the cognate meanings of control under the rubric of learned hopefulness mirroring the Seligman model but emphasizing social participation and empowerment. What Zimmerman, along with others, fails to consider is the possibility that differences may exist between individuals in the need for perceived control in order to feel positively about the future.

Purpose in Life

The attribution of meaning to present experience with its implications for the future is central to the process of hoping. Purpose in life and the capacity to make sense of one's experience are suggested as means of sustaining hope (Fitzgerald, 1979; Frankl, 1978). Antonovsky (1987) uses the notion of coherence as a protective factor against disorganized and fractionating experiences which lead to unpredictability. Attribution (Weiner, 1985), and more specifically explanatory style, have attracted particular interest with regard to depression from those interested in the paradigm of learned helplessness (Abramson, Seligman & Teasdale, 1978). It is a logical development for this group of researchers to focus on learned optimism (Seligman, 1992). In so doing they link the psychology of personal control, explanatory style and future orientation. What is frequently not appreciated is that Seligman and Abramson see attributions of causality as indirect modifiers of behaviour through their impact on expectancy. Despite this, learned helplessness researchers do not usually measure expectancies directly.

Future Support and Leadership

Stotland (1985) believes that there are some people who primarily hope because of their trust in others. The perceived future availability, adequacy and responsiveness of significant others has been described by Henderson, Byrne & Duncan-Jones (1981) as an anxious attachment factor. This work highlights the significant contribution that the perceived future ('the anxious attachment factor') makes to the variance in accounting for the emergence of neurosis. Since anxious attachment involves the fear that others will not be available, it has a relation to both trust and self-reliance.

The perceived *future* availability, and adequacy of significant others, may be more significant than the *current* support. The hopefulness *for* a significant other (i.e. vicarious hopefulness) is an important determinant in the way relatives and therapists behave. The perceived future desirability of an individual to significant others may modify his or her hopefulness (i.e. How much do individuals believe they will be wanted by others?) The perceived adequacy and reliability of leadership figures can be especially significant. In the case of illness, this could be the physician, or a leader in a disaster (Henderson & Bostock, 1977). Stotland & Kobler (1965) have documented the key role played by the administration of a psychiatric hospital in promoting an epidemic of suicide of its in-patients. Wing & Brown (1970) have documented less dramatic effects in psychiatric rehabilitation wards where leadership style characterized by enthusiasm was associated with decreased length of stay of institutionalized patients. Thompson (1965), in his history of 20th century England, sees one of Churchill's main social and leadership functions as a provider of hope during the Second World War. Zimmerman & Rappaport (1988) found that cognitive, motivational and personality measures of perceived control formed one discriminant function and correlated positively with leadership and negatively with alienation. There is evidence that voters are more likely to vote for optimistic candidates (Zullow, Oettingen, Peterson & Seligman, 1988).

View of Future Self and Trajectory

Self-esteem has always held a central place in psychology and psychiatry (Coopersmith, 1967). It has, however, largely been treated with regard to the present view of the self. The explanation of the past determinants of present self-esteem has been foremost. The function of the perceived future self, and with it future trajectory, has received modest attention (Coleman, Herzberg & Morris, 1977). Melges, Anderson, Kraemer, Tinklenborg & Weisz (1971) found that self-esteem and future outlook were highly correlated ($r = .89$). Abramson *et al.* (1989) see lowered self-esteem as a symptom emerging from viewing adversity's causes as internal, stable and global and when inferred negative characteristics about themselves are deemed as less adequate or less desirable in comparison to peers, important to their self-concept and not remediable or likely to change. When this is extrapolated to the future, hopelessness ensues. A hopeful attributional corollary has not been elaborated.

Optimism and Pessimism and the
Theory of Learned Helplessness

Seligman (1992) portrays most people as seeing the world in either an optimistic or a pessimistic manner. Optimists tend to interpret setbacks as temporary, obstacles as surmountable, causes of adversity as circumscribed and defeat as derived externally to themselves. Pessimists, on the other hand, tend to believe negative life-events will produce difficulties for a prolonged period (permanent or stable), that the impact will pervade most of what they do (pervasive or global) and that the events are their own fault (personalized or internal). Seligman identifies underachievement, depression and physical illness as the outcomes of pessimism, and helplessness as the core. Learned helplessness theory has three essential components (Peterson *et al.*, 1993): *contingency, cognition and behaviour. Contingency* 'refers to the objective relationship between the person's action and the outcomes that she/he then experiences. The most important contingency here is uncontrollability: a random relationship between an individual's action and outcomes (p. 8).' *Cognition* 'refers to the way in which the person perceives, explains, and extrapolates the contingency (p. 8).' *Behaviour* 'refers to the observable consequences of (non) contingency and the person's cognitions about it. Typically, helplessness studies measure someone's passivity versus activity. . . . In addition, helplessness theory claims that other consequences may follow as well from the individual's expectation of future helplessness: cognitive, low self-esteem, sadness, loss of aggression, immune changes, and physical illness (p. 8). . . . A pure case of learned helplessness must have all three components: noncontingency between the person's actions and outcomes, the expectation that the outcome will not be contingent in the future, and passive behaviour (p. 9)'.

Abramson *et al.* (1978) reviewed and updated the original theory with their 'attributional reformulation'. They argued that when people find themselves helpless they ask why they are helpless. The causal attribution they make determines the generality, the chronicity of their helplessness, and their self-esteem. The original helplessness theory did not distinguish between those situations in which a person perceived the problem as insoluble and those in which the person perceived that it was soluble but he or she was unable to solve it. They resolved this by distinguishing personal and universal helplessness, using the internal versus external dichotomy. The second inadequacy of the initial formulation was the failure to specify where and when a person who expects outcomes to be uncontrollable will show deficits. Helplessness may be situation specific or more global, chronic or transient. These attributions were seen as predicting expectations, but the expectations were determinative of the helplessness deficits. Further, these attributional tendencies of individuals were hypothesized to be stable over time in the form of an attributional style.

Abramson *et al.* (1978) were also concerned about the implications of inadequacies of the original learned helplessness theory for their model of depression. They were aware that expectation of uncontrollability alone is not sufficient to produce depressive affect. They proposed that affective changes resulted from an expectation that aversive events will occur, irrespective of the perception of uncontrollability. Second, they proposed two types of depression, with and without lowered self-esteem, corresponding to the tendency to internalize the cause. They also clarified the central dilemma: that learned helplessness posited a perceived loss of control in depression while depressives were known to internalize. They proposed that depressives internalized the cause which, because they believe it to be stable and global, leaves them with an expectancy of inability to alter outcome.

Thus, Abramson *et al.*'s (1978) reformulation enabled the fundamental transition from behavioural animal research to cognitive human clinical phenomena. Perceived controllability of the future was moderated by the way the past was explained in time and space. The same sophistication could have been achieved by looking at expectations directly in terms of internality, stability and globality (Scheier & Carver, 1987). However, this would have jeopardized the original formulation more fundamentally, since perceived non-contingency would be neither necessary nor sufficient for helplessness or depression. Despite the richness of the insights, there is an obfuscation of their fundamental caveat, namely, that expectations are the final common pathway to helplessness and their research did not measure expectations directly. In the same year, Brown & Harris (1978) published their classic work on the social origins of depression in Camberwell women. Central to their theorizing was the experience of hopelessness. In particular, they proposed that life-events involving threat, disappointment and loss that led to a *generalized* sense of hopelessness was aetiological in depression. Earlier losses, especially loss of the mother before the age of 11, were presented as pathoplastic in terms of whether a psychotic or neurotic picture emerged. This pathoplastic effect was seen as a measure of severity and related in attachment terms to the earlier experiences of rejection (e.g. with separation by divorce), and abandonment (e.g. with loss by death). This difference was attributed to the difference between threat to hopes that might lead to a clinical picture of protest and the irrevocable loss of hope that might lead to despair. Their position has subsequently been criticized (Tennant & Bebbington, 1978); however, their basic model of depression remains intact. The centrality of the loss of hope emerged more clearly in a paper by Abramson *et al.* (1989), which was specifically directed at depression. They proposed a hopelessness theory of depression and denied that it was an attributional theory. Thus, hopelessness was a proximal sufficient cause of depression rather than merely a symptom of it.

Abramson *et al.* (1989) made several theoretical shifts which paved the way for a fundamental departure from the original learned helplessness model: (1) they replaced helplessness with hopelessness—the crucial expectational component was no longer that of whether the outcome was perceived as controllable but, what the expected outcome would be; (2) hopelessness was no longer a symptom of helplessness but elevated to a proximal sufficient cause; (3) though necessary, helplessness was no longer sufficient to produce depression except insofar as it led to hopelessness; (4) hedonic valance (desirability or importance of the desired or feared outcomes) was included in the contributing factors— thus, conative or motivational factors were considered; (5) hopelessness was a sufficient but not necessary cause of depression—no one phenomenological picture of depression was linked to hopelessness although specific symptomatic links could be made [by way of contrast, Beck (1967) saw hopelessness as a necessary but not always sufficient cause of depression]; (6) attributions, as to cause, consequence and the self, were neither necessary nor sufficient but proximal contributory causes only; (7) attributions of consequences of negative expectancies or non-fulfillment of positive expectancies were emphasized while causal attributions were de-emphasized; (8) negative attributions about the self rather than internalization *per se* were seen as lowering self-esteem—this enables a merging of Beck's views and these authors; (9) attributional style is relegated to a distal contributory cause along with environmental factors such as negative life-events; and (10) the authors postulate a stress-diathesis model of depression analogous to Brown & Harris' (1978) model—however, by way of contrast, the hopelessness theory has less emphasis on self-esteem as the central vulnerability or diathesis. Loss is not seen as the principal stressor. What is perhaps not appreciated is that Stotland (1969) proposed a similar, but wider ranging model of hope in the 1960s. Strangely, Abramson *et al.* (1978, 1989) do not cite him. Further, Abramson *et al.*'s (1989) thesis does not take into account the possibility that expectations, though most determinative, might be easier to access via attributions experientially; causal immediacy and experiential immediacy may not be synonymous. Thus, people may find it easier to discuss their style of attributions than to access their expectations directly.

The hope literature therefore raises a number of key concerns for the helplessness literature. The behaviour of helplessness has been linked to the cognitions of hopelessness. Control or the expectation of no control has been modified to consider expectation of outcome. Optimism and pessimism as measured by the Life Orientation Test (Plomin *et al.,* 1992) and the Attributional Style Questionnaire (Schulman, Keith & Seligman, 1993) have also been shown to have a significant heritable contribution. Helplessness may have 'hardwired' aspects and therefore not be entirely learned. The focus on helplessness has shifted to hopelessness and thence to hope (Nunn, in press).

Morale, Demoralization and Hope

There are many synonyms for hope within the literature. Frank (1985) has elaborated the role of morale and its corresponding notions of demoralization. He has spent a great deal more time elaborating demoralization and the anti-demoralization hypothesis. By demoralization, he means that the person 'suffers from a sense of failure, a loss of self-esteem, feelings of hopelessness or helplessness, of alienation or isolation. These are often accompanied by a sense of mental confusion which may be expressed by a fear of insanity' (Frank, 1985). The difficulties with demoralization as a concept are: (1) the lack of operational definitions for either morale or demoralization and clarification of their interrelationship; (2) the lack of instruments to measure the construct directly—the Psychiatric Epidemiology Research Interview (Dohrenwend, Shrout, Egri & Mendelsohn, 1980) has been put forward as a measure of demoralization, but only insofar as it measures non-specific psychosocial distress; (3) the tendency to include very different experiences, such as alienation and loss of self-esteem, without clear criteria for inclusion or exclusion of other experiences; and (4) the lack of clarity as to the relationship of demoralization to other constructs such as internal/external locus of control, introversion/extraversion, and psychiatric disorder. These objections aside, Frank (1985) has raised the important issue, in passing, that depression has become an over-inclusive concept with poorly defined discriminatory criteria (Snaith, 1993; Thompson, 1989) from other disorders of experience, in particular anxiety and the disorders of morale.

Vulnerability, Coping, Resilience, Hardiness, and Subjective Well-being

Vulnerability has specific implications with regard to hope, with the implied possibility that the 'plaintiff set' represents one variety of the disorders of hopefulness (Brown & Harris, 1978; Tennant & Bebbington, 1978). The perceived future with regard to mastery, meaning, interpersonal support and self-esteem is likely to be a key contributing factor in the development of the 'plaintiff set'. What is unclear is the extent to which a positive perceived future protects against the development of psychopathology. Hope is also implicated in the literature relating to coping behaviour and protective factors (Brown & Harris, 1978; Henderson & Bostock, 1977; WHO Expert Committee, 1977).

Henderson & Bostock (1977) studied the coping behaviour of seven men who survived a shipwreck and were not rescued until 13 days later. The principal behaviours shown by the men were attachment ideation, drive to survive modelling, prayer and hope. Whilst a formulation is attempted in terms of attachment theory, the dominant theme of the paper is one of hope. Each of the behaviours had the effect of expressing or inducing the key elements of hope. Time orientation was towards the future. Desire for reunion, survival and help were expressed. Expectations were buoyed up. Attachment behaviour promoted reunion expectations, but also fuelled determination. The drive to survive prevented 'giving up' except in the one man who died on the fifth day, after having 'given up'. Modelling of a leader 'provided a model of competence, rationality, and hope'. Prayer 'reduced anxiety and allowed the retention of hope'. Finally, in commenting on hope itself, the authors highlight four adaptive characteristics of hope. Hope provides the anticipation of relief, is enhanced through verbalization, sustained by a credible leader, and controls mood to enable survival behaviour. Their study highlights the close relationship between coping responses and the perceived future. Lazarus' (1991) concepts of primary and secondary appraisal style, shaping positive and negative affect in coping, are extremely close to the notion of hope and despair as elaborated in this paper.

Much of psychiatric assessment has focused on the history of developing vulnerability and how it has become realized in psychopathology. Only recently have the discontinuities of development and the formation of personal resilience been recognized as important (Luthar & Zigler, 1991; Nunn, 1995; Rutter, 1981, 1985; Rutter & Quinton, 1984). Kobasa (1979) developed the concept of hardiness of personality to capture those people who tolerate high levels of stress before becoming medically ill. She demonstrated that a higher sense of perceived control, a greater degree of commitment to specific life domains and a greater perception of challenge in response to change were correlated with better health. The processes involved in developing and sustaining personal hopes will require more systematic investigation using the same clearly defined parameters at each stage of the life-cycle without losing sight of the need to adapt those parameters to the unique developmental issues of the study population.

The themes of hope within the literature suggest that hope is a multidimensional concept which, for different individuals, is the final expression of very different determinants. Thus, for some, to be in control may be essential to maintain hope. For others, to make sense of what is happening is more important. For still others, the interpersonal support they perceive will be available is more decisive than either a perception of mastery or meaning. The common theme, irrespective of the particular mechanisms, is the way in which desires and fears become consolidated into expectations.

HOPE AND DISORDER

Loss of hope has been implicated as one of the major features of a number of psychiatric disorders, especially suicide (Beck *et al.,* 1985; Wetzel, 1976) and depression. Hopelessness and depression are often confused. However, it is possible to be depressed but to believe that 'this, too, will pass' and that there is a positive future ahead (Beck *et al.,* 1985; Dyer & Kreitman, 1984; Greene, 1989). It is equally possible not to be clinically depressed, but to have cognitions of despair about the future. In brief, lack of hope and/or despair do not constitute the full syndrome of depression. Nor is it invariably the case that hopelessness accompanies a depressive episode. Depression may have a different prognosis depending upon the presence of high levels of personal hopefulness, high levels of personal despair (Goldney, 1981) or the absence of both. Attempted suicide may be formulated differently if, for instance, it were to be found that those who attempted suicide are characterized by an absence of positive expectancies (hopelessness) rather than the presence of negative ones (despair).

Rholes, Riskind & Neville (1985) found that cognitions of threat were associated with anxiety but not depression while cognitions of loss were associated with both. They also found that transient cognitions at any point in time, as opposed to dispositions, attitudes or traits, were not predictive of depression. However, hopelessness as measured by Beck's Hopelessness Scale (Beck, Weissman & Lester 1974) did predict depression.

Melges (1982) has developed the most comprehensive psychopathology to date based on time and the perceived future. He elaborates a hierarchy in the psychopathology of time with time disorientation (as in dementia) at the top moving through temporal sequence disintegration (as in schizophrenia), rate and rhythm problems (as in depression and mania), temporal perspective problems with overfocus on past, present or future (as in anxiety, antisocial disorders and paranoid disorders) to desynchronized transactions. It is surprising how little his work has been taken up in the research or clinical literature. Stotland (1969) has also developed hypotheses as to how some of these disorders may relate to hope.

Schizophrenia, alcoholism, heroin addiction and the borderline syndrome, have hopelessness as a key feature, either in phenomenology or management (Beck, Steer & Shaw, 1984; Edell, 1984; Fitzgerald, 1979; Ludwig, 1978). But so do illnesses such as chronic bronchitis, ulcerative colitis and malignancies (Engel, 1978; Greer, 1983; Kinsman *et al.,* 1985). Peterson *et al.* (1993) outline (p. 98) a pathway, via the endorphin suppression associated with learned helplessness, to immunosuppression and therefore increased susceptibility to infection and perhaps malignancy. Scheier *et al.* (1989) demonstrated that dispositional optimism predicted problem-focused coping, reduced denial, and was associated with a faster rate of recovery and better post-surgery quality of life in coronary bypass surgery. Visintainer & Seligman (1983) have postulated a causal chain implicating immune function in the association of a wide range of physical disorders and pessimism. Links with such a broad range of conditions and situations suggest that hope and hopelessness may be acting as general mediating or modifying variables.

Disorders of Personal Hopefulness

Are there any conditions that might be seen as disorders of hopefulness *per se*? The syndrome of institutionalization (Barton, 1966) is probably the best example, the principal feature of which is hopelessness. Associated features include apathy, lack of initiative, loss of interest, submissiveness, lack of expression of feelings of resentment at harsh or unfair orders, lack of interest in the future had inability to make plans for it, a deterioration in personal habits, loss of individuality, and a resigned acceptance that things will not change. Other conditions, such as psychosomatic death following voodoo spell, hex and pointing the bone, have as their correlates a powerful belief system in a negative future in association with social isolation and withdrawal of help (Cohen, 1985). In childhood, the pervasive refusal syndrome has helplessness and hopelessness as its core features (Nunn *et al.,* 1996).

So far as personal hopefulness and psychiatric and physical disorder are concerned then, there are at least three main issues. Any disorder may constitute a threat to personal hopefulness. Lack of personal hopefulness may constitute a vulnerability to psychiatric and physical disorder. Loss of hope may constitute disorder in its own right, jeopardizing active survival or predisposing to suicide.

Hope and Recovery

Frank (1973) has argued that placebo is not a non-specific effect of all therapies, but the specific morale restoring effect of any therapy. He argues strongly that all forms of psychotherapy counteract demoralization. Vaillant (1983) and Ludwig (1978) see hope as helpful in recovery from alcoholism and schizophrenia respectively. Brown *et al.* (1992) have linked 'anchoring' experiences with recovery from anxiety disorders and 'fresh start' experiences with recovery from depression. Although they link 'fresh start' experiences with hope, each of their categories represents hopeful changes, as defined in this paper. Thus, anchoring, fresh start, delogjamming, reroutinization and goal adjustment experiences (Brown *et al.,* 1992) all represent a reduction of future threat or the restructuring of future experience.

Melges (1982) has elaborated a future-oriented psychotherapy, Trad (1993) utilizes the notion of provisioning in individual psychotherapy, White (1989) refers to reauthoring in family therapy, while Boscolo & Bertrando (1992) use a time perspective to promote therapeutic change. The role of hope is thus seen as self-evident in behavioural treatments which promote mastery, insight-oriented psychodynamic psychotherapies which provide meaning, supportive therapies which reduce anticipated isolation or alienation, and all forms of therapy that increase one's sense of dignity and self-worth to face the future positively.

CONCLUSION

Despite the extensive use of hope by way of explanation, particularly in clinical settings, it is often diffusely articulated. However, hope is becoming less ethereal, a pervasive and significant correlate of health and disorder, with substantial shifts in current practice and theoretical understanding already beginning to occur. There are some important correlates which flow from these altered notions of the perceived future. First, those therapies which involve exploring the perceived past and vulnerability will also need to consider the perceived future and personal resilience. Second, treatment, particularly for future-sensitive conditions like suicidality and institutionalization, will need to address not merely present needs, but perceived future needs. Third, research methodology often seeks to control for, or exclude, possibly critical intrapersonal effects. The placebo and halo effects, and their relation to the perceived future, would need to be more directly the subject of research inquiry. Fourth, the relation between perceived control and expectation, attribution of causality and expectation, and anxiety and depression will need to be explicated. Fifth, there is the need to develop accurate ways of describing and measuring non-morbid human experience with a view to reformulating afresh the nature of the disorders of experience. The term depression, which has served well in the past, is an imprecise and over-inclusive amalgam of heterogeneous experiences. Uncritical use of the concept should be discouraged to avoid obscurity in an increasingly sophisticated field of inquiry (Snaith, 1993; Thompson, 1989).

Finally, the capacity to assess personal hopefulness in a systematic and comprehensive way will require new skills and a new body of research and clinical knowledge. An accurate method of identifying those dimensions of personal hopefulness that are defective or under threat may provide a more meaningful basis for choosing and integrating various treatment strategies.

Irrespective of the specific developments which emerge, the tendency towards an exclusive preoccupation with the personal past and present, in research and clinical practice, is no longer adequate to provide a comprehensive perspective. The human experience of time, and time in relation to our experience, promises to be of central importance (Lewis, 1932). Temporal experience, which is future oriented and desirable, constitutes a subjective dimension to quality of life which will be increasingly pertinent to psychiatry and the assessment of outcome.

REFERENCES

Abramson, L. Y., Seligman, M. E. & Teasdale, J. D. (1978). Learned helplessness in humans: Critique and reformulation. *Journal of Abnormal Psychology,* **87,** 49–74.

Abramson, L. Y., Alloy, L. B. & Metalsky, G. I. (1989). Hopelessness depression: A theory-based subtype of depression. *Psychological Review,* **96,** 358–372.

Adler, G. (1972). Helplessness in the helpers. *British Journal of Medical Psychology,* **45,** 315–326.

Alloy, L. B. & Ahrens, A. H. (1987). Depression and pessimism for the future: Biased use of statistically relevant information in predictions for self versus others. *Journal of Personality and Social Psychology,* **52,** 366–378.

Antonovsky, A. (1987). *Unravelling the Mystery of Health—How People Cope with Stress and Stay Well.* San Francisco: Jossey-Bass.

Averill, J. R. (1991). Intellectual emotions. In C. D. Spielberg, I. G. Sarason, Z. Kulcsar & G. L. Van Heck (Eds), *Stress and Emotion: Anxiety, Anger and Curiosity,* vol. 14. New York: Hemisphere Publishing Co.

Averill, J. R., Catlin, G. & Chon, K. K. (1990). *Rules of Hope.* New York: Springer-Verlag.

Bandura, A. (1977). Self-efficacy: Toward a unifying theory of behavioural change. *Psychological Review,* **84,** 191–215.

Barton, R. (1966). *Institutional Neurosis.* Bristol: Wright.

Beck, A. T. (1967). *Depression: Clinical, Experimental and Theoretical Aspects.* New York: Hoebner Medical Division.

Beck, A. T., Steer, R. A., Kovacs, M. & Garrison, B. (1985). Hopelessness and eventual suicide: A 10 year prospective study of patients. *American Journal of Psychiatry,* **142,** 559–563.

Beck, A. T., Steer, R. A. & Shaw, B. P. (1984). Hopelessness in alcohol and heroin dependent women. *Journal of Clinical Psychology,* **40,** 602–606.

Beck, A. T., Weissman, A. & Lester, D. (1974). The measurement of pessimism: The hopelessness scale. *Journal of Consulting and Clinical Psychology,* **47,** 861–865.

Bennett, M. I. & Bennett, M. B. (1984). The uses of hopelessness. *American Journal of Psychiatry,* **141,** 559–562.

Bloch, E. (1986). *The Principle of Hope* (3 vols.) Oxford: Basil Blackwell.

Boscolo, L. & Bertrando, P. (1992). *The Times of Time—A New Perspective in Systemic Therapy and Consultation.* London: Norton.

Bradburn, N. (1969). *The Structure of Psychological Well-Being.* Chicago: Aldine.

Brown, G. W. & Harris, T. (1978). *Social Origins of Depression.* London: Tavistock.

Brown, G. W., Lemyre, L. & Bifulco, A. (1992). Social factors and recovery from anxiety and depressive disorders: A test of specificity. *British Journal of Psychiatry,* **161,** 44–54.

Brown, I. & Inouye, D. K. (1978). Learned helplessness through modelling: The role of perceived similarity in competence. *Journal of Personality and Social Psychology,* **36,** 900–908.

Buehler, J. A. (1975). What contributes to hope in the cancer patient? *American Journal of Nursing,* **75,** 1353–1356.

Clark, L. A., Watson, D. & Mineka, S. (1994). Temperament, personality, and the mood and anxiety disorders. *Journal of Abnormal Psychology,* **103,** 103–116.

Cohen, S. I. (1985). Psychosomatic death: Voodoo death in a modern perspective. *Integrative Psychiatry,* **3,** 46–51.

Coleman, J., Herzberg, J. & Morris, M. (1977). Identity in adolescence: Present and future self concepts. *Journal of Youth and Adolescence,* **6,** 63–74.

Colvin, C. R. & Block, J. (1994). Do positive illusions foster mental health? An examination of the Taylor and Brown formulation. *Psychological Bulletin,* **116,** 3–20.

Coopersmith, S. (1967). *The Antecedent of Self-esteem.* San Francisco: Freeman.

Darwin, C. (1890). *The Expression of the Emotions in Man and Animals.* C. Darwin & Francis (Eds), pp. 176–195. London: John Murray.

Diene, E. (1984). Subjective well-being. *Psychological Bulletin,* **95,** 542–575.

Dohrenwend, B. P., Shrout, P. E., Egri, G. & Mendelsohn, F. S. (1980). Non-specific psychological distress nd other dimensions of psychopathology measures for use in the general population. *Archives of General Psychiatry*, **147**, 1229–1236.

Dyer, J. A. T. & Kreitman, N. (1984). Hopelessness, depression and suicidal intent in parasuicide. *British Journal of Psychiatry*, **144**, 127–133.

Edell, W. S. (1984). The borderline syndrome index: Clinical validity and utility. *Journal of Nervous and Mental Disease*, **172**, 254–263.

Elliott, T. R., Witty, T. E., Herrick, S. M. & Hoffmann, J. T. (1991). Negotiating reality after physical loss: Hope, depression and disability. *Journal of Personality and Social Psychology*, **61**, 608–613.

Engel, G. L. (1978). Psychological aspects of gastrointestinal disorders. In S. Arieti (Ed.), *American Handbook of Psychiatry*, 2nd ed. New York: Basic Books.

Eysenck, H. J. & Eysenck, S. B. G. (1970). *Personality Structure and Measurement.* London: Routledge & Kegan Paul.

Fitzgerald, R. (Ed.) (1979). *The Sources of Hope.* Sydney: Pergamon Press.

Frank, J. D. (1973). *Persuasion and Healing: A Comparative Study of Psychotherapy,* pp. 136–164. Baltimore: Johns Hopkins University Press.

Frank, J. D. (1985). Further thoughts on the antidemoralization hypothesis of psychotherapeutic effectiveness. *Integrative Psychiatry*, **3**, 17–26.

Frankl, V. (1978). *The Unheard Cry for Meaning: Psychotherapy and Humanism.* London: Hodder & Stoughton.

French, T. M. (1958). *The Integration of Behaviour,* vol. III. *The Reintegrative Process in a Psychoanalytic Treatment.* Chicago, IL: University of Chicago Press.

Goldney, R. D. (1981). Attempted suicide in young women: Correlates of lethality. *British Journal of Psychiatry*, **139**, 392–390.

Gollin, S., Terrell, F. & Johnson, B. (1977). Depression and the illustration of control. *Journal of Abnormal Psychology*, **90**, 440–442.

Gray, J. A. (1990). Brain systems that mediate both emotion and cognition. *Cognition and Emotion* **4**, 269–288.

Greene, S. M. (1989). The relationship between depression and hopelessness: Implications for current theories of depression. *British Journal of Psychiatry*, **154**, 650–659.

Greer, S. (1983). Cancer and the mind. *British Journal of Psychiatry*, **143**, 535–543.

Henderson, S. & Bostock, P. (1977). Coping behaviour after shipwreck. *British Journal of Psychiatry*, **131**, 15–20.

Henderson, S., Byrne, D. G. & Duncan-Jones, P. (1981). *Neurosis and the Social Environment,* pp. 160–162, 193–199. Sydney: Academic Press.

Hershberger, W. A. (1989). *Volitional Action—Conation and Control.* Amsterdam: North-Holland.

Hull, J. G. & Mendolia, M. (1991). Modelling the relations of attributional style, expectancies, and depression. *Journal of Personality and Social Psychology*, **61**, 85–97.

Kellehear, A. (1984). Are we a 'death denying' society: A sociological review. *Journal of Social Sciences in Medicine*, **18**, 713–723.

Kinsman, R. A., Fernandez, E., Schocker, M. *et al.* (195). Soviet children and the threat of nuclear war: A preliminary study. *American Journal of Orthopsychiatry*, **55**, 484–502.

Kobassa, S. C. (1979). Stressful life events, personality and health: An inquiry into hardiness. *Journal of Personality and Social Psychology*, **37**, 1–11.

Kobler, A. L. & Stotland, E. (1964). *The End of Hope: A Social Study of Suicide.* London: Collier Macmillan.

Kovacs, M. & Beck, A. T. (1978). Maladaptive cognitive structures in depression. *American Journal of Psychiatry,* **135,** 525–533.

Kuvlesky, W. P. & Bealer, R. C. (1966). A clarification of the concept, 'Occupational choice'. *Rural Sociology,* **31,** 265–276.

Lazarus, R. S. (1981). The costs and benefits of denial. In V. F. Dohrenwend & B. P. Dohrenwend (Eds), *Stressful Life Events and Their Contexts.* New York: Prodist.

Lazarus, R. S. (1991). *Emotion and Adaptation.* New York: Oxford University Press.

Lewis, A. (1932). The experience of time in mental disorder. *Proceedings of The Royal Society of Medicine,* **25,** 15–24.

Ludwig, A. M. (1978). Treating the chronically ill hospitalized schizophrenic patient. In W. E. Fann, A. D. Korocan, & R. L. Williams (Eds), *Phenomenology and Treatment of Schizophrenia,* chapter 20, p. 366. New York: Spectrum Publications.

Luria, A. R. (1978). *The Working Brain,* pp. 13–17. New York: Penguin Books.

Luthar, S. S. & Zigler, E. (1991). Vulnerability and competence: A review of research on resilience in childhood. *American Journal of Orthopsychiatry,* **61,** 6–22.

McCarthy, R. A. & Warrington, E. K. (1990). *Cognitive neuropsychology,* pp. 343–370. London: Academic Press.

Meares, A. (1983). Psychological mechanisms in the regression of cancer. *Medical Journal of Australia,* **1,** 583–584.

Melges, F. T. (1982). *Time and the Inner Future: A Temporal Approach to Psychiatric Disorders,* New York: Wiley.

Melges, F. T., Anderson, R. E., Kraemer, H. C., Tinklenberg, J. R. & Weisz, A. E. (1971). The personal future and self-esteem. *Archives of General Psychiatry,* **25,** 494–497.

Menninger, K. (1959). The academic lecture—hope. *American Journal of Psychiatry,* **116,** 481–491.

Moltmann, J. (1967). *Theology of Hope: On the Ground and the Implications of a Christian Eschatology,* p. 25. London: SCM Press.

Murray, J. (Ed.) (1976). *Oxford English Dictionary* being a corrected reissue with an introduction, supplement and bibliography of a new English Dictionary on historical principles founded mainly on the materials collected by the Philological Society. Clarendon Press: circa 1933. 4 supplementary volumes, 2, p. 149.

Norem, J. K. & Cantor, N. (1986). Defensive pessimism: Harnessing anxiety as motivation. *Journal of Personality and Social Psychology,* **51,** 1208–1217.

Nunn, K. P. (1995). Risk, vulnerability and resilience in childhood: The background for prevention. In B. Raphael & G. Burrows (Eds), *Handbook of Preventive Psychiatry,* chapter 23. New York: Elsevier.

Nunn, K. P. (1996). The pervasive refusal syndrome: Learned helplessness and hopelessness. *Journal of Child Psychology and Psychiatry,* **1,** 121–132.

Nunn, K. P., Lewin, T. J., Walton, J. M. & Carr, V. J. (1996). The construction and characteristics of an instrument to measure personal hopefulness. *Psychological Medicine,* **26,** 531–545.

Obayuwana, A. O., Collins, J. L., Carter, A. L., Rao, M. S., Mathura, C. C. & Wilson, S. B. (1982). Hope index scale: An instrument for the objective measure of hope. *Journal of the National Medical Association (US),* **74,** 761–765.

Ornstein, R. E. (1969). *On the Experience of Time,* pp. 15–23. Harmondsworth, Middlesex: Penguin.

Peterson, C. & Bossio, L. M. (1991). *Health and Optimism,* New York: Free Press.

Peterson, C., Maier, S. F. & Seligman, M. E. P. (1993). *Learned Helplessness—A Theory for the Age of Personal Control.* Oxford: Oxford University Press.

Plomin, R., Scheier, M. F., Bergeman, C. S., Pederson, N. L., Neddelroade, J. R. & McClearn, G. E. (1992). Optimism, pessimism and mental health: A twin adoption analysis. *Personality and Individual Differences,* **13,** 921–931.

Ray, C. & Baum, M. (1985). *Psychological Aspects of Early Breast Cancer,* pp. 21–35, 85–97. New York: Springer-Verlag.

Rholes, W. S., Riskind, J. H. & Neville, B. (1985). The relationship of cognitions and hopelessness to depression and anxiety. *Social Cognition,* **3,** 36–50.

Rotter, J. B. (1966). Generalised expectancies for internal versus external control of reinforcement. *Psychological Monographs,* **80,** No. 1.

Rutter, M. (1981). Stress, coping and development: Some issues and some questions. *Journal of Child Psychology and Psychiatry,* **22,** 323–356.

Rutter, M. (1985). Resilience in the face of adversity: Protective factors and resistance to psychiatric disorder. *British Journal of Psychiatry,* **147,** 598–611.

Rutter, M. & Quinton, D. (1984). Longterm follow-up of institutionalization in childhood: Factors promoting good functioning in adult life. *British Journal of Developmental Psychology,* **2,** 191–204.

Scheier, M. F. & Carver, C. S. (1985). Optimism, coping and health: Assessment and implications of generalized outcome expectancies. *Health Psychology,* **4,** 219–247.

Scheier, M. F. & Carver, C. S. (1987). Dispositional optimism and physical well-being: The influence of generalized outcome expectancies on health. *Journal of Personality,* **55,** 169–210.

Scheier, M. F., Magovern, G. J., Abbott, R. A., Matthews, K. A., Owens, J. F., Lefebvre, R. C. & Carver, C. S. (1989). Dispositional optimism and recovery from coronary artery bypass surgery: The beneficial effects on physical and psychological well-being. *Journal of Personality and Social Psychology,* **57,** 1024–21040.

Schmale, A. H. (1972). Giving up was a final common pathway to changes in health. *Advances in Psychosomatic Medicine,* **8,** 20–40.

Schmale, A. H. & Iker, H. (1971). Hopelessness as a predictor of cervical cancer. *Social Science and Medicine,* **5,** 95–100.

Schmidt, R. W., Lamm, H. & Trommsdorff, G. (1978). Social class and sex a determinants of future orientation (time perspective) in adults. *European Journal of Social Psychology,* **8,** 71–88.

Schulman, P., Keith, D. & Seligman, M. E. P. (1993). Is optimism heritable? A study of twins. *Behaviour Research and Therapy,* **31,** 569–574.

Seligman, M. E. P. (1975). *Helplessness: On Depression, Development and Death.* San Francisco: Freeman.

Seligman, M. E. P. (1992). *Learned Optimism.* Sydney: Random House Australia Press.

Simkin, D. K., Lederer, J. P. & Seligman, M. E. P. (1983). Learned helplessness in groups. *Behavioural Research and Therapy,* **21,** 613–622.

Snaith, P. (1993). What do depression rating scales measure? *British Journal of Psychiatry,* **163,** 293–298.

Snyder, C. R., Harris, C. & Anderson, J. R. (1991*a*). The will and the ways: Development and validation of individual-differences measure of hope. *Journal of Personality and Social Psychology,* **60,** 570–585.

Snyder, C. R., Irving, L. M. & Anderson, J. R. (1991*b*). Hope and health. In C. R. Snyder

& D. Forsythe (Eds), *Handbook of Social Clinical Psychology: The Health Perspective.* New York: Pergamon.

Stotland, E. (1969). *The Psychology of Hope.* San Francisco: Jossey-Bass.

Stotland, E. (1985). Letter to K. P. Nunn as a personal communication.

Stotland, E. & Kobler, A. L. (1965). *Life and Death of a Mental Hospital.* Seattle: University of Washington Press.

Taylor, S. E. & Brown, J. D. (1994). Positive illusions and well-being revisited: Separating fact from fiction. *Psychological Bulletin,* **116,** 21–27.

Tennant, C. & Bebbington, P. (1978). The social causations of depression: A critique of the work of Brown and his colleague. *Journal of Psychological Medicine,* **8,** 565–575.

Thompson, C. (1989). *The Instruments of Psychiatric Research,* pp. 87–114. Brisbane: Wiley.

Thompson, D. (1965). *England in the Twentieth Century (1914–1963): The Pelican History of England,* vol. 9, pp. 192–193. Harmondsworth, Middlesex Penguin.

Tonge, W. L., James, D. S. & Hillam, S. M. (1975). Families without hope: A controlled study of 33 problem families. *British Journal of Psychiatry* (special publication No. 11), Royal College of Psychiatrists. Ashford, Kent: Headley Brothers.

Trad, P. V. (1993). Previewing and the therapeutic use of metaphor. *British Journal of Medical Psychology,* **66,** 305–322.

Turnbull, C. (1974). *The Mountain People,* pp. 191–192. London: Picador.

Vaillant, G. (1977). *Adaptation to Life.* Boston: Little, Brown & Co.

Vaillant, G. E. (1983). *The Natural History of Alcoholism: Causes, Patterns and Paths to Recovery,* pp. 193–295. Cambridge, MA: Harvard University Press.

Visintainer, M. & Seligman, M. (1983). The hope factor. *American Health,* **2,** 58–61.

Watson, D., Clark, L. A. & Harkness, A. R. (1994). Structures of personality and their relevance to psychopathology. *Journal of Abnormal Psychology,* **103,** 18–31.

Watzlawick, P. (1983). *The Situation is Hopeless but not Serious: The Pursuit of Unhappiness.* New York: Norton.

Weiner, B. (1985). An attribution theory of achievement motivation and emotion. *Psychological Review,* **92,** 548–573.

Wetzel, R. D. (1976). Hopelessness, depression and suicide intent. *Archives of General Psychiatry,* **33,** 1069–1073.

White, M. (1989). *Selected Papers.* Adelaide: Dulwich Centre Publications.

WHO Expert Committee (1977). Child mental health and psychosocial development. WHO Technical Report Series No. 613. Geneva: WHO Publications.

Wing, J. K. & Brown, G. W. (1970). *Institutionalism and Schizophrenia: A Comparative Study of Three Mental Hospitals, 1960–1968.* Cambridge: Cambridge University Press.

Zimmerman, M. A. (1990). Toward a theory of learned hopefulness: A structural model analysis of participation and empowerment. *Journal of Research in Personalty,* **24,** 71–86.

Zimmerman, M. A. & Rappaport, J. (1988). Citizen participation perceived control and psychological empowerment. *American Journal of Community Psychology,* **16,** 725–2750.

Zullow, H. M., Oettingen, G., Peterson, C. & Seligman, M. E. P. (1988). Pessimistic explanatory style in historical record: CAVing LBJ, presidential candidates, and East versus West Berlin. *American Psychologist,* **43,** 673–682.

12

A Theology of Anger When Living with Disability

Nancy J. Lane

E xpressing one's anger is an important step toward spiritual and psychological growth. However, we do not usually think of expressing our anger at or with God. Many people still think it is wrong. Yet we cannot be in relationship with God if we are unable to express our deepest feelings. Anger is a powerful emotion that can wreak destruction in our lives, or it can become a raw energy that fuels our quest for justice and equality. A theology of anger enables us to question God, wrestling with God as it were, in the quest to find meaning and purpose when living with a disability.

> It is . . . the autonomy of humanity over against God that accounts for one of the most remarkable features of the Hebrew Bible, the possibility that people can argue with God and win. (Levenson, 1988)

The angriest character in the Old Testament is God. The anger of God was expressed as a partner in a covenantal relationship and directed at those who turned away from God. It was an anger born of love and justice for the people of God. This is the difference between anger that is good and anger that is deadly. The first is connected with seeking justice, the second with punishment of others and of ourselves.

> Anger is the antithesis of inertia and death because it is an electrifying *aliveness*. It goes thorough the body like a jet of freezing water; it fills the veins with purpose; it alerts the lazy eye and ear; the torpid lungs grow rich with easy breath. (Gordon, 1993, p. 3)

It is our ability to experience anger which allows us to experience love, joy, and deep caring for life. Anger is the energy which promotes justice and pushes us toward growth. Anger is a fact of life, woven into the fabric of daily living. It

From *Rehabilitation Education, 9*(2) (1995), 97–111. Reprinted with permission.

can be healthy and life-changing, or it can be destructive and death-making. Anger that is denied, repressed or unresolved can cause devastation to our health and well-being. This kind of anger changes nothing and causes love to lose all power (Campbell, 1986).

The anger of people with disabilities is rarely understood or accepted as valid or necessary. Our anger is ignored, denied, or silenced by those who tell us how we should feel and behave. This is one of the many ways which others use power over us. Failure to behave according to standards determined by others is one more way of labeling and stigmatizing us in order to dis-empower us further.

The non-acceptance of who we are as people with disabilities—who are sometimes angry—is death-making to our souls. Labeling us for our anger serves to isolate us and further deny the fullness of our humanity, leaving us frustrated . . . and angry. This may cause us to be locked into a vicious cycle that leads to destructive behaviors, depression and hopelessness. All of this, in turn, makes us even less acceptable to the world of non-disabled people.

When the anger of people with disabilities is denied, we are prevented from being part of a community. Anger is a **protest** against being treated as less than equal. Anger **expressed** is a way of asking to be taken seriously. Anger **heard** is being taken seriously. Anger is a choice we make when faced with the struggles of living. It is a chosen reaction to humiliation (Rohrer & Sutherland, 1981). For people living with a disability, it may be the only appropriate choice in the face of negative attitudes and the barriers of discrimination. However, anger may also be a way of manipulating life, a learned pattern of behavior used to avoid further loss and pain.

How we use the power of anger is also a matter of choice and responsibility (Campbell, 1986). It is not necessary, nor is it always a good thing, to "vent anger" every time we experience it. There has to be a balance, which we find by placing our anger within the context of who we are, our moral values and the choices we prefer. Expressing anger every time we feel threatened or frustrated may not be who we are or how we behave in the world. This is not the same as denying or repressing anger, however. The denial of anger can cause physical and emotional health problems, and the fear of being angry can make these destructive consequences worse. However, expressing that one feels angry is not the same as giving anger free reign to trample on our relationships.

Learning to understand our anger helps us to control our behavior and make responsible choices in how we behave toward ourselves and others. It also helps us to see that how others respond to our anger is their problem and they must deal with their feelings. The exception to this is when our anger is abusive and destructive. We have a responsibility to "be angry but sin not" (Ephesians 4:26).

In order to examine the role of anger in the lives of people with disabilities, we will first review the psychology of anger in relationship to psychological and spiritual growth. Next, we will discuss the Biblical paradigms for expressing anger to God and why doing so is necessary if one is to have a relationship with God.

THE MEANING OF ANGER

Whenever we are prevented from achieving our goals and desires, we are frustrated and have a need to change the situation. The emotional response to frustration is anger. There is "a distinction between feelings of anger and the emotion of anger" (Campbell, 1986, p. 25). A response to a threat or to frustration causes bodily change, thus we "feel angry." The "emotion of anger is a state of mind of a more complex nature in which we have associated those feelings with various perceptions, thoughts and . . . fantasies" (Campbell, 1986, p. 25).

Anger as an emotion is expressed in a variety of ways: teasing, practical jokes, sarcasm, prejudice, gossip, domination, suicide, rape, tickling, arguing, shooting, killing, and destroying. Anger as an element of passive behavior is expressed in: depression, guilt, withdrawal, the "super-sweet" personality, pouting, silence, and moodiness (Rohrer & Sutherland, 1981).

Anger can be destructive if we do not understand our emotions and feelings as people living with disabilities. "Accepting" one's disability is not the same as "liking" it. I have no choice in accepting or not accepting my disability. I do have a choice in liking or disliking the disability itself. Note that I am referring to liking or disliking "the disability" and not my person. Destructive anger occurs whenever we feel the following: we feel powerless over other people and circumstances; we do not feel self-sufficient; we have a diminished feeling of importance; or we feel frustrated in the face of what cannot be achieved (Rohrer & Sutherland, 1981).

Sources of Anger

1) Anger is a component of the grief cycle, experienced whenever there is loss. Disability creates loss, usually for a life-time. 2) In addition to our actual limitations, society imposes additional limitations on us through the lack of equal access to life at every level (e.g. medical, financial, employment, education, recreation, socializing, community, worship). 3) If we feel we lack power, we may substitute anger for feelings of weakness. 4) When we fear our own desires and needs, we retreat into anger as a way of restoring a sense of self-sufficiency (Rohrer & Sutherland, 1981). For example, if we deny our need for assistance, we may tell people that we do not need them or anybody else! The truth is that we do, but our *fear* of having needs is too frightening so we retreat into anger. 5) We may use anger to keep from feeling unimportant. I see this as a two-edged sword for persons with disabilities. On the one hand we may be treated as less than equal, our human and civil rights often denied. In these instances, the energy of anger may be necessary to protect our rights and dignity and to bring needed change. On the other hand, there are many people with disabilities who use their anger to demand importance in situations that do not warrant their being treated as more special than the next person. 6) Anger is often used to hang on to the illusion of perfection. Rather than admit to any personal inadequacy, people

sometimes place the blame outside of themselves. The illusion of perfection in people with disabilities may be lived out as a denial of one's limitations. We may try to live without asking for needed access, reasonable accommodation, or the assistance which would make life easier. We may expend enormous energy trying to cope as if nothing were different, when in fact something is. Since this is not being honest or truthful about our reality, we are feeding both the illusion and our anger. 7) Anger is often the reaction to physical, emotional, psychological and spiritual abuse of vulnerable persons. Sobsey (1994, p. 35) says ". . . people with disabilities are often repeatedly and chronically abused . . . the relative risk may be five or more times higher than the risk for the general population." Additional research suggests that 90-95% of women with disabilities are repeatedly abused but seldom receive the needed help to either end the abuse or recover from its effects (Lane, 1993).

Identifying Anger

"Body language" tells others if we are angry. If we sit with arms folded across our chest, bouncing our feet, or are frowning, our body is conveying what our words may not be saying. Our bodies also tell us if we are angry, through headaches, colitis, ulcers, hypertension, skin rashes, and chronic fatigue.

Unacknowledged and unresolved anger causes physiological changes even if we are unaware of them. Our bodies experience anger in chemical changes which affect the autoimmune system. Many physical illnesses have been attributed to "bottled up" anger. However, it is important to say here that anger is inseparable from other emotions. Many illnesses are the result of "unresolved conflicts associated with a range of emotions, of which anger would be one" (Tavris, 1982, p. 117). It is not the emotion, but our *fear* of the emotion which causes us habitually to avoid acknowledging them and thus to become ill. Our actions or behavior also convey our anger—swearing, arguing, walking away abruptly, and using the silent treatment. These are abusive behaviors, indicating that one's anger has become destructive.

Various situations affect the intensity of one's anger: 1) The mood at the moment—loss of security, feelings of inadequacy, and poor body-image lower one's threshold for anger. 2) Issues involved with abuse, Post-Traumatic Stress Disorder, or depression. 3) Other stresses in your life—the greater the areas of frustration, confusion and loss, the less one is able to adapt to additional stress.

> One measurement of emotional stress in a changing situation is the depth of anxiety, fear, anger and guilt. Stress . . . increases the more we feel that the change is out of our control (anxiety), that there is nothing anyone can do about it (fear), that someone else could have changed the situation and didn't (anger), or that we could have changed the situation and didn't (guilt). (Linn & Linn, 1978, p. 39)

4) How you interpret the situation: we see things through the filter of our self-image. 5) Our needs and desires of the moment: if we are ignored or not heard,

overworked, unloved, or lacking security; unmet needs affect our mood. 6) One's ego strength at the moment: our ego strength is based on our opinion of ourselves—are we okay in our own eyes? 7) The status of one's body chemistry: fatigue and illness cause psychological stress and anger. What we eat, the medicines we take, and how we care for our bodies in general affect our emotions. For example, excesses of sugar, alcohol, caffeine and drugs rob our bodies of the essentials which affect the nervous system. Disability adds an additional stress to each of these situations. If one's hierarchy of needs (as defined by Maslow) is also compromised, these situations are further burdened.

In deciding to identify the sources of our anger from prejudice, discrimination, denial of our rights, losses or abuse, we have three choices: "to remain silent, to leave, or to confront" (Christ, 1987, p. 29). Confrontation has a high price, but these struggles are often necessary in order to eliminate the barriers which we face and which exclude us from full participation in life.

Anger and Loss

We experience pain and vulnerability whenever we experience loss. People with disabilities usually experience continuing loss. There is the loss of idealized self-images and hopes; the loss of abilities, of dreams and expectations, of limbs or senses; the loss of opportunities, friends, and lovers. Each time we come up against an occasion which reminds us of a loss, we experience the loss again.

Anger in times of overwhelming grief can cause many physical reactions, leaving us with an ever greater sense of helplessness and loss of control (Campbell, 1986). If we endure the pain of a severe loss, we may enter a chronically depressed state in which we withdraw in order to protect ourselves from further loss. As the years pass, the loss will create a powerful screen of defensiveness (Campbell, 1986). We will need to recover our anger in order to heal and live again with feeling and hope.

We can group many of the losses we feel into four categories.

1. Power: power is a means of being free to make our own choices. It is the opposite of feeling weak or powerless. Power comes from how we see ourselves. However, persons with disabilities are often **dis-empowered** by service systems and political structures which deny them access to economic and medical opportunities. Anger is often necessary to maintain our freedom and autonomy. Our *loss* is felt in the frustration of being dis-empowered and denied the benefits others take for granted. For example,

   The demeaning and increasingly fruitless nature of the application and renewal process for Social Security and other entitlements can be one of the most anger-provoking barriers experienced by [persons with disabilities] . . . So [we] find [ourselves] doubly frustrated and angry both at the system itself and others who refuse to understand [what we are put through]. (Thompson, 1985, p. 84)

Helplessness reminds one of one's powerlessness. Anger can be a screen to hide feelings of helplessness. Anger can also be an appropriate reaction to our inability to defend ourselves from the violations of abuse and exploitation. Both of these point to the power differential which creates an on-going *loss* for people with disabilities. Being treated as a child is a familiar experience for people with disabilities. Others make decisions for you regardless of your wishes and desires, thereby dis-respecting your need for autonomy and your independence as a person. This *loss* of independence and autonomy is another frustration of goals and desires.

2. Self-sufficiency: many people assume that people with disabilities are inadequate or unable to do many tasks or jobs. This is yet another *loss,* a frustration of hopes and desires. The appropriate response is anger which will educate others and seek change. It means being assertive and demanding one's equal rights.

3. Wanting to be important: the less secure we are about ourselves, the more we need to be important to others. If our importance is threatened, we become angry. A secure sense of self is made difficult when there are so many losses. Until we know that we are accepted by another, loved by another, and heard by another—we will continue to be angry. Our sense of importance comes from *being understood.*

4. Loss of self-esteem: low self-esteem originates in our being ignored and not being heard. It is often assumed that people with disabilities do not have the same feelings as others, or that somehow our feelings are of less importance. "Loss of self-esteem comes when our feelings are not important enough to be heard" (Rohrer & Sutherland, 1981, p. 69). When our feelings are dismissed or we are told we should not feel what we feel, *who we are* is denied. The real work of healing lies in others' *listening* to our stories, feelings, desires and fears. Until our feelings are acknowledged, we have not been acknowledged as persons.

Many of us become angry when we are not heard. All too often we are told not to express our anger because non-disabled people simply cannot handle it (Thompson, 1985). It is alright for people to be angry about every issue from gay rights to the environment; but it is not alright to be angry because others refuse to hear us or refuse to accept that many of our problems result from barriers others continue to erect (Thompson, 1985).

Each loss prevents one from having a sense of autonomy or power over her/his own life. Anger is the attempt to retrieve choice, freedom, autonomy, equality and respect for our adulthood. The problem lies in how we use the anger associated with these losses and how we become empowered.

Anger and Depression

Anger is also a *response* to the losses we experience and is part of the on-going grief cycle in people with disabilities. Some depressions are reactions to crisis in which there has been a failure to express anger. If you cannot express anger, you cannot move through it, nor can you move through the grief cycle. You remain stuck in a cycle of loss, frustration and depression. Excessive or prolonged grief leads to depression, "an unhealthy condition that has gone beyond the bounds of normal mood changes and situational reactions" (Berg & McCartney, 1981, p. 3). We feel so hopeless, lonely, deprived or frustrated that we seek to escape the pain by withdrawing inside ourselves.

Freud saw depression as anger turned inward, "creating guilt, depression and the urge to self-destruction" (Campbell, 1986, p. 55). However, this is not the case with the universal experiences of loss and vulnerability. ". . . anger and depression are not mirror images of one another. Depression is not simply . . . *anger turned inward*" (Martin, 1986, p. 32). Both anger and depression may be learned coping strategies [cf. Seligman's work on learned helplessness]. Learned patterns of behavior may go back to childhood when something needed was not provided. The scars of deprivation cause us to defend ourselves against the fear of abandonment. Anger, anxiety and depression are closely connected and feed one another. Anger may not even be a possibility here as there is an established pattern of guilt and withdrawal (Campbell, 1986). We withdraw from danger by blaming self. Guilt and self-blame are often the result of loss. This creates a vicious cycle of seeing ourselves as worthless and erodes our self-image. One gets sucked into a black hole of helplessness and meaninglessness.

Even if we learn how to use anger creatively to address issues of injustice and to bring about change, we can experience depression from burnout. There is a "disability fatigue," an inescapable burden which comes from living with a dis-ability *and* needing to fight for equal opportunity, educate, explain, demand rights, and never having a rest from the effects of the disability itself. This fatigue can cause us to become very frustrated; when there is no outlet for the frustra-tion, the fatigue settles in on us like a heavy weight, exacerbating our sense of helplessness. Frustration can cause one to give up hope or turn to violence (McClosky, 1986).

Suffering is one more of the frustrations we do not know what to do with. The root cause of most anger at God has to do with our trying to find meaning in the problem of suffering. If we are to find meaning in our frustrations and anger, we need to come before God and with glaring honesty name the anger about our suffering and disability. Until we put the pain of our anger before God, it cannot be healed. Repressing anger in a relationship causes the relationship to die. We cannot be present to God without being honest about our feelings. If our anger is repressed from God, then God cannot know us in the fullness of our being. In order to understand the significance of expressing one's anger to God, we will examine the meaning of a covenantal relationship with God.

Discussing anger within a relationship with God raises questions about God's anger. However, it is not the purpose or intent of this paper to discuss God's anger, which is appropriately a question of Biblical hermeneutics. The Old Testament has many examples of God's anger at the people of God. My personal understanding of this issue is that when we turn away from God through negligence, disobedience or sin, God is angry, but in creative ways which are meant to call us back to God (especially found in the Psalms). Moltmann (*The Crucified God,* 1974, p. 272) says the wrath of God is injured love, which is not inflicted, but is a divine suffering of evil. However, the wrath of God, as seen in the Old Testament, is a current topic of debate among many feminist theologians who see it as a form of patriarchal abuse. I suspect the theology of a wrathful God will have to be deconstructed before it can be reconstructed into an understanding which will be helpful.

Anger at God

Part of our faith journey and the healing of our anger lies in our ability to question God. What God do we worship if we are afraid to challenge God with our questions of why? Do we follow a God born of our own fear or a God of love who leads us from self-hatred into acceptance? One's relationship with God may be broken out of fear of expressing anger. Yelling at God will help re-establish the relationship. It may be that we only pray when shaking our fist at God.

The establishment of both the Old and the New Covenant created a relationship between God and the people of God.[1] A covenant formulates a dialectical theology in which there can be a dialogue of questions and answers. One can both argue with God and yet obey God. Both are spiritual acts; discovering when each is appropriate in the life of faith requires discernment.

The point of this is to show that when we have a relationship with God, dialogue is expected and warranted. At the same time, we can acknowledge that the ways of God are a mystery; there is paradox. Our "answers" may be in the silence—in the mystery—or in discerning what it is that is being asked of us. Answers require questions, and many of our questions are rooted in the anger of our limited understanding. The same devastating questions which we ask of each other must be asked of God. At the same time, to question is to affirm.

Suffering is a radical challenge to the meaning of human existence. The problem of suffering raises the questions about good and evil, and the source of evil. Much of our anger at God may come in the form of asking hard questions, for which there may be no answers. Most of the questions have to be asked in order for us to struggle toward the answer—which will be different for each of us. We find God in our questioning, not in ready-made answers from those who know nothing of suffering. We discover God in seeking to question the meaning of life, the meaning of suffering, and the meaning of evil. Questioning is costly: it can be as painful as the suffering itself.

Paradigms of Expressing Anger at God

Job seemed to be familiar with the meaning of covenant as described above. He says: "But I would speak to the Almighty, and I desire to argue my case against

God" (Job 13:3). Job's anger at God comes out of his internal conflict with God, thus "Job feels free to call upon God for an advocate against God" (Garrison, 1982, p. 169). Job recognizes the total opposites within God which create a dialectical tension. Further, this encounter with God shows that "if it is God who gives and who takes away, the believer is irresistibly pushed again and again toward God" (Garrison, 1982, p. 169).

Job angrily challenged God to explain the cause of his suffering. He did not really expect an answer, nor did he get one. "The God who responds to Job with a magnificent description of his power and creativity and who angrily rebukes his comforters for their lack of understanding, is a God whom Job can continue to obey" (Campbell, 1986, p. 86). This is a God of creation and order, not chaos and destruction. God's anger can be seen as a love with creative purposes. In challenging a God, Job came face to face with God and entered into God's mystery, in which we see that there are no answers for now. Yet, like Job, we can go on in faith, trusting that the God of Love will never abandon us.

There is great liberation in expressing anger at God because we are acknowledging the reality and the depths of pain and suffering. The book of Job and many of the Psalms express this realistic anger. "If anger is the other side of love, then it must at times be a feature of living faith . . ." (Campbell, 1986, p. 49). We are not offending God but we are expressing our sense of betrayal from the One whom we trusted as loving us. Campbell (1986. p. 77) says that ". . . such anger is best understood as the cry of someone who will not despair of God. . . ." We come face to face with the dark side of God, yet continue to trust in God's mercy by virtue of our crying out. Campbell writes that "Anger is the undefeated messenger of hope" (Campbell, 1986, p. 78). I suggest that those who fear expressing anger at God live in a state of hopelessness, unable to move through the anger toward liberation.

There are no answers as to how one finds the way to God. There are only pointers, which is the message to be found in Job. In humility we have to acknowledge the greatness of God, which is beyond our mortal comprehension. It is the intervention of God which opens Job's eyes. In other words, only as we invite God into relationship with us does God dialogue with our suffering and our questions of meaning.

The anger of Jesus in his final hours is reminiscent of Job. Jesus is tested beyond what is fair and reasonable as he speaks these bitter words of anger and despair: "My God, my God, why have you forsaken me?" (Matthew 27:45).[2] With these words, Jesus enters into the depths of the mystery which is God. Campbell (1986, p. 48) argued: "The road to Calvary, entered out of love and passion for the truth, leads to a darkness where all that is left is anger against God . . ., a final and terrible defeat of faith, before the words of trust can be uttered: *Into your hands I commend my spirit* (Luke 23:46) and the words of acceptance, *It is finished* (John 19:30)."

It is in this abandonment experienced by Jesus that God enters fully into the depths of human suffering and experiences the absence of God. The abandonment and the silence of God are characteristics of God's non-intervention, where in our estrangement from God, we experience the nearness of God (Rosse, 1987). It is here that we are surrounded by the love of God. When we enter into a deeper relationship with God, we come to know an unconditional love and acceptance, which can empower us to love and accept ourselves as we are. As we accept our life *as it is* before God, we open ourselves to God and to our own deepest self (Rosse, 1987).

God *suffers* with us, and certainly that is the message of the Cross. The New Testament makes it very clear that God does not ever will suffering for us, nor does God send suffering to test us.[3] Often scriptures are misinterpreted and God becomes a sadist. Scriptures indicate that God *permits* evil and suffering (cf. the Psalms; Job; Ecclesiastes 6:2; Matthew 5:45; I John 5:19). Perhaps our anger at God is because God's power was self-limited when we were given freedom to choose between good and evil. It is not always easy to live with the consequences of freedom.

There can be no doubt as to the incomprehensibility of the ways of God. God does not exist for us, but we exist for God, to reveal God at work in the world. Certainly the mature life of faith requires that we obey God. Arguing with God could be regarded as a refusal to obey. However, if we live in covenant with our God, then we have the freedom and the responsibility first to argue—and then to *listen*. Expressing our anger at God involves enormous risk. Our questions will invariably lead us deeper into the life of faith, where the answers (which are often in the *silence*) may require of us far more than we anticipated.

Forgiving God

We have said that expressing anger at God is part of being in relationship with God. One cannot be in a relationship where there is no forgiveness. Further, it is not a covenantal relationship if forgiveness is offered by only one partner.

In the play *J.B.* by Archibald MacLeish, Job's response is to forgive God for not making a better world. It is a response born of love, which is a gift.

> Man depends on God for all things, God depends on man for one. Without man's love, God does not exist as God, only as creator, and love is the one thing no one, not even God . . ., can command. It is a free gift or it is nothing. And it is more itself, most free, when it is offered in spite of suffering, of injustice, and of death (MacLeish, "God has need of Man" in Glatzer, 1969, p. 285).

Glatzer considers this to be a humanist rendering of what was originally conceived to be an issue of faith. I note this only to show that I am aware of the criticism. However, I believe the points made about covenant and dialectical theology point to a *relationship* with God. Relationships require that we either are indifferent or we love the other. Anger arises because we care deeply, we love. I therefore see love as the reason and the source of our ability to forgive God.

Rabbi Kushner carries MacLeish a bit further when he speaks about forgiving God:

> Are you capable of forgiving and loving God even when you have found out that [God] is not perfect, even when [God] has let you down and disappointed you by permitting bad luck and sickness and cruelty in [God's] world, and permitting some of those things to happen to you? Can you learn to love and forgive [God] despite [God's] limitations as Job does, and as you once learned to forgive and love your parents even though they were not wise, as strong, as perfect as you needed them to be?
>
> And if you can do these things, will you be able to recognize that ability to forgive and the ability to love are the weapons a God has given to us to enable us to live fully, bravely, and meaningfully in this less-than-perfect world? (Kushner, 1981, p. 148).

To talk about forgiving God may seem to imply blame. God's reply to Job makes it clear that the ways of God are mysterious to us, and to blame God would be arrogance and blasphemy. However, holding God accountable for what is allowed is to hold God accountable for God's love in the relationship.

Acceptance of God's will without love is not enough. The only answer against injustice is *love*. To forgive God is to require that we be treated fairly, which is to obey the commandment to love ourselves as we love God (Glatzer, 1969). Thus, when we forgive God for the injustices of the world, we speak out of love for God and love for ourselves as created in the image of God.

Just as anger is necessary in the face of societies' non-acceptance of people with disabilities, forgiveness is required to *let go* of the pain which caused the anger. In the splendid film, *My Left Foot,* Christy Brown never internalized the appalling messages of society or the Church. He recognized accurately how people—unconsciously but insensitively—manipulated him, often overpowering him in order to control him. Christy was deeply wounded by the lifelong struggle against prejudice. He ached with the sense of being excluded. His infuriation, his rage, forced people to deal with him. Like the current generation of persons with disabilities, Christy asserts that prejudice is a far greater problem than any impairment. He reflects our demands for dignity, self-determination and equal access to society, the Church, and life (*Disabilities Study Quarterly,* Fall 1990, p. 23–25).

Christy's anger is often interpreted by others as a deadly power, unleashed unfairly and certainly in ways that made others very uncomfortable. ". . . the heavy topsoil of repressed injustice breeds anger better than any other medium" (Gordon, 1993, p. 31). The only way to stop this anger-turned-to-rage is by forgiveness. How difficult it is to forgive those who have killed our soul and thwarted our goals and desires for equality. However, we recover our soul and our life only when we forgive and in forgiving, *let go* of the hurt inflicted on us. In the silence and emptiness which follow, we put to rest anger turned deadly. This is justice too, for life is restored in us and we begin to experience "the peace which passes all understanding."

Anger that has turned deadly may have severed one's relationship with God. Hating God is much healthier than turning hatred in upon ourselves. It takes courage and a *knowledge* of God. Hating yourself is simply hating God in disguise because you lack courage to do otherwise. Expressing this strong feeling allows us to be honest and break down the barriers between us and God.

Forgive God for the pain and suffering which you feel is unfair and deep. We are not suggesting that you forgive God for not getting your own way in life. No one does. Nor should we forgive God for what we bring upon ourselves . . . addictions, bad habits, irresponsible living. Rather, forgive God for those things which cannot be changed or over which we have no control.

Once we have forgiven God, we are changed in ways which open us to accepting the realities of life which cannot be changed. Life is not perfect—it comes with pain and suffering. It also comes with things which give us happiness and meaning. We come to understand that God suffers with us and know that we are not abandoned. We know God forgives those who have brought pain and destruction into our lives. We accept that the love of God forgives us for the pain and destruction we cause others or ourselves.

Anger as a Creative Power

Beverly Harrison (1981, p. 50) writes that "Anger directly expressed is a mode of taking the other seriously." Too often it is we who are not taken seriously, so it is difficult for our anger to be *heard* and understood as necessary for our inclusion. It is imperative for us to find creative and meaningful ways of dealing with the threats and frustrations of living with a disability. Our anger must become a constructive tool for communicating clearly and truthfully what we need and what we feel.

"The gospel of anger" can be found in the anger of Jesus, who sided with the rejected of society and who spoke out fearlessly against the authorities. Jesus had no patience with those whose piety overlooked justice and mercy. His anger was to speak truth to falsehood and hypocrisy. The gospel of anger is about truth, love and justice (Campbell, 1986). This is anger which identifies and articulates clearly what is needed. It speaks out of love and seeks to bring change where it is needed.

Much of the injustice we face is created and sustained by political structures. It is difficult to address an entire system in an effort to create change and effect justice. Personal communication usually has no effect, and political communication by persons with disabilities has brought too little too late for too few. We can use our anger in positive ways to insist upon change by seeking love and not destruction. This is the hard path as it makes no concessions to injustice and requires a spiritual discipline which will keep us from becoming the oppressor.

When anger is because of oppression and social injustice, we usually feel alienated from others. However, failure to express our anger at the injustices which threaten the quality of our lives results in apathy and diminishment of who we are (Campbell, 1986). People tend to feel angry and guilty when the oppressed "spill their guts." It requires courage and boldness to confront with honesty and clarity the injustices which undermine our lives. This is another place where expressing our anger to God can protect us from apathy.

Once we come to understand our anger and move through it, we can begin to synthesize it with other aspects of who we are: 1) We may combine it with intelligence and reasoning so that we develop a sharp mind. 2) Anger may motivate our ambition and we will achieve our goals. 3) Anger may stir us to work for justice where there is injustice. 4) Anger may drive us to work tirelessly on behalf of others who suffer (Rohrer & Sutherland, 1981). 5) We can turn anger into compassion through support groups which break down our sense of isolation (McCloskey, 1986).

All that has been outlined and discussed demonstrates the many vicious cycles which "tend to turn inward and downward, perpetuating and often deepening the anger felt by [people] with disabilities. . . . This anger grows strong as the cycles continue and it is not going to disappear either quickly or easily" (Thompson, 1985, p. 84). Healing begins as we who live with disabilities recognize our anger and give credibility to it. It *is* what we feel; it is based on what we *have* experienced. Our losses are real. Our reality is not changed by the latest euphemism or any other denial of our experiences, feelings and emotions. It is normal to be affected by loss, grief, and the injustices which frustrate our achievable goals. "No one should be asked to accept discrimination from anyone" (Thompson, 1985, p. 85). Our anger is rational and justified.

Anger is a basic, human experience, and vital to the process of the inner transformation which leads to our wholeness (Martin, 1986). Campbell (1986, p. 65) writes that ". . . love is better served when anger is neither feared nor denied, but is given its place in our lives." We must learn to cope creatively with accepting the reality of our disabilities and the limitations which they impose on our lives. We can choose to remain angry over what has been lost or never realized, or we can find joy and grace in what has been given and in what can be. We can focus on our weaknesses or we can develop our strengths into their fullest potential. Perhaps the words of William Sloan Coffin (1989) are the best reminders of the positive role anger can play in our lives: "Anger keeps you from tolerating the intolerable."

NOTES

[1] *cf. Exodus 6:7; Jeremiah 7:23; 11:4; 30:22; 31:31; Exekial 36:28; Luke 22:20; 1 Corinthians 11:25; II Corinthians 3:6; Hebrews 8:8; 9:15; 12:24.*

[2] *New Revised Standard Version.*

[3] *The expression "the will of God" occurs 15 times in the New Testament, 8 times in the Pauline corpus. The "will of God" is linked to suffering in only 3 of those instances. It occurs once in the Old Testament in Tobit (12:18) in the context of healing.*

REFERENCES

Berg, R. F., & McCartney, C. (1981). *Depression and the integrated life.* New York: Alba House.

Campbell, A. V. (1986). *The gospel of anger.* London: SPCK.

Christ, C. P. (1987). *Laughter of Aphrodite: Reflections on a journey to the goddess.* San Francisco: Harper & Row.

Coffin, W. S. (1989, Fall).

Pax Christi. Disabilities Study Quarterly. (1990, Fall). pp. 23–25.

Fiddes, P. S. (1988). *The creative suffering of God.* Oxford: Clarendon Press.

Furey, R. J. (1986). *So I'm not perfect.* New York: Alba House.

Garrison, J. (1982). *The darkness of God: Theology after Hiroshima.* Grand Rapids, MI: Wm. B. Eerdmans.

Glatzer, N. N. (1969). *The dimensions of Job.* New York: Schocken Books.

Gordon, M. (1993, June 13). Anger: The fascination begins in the mouth. *The New York Times Book Review.*

Harrison, B. W. (1981). The power of anger in the work of love: Christian ethics for women and other strangers. *Union Seminary Quarterly Review, 36* Supplement.

Heyward, I. C. (1982). *The redemption of God.* New York: University Press of America.

Kushner, H. S. (1981). *When bad things happen to good people.* New York: Avon.

Lane, N. J. (1995). *The abuse of power by church and society toward women with disabilities: The theological and spiritual implications of sexual abuse of the vulnerable by the powerful.* Ph.D. Dissertation, The Union Institute, Cincinnati, Ohio.

Leon-Dufour, X. (1962). *Dictionary of biblical theology* New York: The Seabury Press.

Levenson, J. D. (1988). *Creation and the persistence of evil: The Jewish drama of divine omnipotence.* San Francisco: Harper & Row.

Linn, M., & Linn, D. (1978). *Healing life's hurts.* New York: Paulist Press.

Martin, S. A. (Spring, 1986). Anger as inner transformation. *Quadrant, 19*(1).

McCloskey, P. (1986). *When you are angry with God.* New York: Paulist Press.

McGinnis, J. (1993, May/June). Living the vulnerability of Jesus. *Weavings,* pp. 37–44.

Moltmann, J. (1974). *The crucified God.* San Francisco: Harper & Row.

Rohrer, N., & Sutherland, P. (1981). *Facing Anger.* Minneapolis: Augsburg.

Rosse, G. (1987). *The cry of Jesus on the cross: A biblical and theological study.* New York: Paulist Press.

Smedes, L. B. (1984). *Forgive and forget: Healing the hurts we don't deserve.* San Francisco: Harper & Row.

Sobsey, D. (1994). *Violence and abuse in the lives of people with disabilities.* Baltimore: Paul Brookes.

Tavris, C. (1982). *Anger: The misunderstood emotion.* New York: Simon and Schuster.

Thompson, R. D. (1985). Anger. In S. E. Browne, D. Connors, & N. Stern (Eds.), *With the power of each breath: A disabled women's anthology.* Pittsburgh: Cleis Press.

Wiesel, E. (1960). *Night.* New York: Avon.

13

No Blood, It Doesn't Count

Susan Buchanan

She was a small brown-skinned child with eyes as liquid brown as chestnuts. These features and her dark hair confirmed her Acadian ancestry. In the beginning, she stood up to me and the others in the wild pack of children who claimed the trailer park we all lived in as "our land." She would scream defiance at us and we would respond with more taunts, more cruelty. I don't even remember her name but I do remember her difference. And I remember how I and my fellow pint-sized tyrants treated her.

One hand was *normal,* nimble and deft as it threw gravel at us. The other hand had a tiny thumb and only two fingers. The fingers were fused together so they appeared as one wide finger. Otherwise she was the same as any other child. However, this one difference seemed to justify our behaviour towards her. We would scream names at her—"hook-girl" or "weirdo" or "freak."

Soon she would not leave her yard. That didn't stop us. We would line up on the edge of her driveway and torture her until her responding screams dissolved into angry tears. One day she took her mother's kitchen scissors and tried to cut her webbed fingers apart. After that we never saw her and convinced ourselves she had moved away.

When I proudly started Grade One that fall I took the bus to school. One of the first things I learned was that hook-girl's family had not moved. Instead, her mother would drive her to and from school. This was "sissy" behaviour and gave us more ammunition to use against her.

In Grade Three, my class raised money for people with disabilities. Our reward was that we could be part of the audience when that year's poster child came to visit our school. He wore heavy braces on his legs and ugly mud-brown orthopaedic shoes. We were told that he was a "brave little man" and we should consider ourselves blessed that we were not in his position.

Years later, I would meet a young woman who confided in me that her dream to be a poster child had never come true and this must have been because she was

From *Rehabilitation Digest, 26*(2) (1995), 3–4, 24. Reprinted with permission.

not "cute" enough. I was stunned that this young woman had wanted something so pathetic (in my mind), so badly. I could not imagine a need that involved being exploited.

By this time, I was also disabled and was struggling for an identity that did not engender sympathy and benevolence in others. I was beginning to understand that I had grown up and was influenced by an attitude that endorsed the idea that people with disabilities had little or no value in society, that they should consider themselves lucky even when attention came in the form of exploitation.

I was 16 when I was in a car accident and sustained a cervical spinal injury. At 16 I was uneasy about who I was. I was shy and embarrassed about my young woman's body and often longed for the androgenous shape of childhood. I was uncomfortable and awkward around others in my peer group. And suddenly my body was in revolt. It had no movement or sensation from just below my collar bones and no voluntary control of bodily functions.

The nurse who now dealt with "managing" these functions jokingly reassured me that "we all left our modesty at the door of the hospital." It was curious to me that "we" did not mean that they were part of this experience. The "we" seemed to be an effective strategy to depersonalize me and my "condition," to take away my identity so that no one had to deal with the reality of my accident. Perhaps it was a self-protective measure, designed to keep their emotions and personal feelings from shaping their professional concern for me.

I know they meant no harm, but my fragile self-esteem was crushed, and I felt helpless and out of control. I was appalled that my urine output and my bowel movements were discussed in a casual manner. I remember having friends from school visiting me and a nurse coming in to ask me if I had a suppository scheduled for later that evening!

Others had even less respect for me and my new body. Each day following the accident, a doctor would come by for another pinprick test. He would pull back the light sheet and my johnny shirt to reveal my naked chest. Starting at my rib cage, he would make tiny stabs with a pin, moving upwards until he had elicited a response from me. Often he was accompanied by an intern and the two would discuss my "case" as though I was not in the room.

I know that none of this was intentional. It was a far less deliberate disregard than we had had for "hook-girl." However, it was a damaging, subtle abuse, made all the worse because the scars it left behind were invisible. It continues to be difficult to describe because while it was happening I was receiving excellent medical attention and nursing care.

It took me many years to recognize the damage and several more to resolve it. My past had left me ill-equipped to acknowledge my own role in this most subtle form of abuse. A wounded self-esteem is like a scab. It is sometimes easier to pick away at it and cause more harm than it is to take care of it and let it heal.

My memories of my early years are more like bits of shattered glass than pieces of a puzzle that can be put together to make a sensible whole. Hard-edged, brittle and sharp, they have often made it dangerous for me to reach into the past and not cut open my old wounds again. My father was an angry, violent man who tried to own our fear. He never hit me or my two sisters, but he beat my mother and roared abuse at her. I wanted him to beat me so that maybe he would stop hurting my mother. My guilt was unbearable and stifling. I learned at a young age that it would be helpful if I could find a way to protect those I loved from pain.

I grew up with conflicting messages relayed to me by the adults around me. For example, punishment was often "for my own good." In my child's mind, I sometimes thought that my father was beating my mother "for her own good." Years later, when I was in the hospital and rehab centre, I would often hear a variation of that message. Nurses, doctors, therapists, social workers, frequently tried to persuade, and sometimes order, reluctant patients to do something the patients did not want to do. "This is for the best," "your family only wants the best for you," and "this is for your own good," were words used on patients labelled "noncompliant."

As a child, I was also told that if there was "no blood, it doesn't count." An injury to me, physical or emotional, was measured against its visibility. I came to believe this to be true. Even the injury that left me a quadriplegic was bloodless—I didn't even have an obvious bruise. It took me a long time to understand the difference between being a stoic martyr and being a woman grounded in the reality of my disability and appreciative of my many gifts.

The emotional abuse that so many people with disabilities experience in hospitals and rehab centres is "institutionalized benevolence." In and of itself, it is not an act of violence. But when encounter after encounter leaves a person diminished in spirit, damaged in self-esteem, altered in body image as the result of another surgery, then a person does feel violated and betrayed.

This is what happens to so many people, boys and girls, who grow up with a physical disability. A promise is held out that "one more surgery" will fix the child's gait, straighten a twisted spine, lengthen a shortened tendon. Parents want the best for their child and sometimes they hold on to a dream that the child can be "fixed." Can you imagine how inadequate that child may begin to feel? How worthless, powerless, confused and, eventually, angry? The child's self-esteem is profoundly challenged.

For girls with disabilities, childhood may not be too troubling, but a major task of teenage and early adult years is the development of a healthy self-esteem and role recognition. Girls with disabilities are not usually seen as potential mothers, wives, partners, lovers. And often, they continue to be seen as burdens or angry people who cannot deal with being disabled. Our culture maintains its vision of what a woman should look like, act like, and what roles she should fulfil. A girl with a disability, who has spent extensive time being "medicalized", can have a more difficult time dealing with her apparent "rolelessness."

Lindy (not her real name) remembers when she was 23 and being hospitalized for "one more surgery." At a time when most 23-year-old women are forging their adult lives, she was being admitted to a children's hospital. The surgeons and other medical staff knew her well; she had been hospitalized more than 30 times as a child and young adult. Lindy's parents were encouraging her to have an operation to put rods in her back so that she would "look better." A year later, those rods were taken out because they had caused more discomfort than good.

This time Lindy promised herself she would never be admitted to a children's hospital again. And she would not have another surgery unless her life was in danger. This is the first time she remembers taking an "adult" action. She was tired of her extended childhood.

A basic human tendency appears to be the need for autonomy. Children grow up and struggle to assert their autonomy, men go to war so that countries can be free and independent. The examples are vastly different but the motive is similar. In a hospital, a person quickly loses her autonomy. The royal "we" is used over and over. Lindy says she never knew who she was all those years. Only now, more than 10 years later, does she see herself as a woman. "This is the first time I have ever been loved and appreciated for who I am. My boyfriend loves me—scars, crooked back and all."

Amanda (not her real name) also remembers her struggle to assert herself as an adult. She says, "My mom was a nurse and I always felt I couldn't please her. I guess I thought that because she was a nurse she would be more understanding towards me. Instead, she would tell me I smelled bad when I was having bowel problems or she would punish me when I got another pressure sore."

At 20 years of age, Amanda moved away from home but she says it has taken almost 20 more years to begin to love herself for who she is. She believes that she had so many problems related to her disability because she "really hated" herself and her body. "I was cut up and cut open so many times I started seeing my body as nothing more than a piece of flesh covered with scars." Avoiding "traditional, mainstream" medicine as much as possible these days, Amanda has been exploring holistic alternatives. She believes she is beginning to find peace within herself.

Not all girls and women with disabilities experience a battered self-esteem. Not all doctors, nurses and other medical professionals are insensitive and disrespectful of a woman's self-worth. But the experience of frequent hospitalizations combined with the devalued role many women with disabilities have in our culture is powerful medicine—the kind of medicine that tastes bad, is hard to take over and over, and does not seem to ease the pain.

Part III: *Study Questions and Disability Awareness Exercise*

1. Are there any situations that you can think of in which the removal or reduction of a disabling condition may not result in the happiness or independence of that person?
2. Explain why a person who loses one arm may have a more difficult time adjusting than a person who loses two arms and one leg?
3. Are there situations in which you believe that acquiring a disability may result in increased happiness or independence for a person?
4. What are the differences between adaptation to a sudden onset of a disability (spinal cord injury) as compared to a gradual onset (multiple sclerosis)?
5. Are the stages of adjustment to a physical disability similar to the adjustment to an emotional disability?
6. Are the principles and assumptions related to the adaptation to disability applicable to AIDS?
7. Can denial ever be helpful in the adjustment to a disability? Give an example.
8. What do you think is the most commonly held "myth" regarding persons with disabilities? What suggestions do you have regarding the reduction of that myth in our society?
9. You've just been told you have only one month before you experience a lifestyle-changing disability. How would this information affect you? Would you benefit from a group experience with other people with similar disabilities?
10. Imagine that one week from now a severe myocardial infarction will result in your living under major limitations, e.g., no sexual activity for 1 year, no working, and the knowledge that your next attack could be your last. Discuss your activities for this week.
11. You have been told that chances are very good that you will have a heart attack in 6 months unless you drastically change your lifestyle. Develop a program designed to help you delay or avoid having a heart attack. Can you follow through with this program? What would be most difficult for you to change?
12. You have just been informed by your physician that due to your heart condition you must change your occupation. What would you do?
13. How do Wright's four major changes in a person's value system apply to people who have mental disorders ? What about to persons with AIDS?
14. What are the methodological problems related to research on acceptance of loss and value change?

15. Should hope be a factor in the treatment and rehabilitation process? Why? Why not?
16. Do certain disabilities promote learned helplessness? If so, which ones?
17. Does hope have more of a role in psychiatric rehabilitation than physical rehabilitation? Explain.
18. How does the health care and rehabilitation system encourage or discourage the expression and resolution of anger?
19. Explore how anger relates to loss.
20. How can anger facilitate creativity?
21. What are the unique issues faced by girls and young women with disabilities?
22. What does Buchanan mean by a "battered self-esteem?"
23. What can each of us do to make the rehabilitation system more user-friendly?

HERE TODAY, GONE TOMORROW

Personal health is frequently taken for granted. In order to provide the reader with a perspective on his or her personal values related to physical or psychological well-being, this experience focuses on the impact of disability from a personal frame of reference.

Goals

1. To heighten awareness of the role good or poor health plays in a person's life.
2. To stress the importance and temporality of a person being "able-bodied."
3. To put into perspective the values of people faced with limited time frames regarding loss of physical and emotional functioning.

Procedure

1. The leader begins by asking "Have you ever considered what a loss of health would mean to you?"
2. Cards are distributed to each member. They contain one of the following statements: "You have just been informed that you have a degenerative disease and you will be very functionally limited in: (a) 5 years, (b) 1 year, (c) 6 months, (d) 3 months, (e) 1 month.
3. Participants are instructed to write what they would do for each of these time frames (Time: 10 minutes).
4. When completed, one person is asked to read his response for a specific time frame. This is done until each time frame is covered.
5. Discussion may focus on the quantitative and qualitative aspects of the responses. Does a respondent stress doing for self or for others?
6. Explore the differentiating effect of time and relate this to the reality that some people do not have the opportunity to be aware of a degenerative condition and must deal with a traumatic event, such as immediate loss due to trauma.

Part IV

The Interpersonal and Attitudinal Impact of Disability

The societal response to disability is, in part, a reflection of the beliefs of others toward disability and persons with a disability. These beliefs are often negative and affect the interpersonal relationships between persons with disability and those without disability, as well as society's attempts to rehabilitate persons with disabilities.

Interactions that are not constructive are typically described as strained or anxiety provoking for both participants. In some cases this strain, in combination with negative attitudes, contributes to persons with disability being socially excluded from others. In other cases, they may be intruded upon through stares or questioned out of curiosity.

Individuals with disabilities and persons from minority racial and ethnic groups often face common problems of stigma and discrimination. The treatise presented in chapter 14 by Syzmanski and Trueba is that these problems are contributed to by a castification process embedded in education and rehabilitation service systems. These systems which are intended to assist and empower often contribute to social exclusion and disempowerment. Models of disability and disability services, castification process and theories, castification in disability services, and professional power considerations in castification and an example of the castification process are addressed. Recommendations for changes are presented.

Portraying persons with disability as "victims" is common in our society. Lynch and Thomas discuss in chapter 15 the damaging effects of this portrayal and urge that a perspective be adopted which will eliminate this concept, empower clients and de-emphasize the differences between persons with and without disabilities. Implications for research and practice are provided.

Three perspectives on the social lives of persons with schizophrenia: those of the person with the disability, those of the family members and those of clinical investigators are presented in chapter 16. Images which portray the essence of each perspective are described with supporting evidence. The legitimacy and validity of each perspective and the role they each play in understanding, treating, and improving the social lives of individuals with severe mental illness are discussed.

Part IV enables the reader to more clearly understand the interpersonal impact of disability, how the lives of persons with disabilities are affected, and how they may be changed.

14

Castification of People with Disabilities: Potential Disempowering Aspects of Classification in Disability Services

Edna Mora Szymanski and Henry T. Trueba

P eople with disabilities are a heterogeneous group of individuals whose disabilities affect their lives in different ways. Similarly, people of racial and ethnic minority groups demonstrate considerable within group and between group variability. Nonetheless, both individuals with disabilities (Fine & Asch, 1988) and persons of racial and ethnic minority groups (Trueba 1993a) may face common social problems of stigma, marginality, and discrimination. A central tenet of this discussion is that at least some of the difficulties faced by persons with disabilities are not the result of functional impairments related to the disability, but rather are the result of a castification process embedded in societal institutions for rehabilitation and education and enforced by well meaning professionals. To develop this premise, we will examine issues related to the social impact of both disability and minority status through the following topics: (a) models of disability and disability services, (b) castification process and theories, (c) castification in disability services, (d) professional power considerations in castification, and (e) an example of castification through a campus disability policy.

MODELS OF DISABILITY AND DISABILITY SERVICES

Disability and related terms (e.g., stigma) are broad concepts that are constructed differently by various stakeholders (Goffman, 1963; Skrtic, 1991; Stubbins, 1991).

The authors wish to acknowledge the contribution to our thinking of the excellent students at the University of Wisconsin-Madison, who participated in a class on Race, Ethnicity, and Disability during the Spring semester of 1993.

From *Journal of Rehabilitation, 60*(3) (1994), 12–20. Reprinted with permission.

The particular construction or definition of disability applied by a group appears to relate to the special interests of skills of the defining group (McKnight, 1977; Stubbins, 1991). For example, rehabilitation psychologists tend to define disability in terms of specific psychological aspects that are diagnosable and can be addressed by therapy; independent living specialists often define disability in terms of the environmental barriers (physical or attitudinal); and special educators may consider disability in terms of the difficulties encountered in learning.

A variety of approaches to understanding disability currently exist. Hahn has suggested the sequential evolution and current existence of (a) the medical model, which focuses on functional impairments; (b) the economic perspective, which emphasizes vocational limitations; and (c) the socio-political model, in which disability is viewed as a product of the interactions of the individual with the environment (Hahn, 1985, 1989). In addition to those identified by Hahn, socio-cultural and legal models of disability are suggested by recent literature. Specifically, the recent rediscovery of Vygotsky's socially-based learning theories has suggested cultural and social components in the construction of disability (Trueba, 1993a; Trueba, Rodriguez, Zou, & Cintron, 1993; Trueba, Cheng, & Ima, 1993). Similarly, federal legislation and regulations, including the early white cane laws, the recent Americans with Disabilities Act, and Workers' Compensation laws have added legal aspects to the definition of disability (Cook, 1991; Jenkins, Patterson, & Szymanski, 1992).

Different definitions of disability currently coexist (Hahn, 1985), and, unfortunately, professionals are often unaware of those perspectives that lie outside their specific discipline (Stubbins, 1991). On a disciplinary level, different definitions appear to inhibit the multidisciplinary collaboration necessary to address the broader social aspects of disability that affect the daily lives of individuals (Stubbins, 1991). On a programmatic level, the result of these multiple orientations is "disabled policy" (Berkowitz, 1987), characterized by often conflicting programs, which are part of an "institutional landscape and make the process of reform more difficult" (Berkowitz, 1985, p. 11). Three currently existing programs, which reflect different definitions of disability, are the state-federal rehabilitation program, the special education program, and the independent living movement.

The state-federal rehabilitation program follows a traditional rehabilitation process model, which is characterized by four phases: evaluation, planning, treatment, and termination (Rubin & Roessler, 1987). The evaluation phase includes documentation of a disability and determination that the disability is likely to present an impediment to employability (Mandeville & Brabham, 1992). Although recent legislation and philosophical stances in the rehabilitation counseling profession have suggested that rehabilitation consumers should have an active role in the process (Mandeville & Brabham, 1992; Rehabilitation Act Amendments, 1992; B. Wright, 1983), the process still appears to remain firmly under the control of the professional who often has the power to determine whether a person with a disability is eligible to participate in a program or receive some form of benefit.

Federally legislated special education programs follow similar processes to rehabilitation (e.g., evaluation, planning, intervention). However, unlike rehabilitation services, special education is considered to be an entitlement program open to any school age person with a disability who needs special instruction as a result of the disability (Szymanski, Hanley-Maxwell, & Asselin, 1992). As in rehabilitation, the special education process remains under the control of the professional (Nisbet, Covert, & Schuh, 1992; Skrtic, 1991).

The independent living movement, which emerged from multiple social movements of the 1970s, including civil rights, consumerism, and demedicalization, differs significantly from the rehabilitation and special education programs. Independent living services are consumer driven with a focus on access to societal benefits and independence (DeJong, 1979).

> According to the independent living paradigm, the problem does not reside in the individual; it often resides in the solution offered by the rehabilitation paradigm, which contains the dependency inducing potential of the physician-patient or professional-client relationship. The locus of the problem is not the individual, but the environment that tends to limit the choices available to people with disabilities. (Nosek, 1992)

Two key differences emerge in the three models described—the underlying view of disability and the role of the professional. The special education and rehabilitation models are clearly based on the medical and economic models of disability, which address objectively definable disability states that can only be diagnosed and remediated by qualified professionals (Salifos-Rothschild, 1976; Skrtic, 1991). In contrast, the independent living model is based on a socio-political view of disability as a problem residing outside of the individual that must be understood from an individual frame of reference (Roth, 1985) and that is often exacerbated by professional control (Nosek, 1992).

Interestingly, however, despite differences in perception of the nature of disability and the value of professional interventions, the models appear to share a common approach. Whether the discussions emanate from the positivist approaches of rehabilitation and special education or the more phenomenological approaches of independent living, they often focus on the individual as a unit of analysis with tangential consideration of the interaction of individuals in societies and cultures. The problem with these approaches is that such specificity of focus often misses the dynamic nature of action in which actors (e.g., individuals with disabilities, professionals) cannot be considered separately from their actions, the audiences or recipients of the actions, the cultural and social context of the action, and other current and historical contexts surrounding the action (Wertsch, 1991).

Disability is known to be very much of a social and cultural phenomena (Arokiasamy, Rubin, & Roessler, 1987; Scott, 1969; Skrtic, 1991; B. Wright, 1983). And, many people with disabilities share a common status of disadvantage with racial and ethnic minority groups (Hahn, 1988; Stubbins, 1988). Thus, it seems that disability and disability services must be examined in the larger context of social and cultural forces. For this reason, the next section is devoted to discussion of the anthropological theories relating to castification.

CASTIFICATION PROCESS AND THEORIES

People with disabilities often share a common status of marginality with members of racial and ethnic minority groups. In fact, this common status was part of the rationale for Hahn's introduction of the minority group model of disability (1985, 1989). When considering the disadvantaged or marginal state of specific minority groups, the question arises as to why some groups are marginalized and other groups are not. Castification is a construct that has been used in anthropology to explain the process of differential marginalization. Although, like disability, castification can be defined in different ways, we have chosen the following definition for the current discussion.

> Castification is fundamentally an institutionalized way of exploiting one social group (ethnic, racial, low-income, or other minority group), thus reducing this group to the status of a lower caste that cannot enjoy the same rights and obligations possessed by the other groups. (Trueba, 1993a, p. 30)

The cultural myths invented to castify and thus rationalize abuse of power are nothing new in history. The Europeans who conquered the new world attempted for centuries to defend the notion that natives from the American continent did not have the same human value (human soul) comparable to those of the Europeans. Slavery, rape, and forced labor become permissible on the grounds of the fundamental "spiritual difference" between Europeans and non-Europeans, as well as on the grounds that civilization and redemption (cultural and religious beliefs) would eventually result from European conquest and domination (Trueba, 1993a). Similarly, policies of institutionalization and sterilization of persons with disabilities were often justified by myths about the value of people with disabilities and the need to protect society (Arokiasamy et al., 1987; Cook, 1991).

Racial and ethnic problems and debates in Europe and in America seem to repeat history. Consider, for example, the waves of hatred in Europe and the myths of racial superiority among certain Europeans. The roots of the myth of Aryan superiority that eventually produced the Jewish Holocaust of Hitler's Germany are found in the "unilineal cultural evolution" themes of nineteenth century social evolutionary theories (Suárez-Orozco, 1993), which are still evident in European and American society. For example, the majority of poor children in the United States are victims of xenophobia, which has many expressions and reflects a profound racism of white America.

Expressions of xenophobia are often at the root of social movements, such as Neo-Naziism, monolingualism and monocultural policies (e.g., the English Only Movement), the Klu-Klux-Klan, and the Moral Majority. In the view of many members of these movements, pluralistic policies, such as, the funding of education in the home languages of ethnic groups and the use of affirmative action criteria to implement fair employment policies (policies that reflect the ethnic composition of the labor force) are unacceptable (Trueba, 1993a). It is suspected that similar sentiments accompany implementation of the Americans with Disabilities Act.

Poverty in the United States is not only a disgraceful manifestation of castification processes, but a clear example of how lack of equity in employment, education, and social services condemns generations of ethnic minority children and their families to a status of underclass, of second class citizenship. For example, in 1989, 2.6 million Latino children (out of the total 4.2 million Latino children) were under the poverty level, and lived in urban and suburban areas (not in rural areas). The 1989 frequency of children living in poverty among the various Latino groups was 48.4% for Puerto Ricans, 37.1% for Mexicans, and 26.1% for Central and South Americans (Trueba, 1993a). Similarly, although people with disabilities "account for 13.5% of the population, [they] are represented at the lowest income group at nearly double this proportion, and are severely underrepresented in the highest income group" (Storck & Thompson-Hoffman, 1991, p. 31). Although ethnic minorities are overrepresented in populations of persons with disabilities (Storck & Thompson-Hoffman, 1991; T. Wright & Leung, 1993), this overrepresentation does not appear to fully account for the concomitant poverty.

The tolerance that Americans demonstrate for poverty is related to biological determinism. According to Jonathan Kozol, many white Americans stereotype blacks as being intrinsically inferior:

> When they hear of all these murders, all these men in prison, all these women pregnant with no husbands, they don't buy the explanation that it's poverty, or public schools, or racial segregation. They say, "We didn't have much money when we started out, but we led clean and decent lives. We did it. Why can't they?" . . . "They don't have it." (Kozol, 1991, p. 192).

The flat and direct statement, "They don't have it," is the most emphatic return to a biological determinism, perhaps under the cover of a new cultural determinism. This is important to consider in the light of the most popular literature regarding low achievement of minority groups, groups described as "caste-like." Following the refutation of last century's biological determinism (based on "unilineal cultural evolution") led by Franz Boas (1916, 1928) and his colleagues, anthropology saw a kind of psychological determinism creep in and then be refuted. Is this new "cultural" determinism creeping once more into theoretical discussions of differential minority achievement?

Cultural ecology, one of the most vigorous and visible statements on castification coming from cultural anthropologists, has paradoxically evolved into a kind of cultural determinism (Foley, 1991; Trueba, 1988b, 1991, 1993a). John Ogbu and his colleagues (1974, 1978, 1987, 1989, 1991a, 1991b, 1992; Ogbu &

Matute-Bianchi, 1986; Matute-Bianchi, 1991; Gibson & Ogbu, 1991) developed a typology to explain deferential performance of minority groups through classification according to the following categories: autonomous, immigrant, and castelike. Small groups who may or may not have a "distinctive" ethnic identity and who are successful in school (e.g., Jews, Mormons) were considered to be autonomous minorities. Minority groups who came to the United States for better economic, political, or overall situations, and who, despite cultural differences, did not demonstrate lasting, disproportionate school failure were classified as immigrant minorities (e.g., Chinese in Stockton, California; Punjabi Indians in Valleyside, California). And, minorities "who were *originally brought into United States society involuntarily* through slavery, conquest, or colonization" (Ogbu, 1987, p. 321) were classified as castelike (Ogbu, 1987).

Although Ogbu's typology helped to explain the barriers faced by castelike minorities, his major flaw was the circular reasoning that accompanied the use of the hypothetical construct, *castelike personality,* to explain the behavior of entire groups. The circularity of this explanation was similar to that noted in psychology by Ebel (1974) in the use of the hypothetical constructs of intelligence and motivation to explain behavior. *When hypothetical constructs grounded in a dominant culture are used to explain the behavior of members of a minority group, it is not surprising that the results emphasize difference and deviance.*

The flaw of circular reasoning in cultural ecology is exemplified when one considers the achievements of many members of involuntary groups who indeed succeed and retain their ethnic identity. In this respect, the assumptions presented in Ogbu's typology seem theoretically weak or even faulty, and historically undemonstrable, especially if applied to highly heterogeneous ethnic groups such as African Americans, Latinos, Hawaiians, and American Indians, among many others in the United States.

The discussion of castification in this paper was predicated on the observation of the authors that people with disabilities often experience the same types of differential social exclusion experienced by members of racial and ethnic minority groups. Indeed, as demonstrated in the next section, many scholars have discussed the disempowering or castifying roles of the social institutions addressing disability (see e.g., Gove, 1976; Salifos-Rothschild, 1976; Scott, 1969; Stubbins, 1988). Interestingly, it seems that cultural determinists defend their positions as dogmas with the same passion that disability professionals defend their taxonomies of disabilities and therapeutic interventions.

CASTIFICATION IN DISABILITY SERVICES

Castification processes, as described in the previous section, seem to have their roots in a determinist view in which people who are different are viewed as somehow less "human" or less capable (Trueba, 1988a, 1988b, 1991; Trueba, Cheng, & Ima, 1993; Trueba, Rodriguez, Zou, & Cintron, 1993). Cultural ecology encountered problems of castification when a version of the same construct used to explain the differential status of minority groups (i.e., castification) was used to explain the behavior or lack of achievement of whole groups of people (i.e., through castelike personality). Similar problems of castification may plague disability services when the same categories of impairment and functional limitation (constructed mostly by people without disabilities) are used to determine eligibility for services, to prescribe interventions, and, on occasion, to explain failure.

The common problem in both disability services and cultural ecology is that some of the theoretical classification systems and societal institutions that have been invented to assist minority individuals can also serve to oppress those individuals. Hypothetical constructs, such as castification and the functional limitations of disability, can help us to understand the processes of social reaction to persons who are different. However, when such hypothetical constructs produce classification systems that are then used to impose limiting explanations of the behavior of "classified" individuals, the process becomes circular. *The constructs and those who use them then become agents of castification.*

The detrimental effect of such castification has been documented in anthropology, where the limiting impact of culturally-determined degradation incidents has been studied among the Japanese and other ethnic groups (DeVos, 1973, 1982, 1992; DeVos & Wagatsuma, 1966; DeVos & Suárez-Orozco, 1990). In the disability literature, the oppressing impact of castification has been referred to as stigma (Goffman, 1963), which affects interpersonal interaction (Gove, 1976) and may mitigate against political activism (Scotch, 1988; Scott, 1969). Consider, for example, the following description of castification of people with disabilities by rehabilitation professionals.

> A serious overall curtailment of options occurs when professionals adhere to a stereotyped role for . . . [people with disabilities], which, like sex-appropriate roles, offers a single "appropriate" model of thinking and behaving for the . . . person and precludes a whole range of "inappropriate" options, regardless of the individual's abilities, talents, and inclinations. (Salifos-Rothschild, 1976, p. 41)

In the account by Salifos-Rothschild (1976), we see a circularity of reasoning whereby the same construct (i.e., disability), which is used to explain the individuals' situation, is also used to explain the limits of acceptable behavior. This circularity and its resulting limiting effects on individuals parallels Trueba's (1993a) criticisms of the use of Ogbu's typology in cultural ecology. While considerations of type, age of onset, and severity of disability may contribute to understanding the situations of persons with disabilities, they cannot be used as primary explanations of behavior.

The disempowering nature of these classification systems is often all too apparent to people with disabilities applying for rehabilitation services in an effort to enhance self-sufficiency and personal independence. Rather than being treated as adults with free or equal status, they may be confronted by able-bodied persons asserting a right to determine what kinds of services they need

(Stubbins, 1988). Such able-bodied individuals are often acting in accord with deterministic beliefs that, like those of cultural ecology, suggest that the behavior or needs of groups of individuals can be understood by their common attributes (e.g., disabilities, ethnic identification).

It is important to note that many professionals reject paternalism and actively work to foster empowerment. Nonetheless, professionals are in pivotal positions in which they can either facilitate empowerment or present additional barriers (Szymanski, 1985, 1994; Szymanski, Rubin, & Rubin, 1988). Further, professionals are in positions in which they are vulnerable to the implicitly deterministic castifying policies of the social institutions for whom they work. The implicit power of deterministic policies presents a particular professional dilemma. We suspect that the nature of use or abuse of power by professionals contributes to the extent to which disability services can actually castify rather than empower persons with disabilities.

PROFESSIONAL POWER CONSIDERATIONS IN CASTIFICATION

The abuse of power by professionals can contribute to castification of minority groups by the same social institutions created to help those individuals. The determinant role of agencies and institutions (including third party payers) in handicapping persons with disabilities has been pointed out by sociologists and anthropologists discussing empowerment processes (see e.g., Mehan, Hertwick, & Meihls, 1986; Trueba, 1988a; Trueba, Spindler, & Spindler, 1989; Delgado-Gaitan & Trueba, 1991; Trueba Rodriguez, Zou, & Cintron, 1993) and those studying rehabilitation (see e.g., Albrecht, 1992; Illich, 1977; McKnight, 1977).

Power is at the root of the potential handicapping nature of interventions. However, according to Stubbins (1988),

> rehabilitation practitioners [are not] necessarily aware of how their choice of techniques is tied to power considerations—both by the influence exerted upon them by political and ideological interests and by the influence they exert on their clients in carrying out their assigned mandate. (p. 2 6)

Another dilemma for professionals in disability services is the implicitly deterministic foundations of professional practice, which may actually conflict with some models of disability. The conceptualization of professional knowledge is based on a logical positivist approach to inquiry (Skrtic, 1991), which "seeks facts or causes of social phenomena apart from the subjective states of individuals" (Taylor & Bogdan, 1984, p. 1). Clearly, the positivist nature of professional knowledge contributes to castification. Further, it is quite at odds with some descriptions of disability, particularly that of W. Roth (1985), who indicated that "a disability characterizes the experience of anyone who experiences the world mediated through a different body than others" (p. 44).

Professional autonomy, which is considered to be the ultimate criterion of professionalism, "implies that professionals know best what is good for their clients because they have access to the profession's specialized knowledge and skills" (Skrtic, 1991, p. 90). Although some (e.g., Szymanski, 1985, 1994) have suggested that professionals must work in partnership with people with disabilities and their families, others (e.g., Rubenfeld, 1988) have questioned whether such partnerships were really possible due to the implicit power differentials in the relationship. The issue of professional autonomy seems to be at odds with phenomenologicl conceptions of disability (Skrtic, 1991) and may contribute to castification.

The advent of credentialing and opportunities for third party payment have appeared to coincide with increased emphasis on a medical or functional limitations approach to disability and related classification schema (D. Linkowski, personal communication, January 25, 1993). In this approach, professionals diagnose the source of the problem, which is clearly attached to the individual, and deliver interventions designed to "fix" the individual so that they can function more effectively in society. In order to receive services, individuals must accept their disabilities as sources of personal inferiority and relinquish majority status and self-determination (Salifos-Rothschild, 1976; Scott, 1969). "What is commonly considered realistic by professionals is that [social] construction which helps to enhance their own regards and their control over other people" (J. Roth, cited in Salifos-Rothschild, 1976, p. 40). Strong sanctions are applied to persons with disabilities who do not willingly relinquish their majority status. They are often additionally labeled as deviant, uncooperative, or ungrateful (Salifos-Rothschild 1976; Scott, 1969). According to Scotch (1988)

> The stigmatization of . . . persons [with disabilities] is reinforced and even created by the attitudes of providers of rehabilitation services. . . . By promoting the image of . . . people [with disabilities] as dependent and in need of professional help, medical and rehabilitation professionals retain control over program beneficiaries at the cost of severely constraining the . . . person . . . (p. 162)

It seems that the movements toward professionalism, third party payment, and managed care may be reinforcing the castifying nature of the classification schemes that were originally invented to help us to understand the situations of people with disabilities. We are now using these same schemes to determine what services and how much services are needed by individuals. Somehow, the complex nature of individual action in a social and cultural environment is reduced to billable, diagnostic categories.

This cycle of castification in disability services is likely to continue due to the roles of professionals and the extent to which their increased avenues of remuneration reinforce castification of people with disabilities. The identification and remediation of disability provides a good living for disability professionals who might not be needed if disability were regarded as a simple, acceptable, manifestation of human diversity (Amado, 1988).

The disempowering processes discussed in the previous sections of this paper are very much in evidence today. In the next section, we illustrate castification through current policy for students with disabilities on a large university campus.

AN EXAMPLE OF CASTIFICATION
THROUGH CAMPUS DISABILITY POLICY

Special education, as it is usually delivered in public schools, has been considered by many critics to be seriously flawed. One of the major flaws has been the creation of a separate system, complete with multitudes of professionals who may effectively isolate students with disabilities from the mainstream educational community (Lipsky & Gartner, 1989; Skrtic, 1991; Will, 1986). Another flaw, was the disempowerment of people with disabilities and their families by professionals (Ferguson, Ferguson, & Jones, 1988; Nisbet et al ., 1992; Szymanski, 1994).

Unfortunately, models similar to special education, which are based on positivist, medical and functional limitations approaches to disability, have developed on college campuses. In the post-secondary setting, such traditional service delivery models, which promote dependence on professionals, exist in sharp contrast to the student development model, which is directed toward acquisition of student independence (Brown, Clopton, & Tusler, 1991).

The limitations of the special education model on college campuses are evident in the extent to which students are included in mainstream processes. Problems certainly exist when the very services and structures that have been put into place to facilitate the education of students with disabilities often serve to isolate them from other students and from normal university processes (K. Al-Ashkar, personal communication, November, 1992). Consider, for example, a recent memo (which has since been changed) from a university office serving students with disabilities that advised students, who used alternative testing services, to:

A. Obtain a letter from us describing the accommodations that you are approved for and the role of the faculty in meeting your needs (available from the counselor who developed your service plan).

B. Meet with your professors as soon as possible. Provide them with the letter describing your approved accommodations. Explain to them the effects of your disability on taking examinations and how the accommodations you are approved for attempt to equalize your ability to take examinations. (McBurney Disability Resource Center, 1993)

The proposed procedure demonstrates the castifying effect of a disability service on at least two dimensions. First, it implies that the counselor, rather than the student and the professor, knows what is best for the student in a particular class. Second, the procedure bypasses the most productive method of accomplishing accommodation, that is, for the student to communicate directly with the professor before the class starts. In so doing, the policy appears to imply that because students have a disability, they are to be isolated from normal social interactions and required to present a letter (scarlet?) from a professional when communicating with faculty members about that very subjective experience of disability.

The point of the example presented in this section was to demonstrate that the practice of castification is alive and well. Fortunately, in this example, reaction by students with disabilities and interested faculty resulted in change. However, many other examples could have been offered, and the point remains. People with disabilities are often, unintentionally, relegated to inferior statuses by human service and education professionals. Not only does this castification profoundly affect the individual's self determination, but it also affects their interpersonal relations. For example, although the proposed accommodation letters could have been helpful to students who are not articulate or to hesitant faculty members, such letters also could have had the appearances of bringing an "excuse from home". Excuses from home are not commonly accepted practices with many university level professors who view students as responsible adults.

Obviously, disability services present complex challenges. The same constructs that we use to better understand the situations of people with disabilities can be inadvertently used to disempower them. The potential for misuse is subtle as was illustrated by the campus policy. On one hand, the campus policy facilitated access of students with disabilities. At the same time however, the policy had a potentially castifying effect in that it could be interpreted to infer inferiority and the need for professional assistance from classification as having a disability.

CONCLUSION

In summary, many professionals consider empowerment of people with disabilities as a goal of education and rehabilitation. However, some of the processes of rehabilitation and special education have inherent castifying elements. They reflect some of the deterministic elements that are also problematic in cultural ecology. Examination of the role of professionals and service delivery programs in castification provides us with a potentially disturbing picture.

The answer, however, is not simple. All professionals and all disability services do not necessarily contribute to castification of persons with disabilities. However, the potential for negative consequences of disability policies and practices is very real. These potential consequences relate to the fact that disability is a multi-faceted phenomena that is constructed differently by various stakeholders. In addition, while the somewhat hypothetical constructs of disability and functional limitations can help us to understand the situations of people with disabilities, these same constructs cannot be used to explain behavior or to determine type and amount of needed services. Such practices are inherently deterministic and reflect lack of consideration of the complex social and cultural nature of human behavior.

The solution would seem to involve two fundamental alterations in the ways disabilities and disability services are understood. First, we must recognize the limitations of classification schemes, which reflect implicit determinism (Trueba, 1993a). Second, we must embrace Wertsch's (1991) dynamic concepts of socially mediated action, and realize that people with disabilities, the professionals who serve them, the interventions provided by those professionals, and the social and cultural contexts of the interventions are all interconnected and cannot be analyzed separately. In other words, we cannot understand the forest of the social impact of disability if we only focus on individual trees.

We propose that disciplines studying disability and disability policy examine some of the multi-level, multi-disciplinary approaches that are emerging in the study of minority empowerment (see e.g., DeVos (DeVos, 1973, 1982, 1992; DeVos & Wagatsuma, 1966; DeVos & Suárez-Orozco, 190; and especially, DeVos, 1990, pp. 208–214), Trueba, 1991; Trueba, Rodriguez, Zou, & Cintron, 1993; Trueba, Cheng, & Ima, 1993). It would seem that our understanding of the impact of disability would be significantly enriched by multi-disciplinary investigations that address various levels of specific disability services or policies (e.g., individual, interpersonal, institutional/organizational, societal) from the framework of different stakeholders (e.g., people with disabilities, families, communities, different professional groups, front line service providers, employers). Such investigations will not yield simple or easy solutions to issues in disability policy and practice. They will, however, provide us with the contextual information with which to better understand people with disabilities and the impact of disability policies and services.

REFERENCES

Albrecht, G. L. (1992). *The disability business: Rehabilitation in America.* Newbury Park, CA: Sage.

Amado, A. R. N. (1988). A perspective on the present and notes for new directions. In L. W. Heal, J. I. Haney, & A. R. Novak Amado (Eds.), *Integration of developmentally disabled individuals into the community* (2nd ed.) (pp. 299–305). Baltimore: Paul H. Brookes.

Arokiasamy, C. M., Rubin, S. E., & Roessler, R. T. (1987). Sociological aspects of disability. In S. E. Rubin & R. T. Roessler, *Foundations of the vocational rehabilitation process* (3rd ed.) (pp. 91–119). Austin, TX: Pro-Ed.

Barth, F. (1969). *Ethnic groups and boundaries.* Boston: Little, Brown.

Berkowitz, E. D. (1985). Social influences on rehabilitation: Introductory remarks. In L. G. Perlman & G. F. Austin (Eds.), *Social influences in rehabilitation planning: Blueprint for the 21st century,* (pp. 11–18). A report of the Ninth Mary E. Switzer Memorial Seminar. Alexandria, VA: National Rehabilitation Association.

Berkowitz, E. D. (1987). *Disabled policy: America's programs for the handicapped.* London, England: Cambridge University Press.

Boas, F. (1916). *The mind of primitive man.* New York: Macmillan.

Boas, F. (1928). *Anthropology and modern life.* New York: Morton.

Brown, D., Clopton, B., & Tusler, A. (1991). Access in education: Assisting students from dependence to independence. *JPED, 9,* 264–268.

Cook, T. M. (1991). The Americans with Disabilities Act: The move to integration. *Temple Law Review, 64,* 393–469.

Cummins, J. (1984). *Bilingualism and special education: Issues in assessment and pedagogy.* Clevedon, Eng.: Multilingual Matters.

DeJong, G. (1979). Independent Living: From social movement to analytic paradigm. *Archives of Physical Medicine and Rehabilitation, 60,* 435–446.

Delgado-Gaitan, C., & Trueba, H. (1991). *Crossing cultural borders: Education for immigrant families in America.* London, England: Falmer.

DeVos, G. (1967). Essential elements of caste: psychological determinants in structural theory. In A. DeVos & H. Wagatsuma (Eds.), *Japan's Invisible Race: Caste in Culture and Personalty* (pp. 332–384). Berkeley: University of California Press.

DeVos, G. (1973). Japan's outcastes: The problem of the Burakumin. In B. Whitaker (Ed.), *The fourth world: Victims of group oppression* (pp. 307–327). NY: Schocken.

DeVos, G. (19890). Ethnic adaptation and minority status. *Journal of Cross-Cultural Psychology, 11,* 101–124.

DeVos, G, (1982). Adaptive strategies in U.S. minorities. In E. E. Jones & S. J. Korchin (Eds.), *Minority Mental health* (pp. 74 117). New York: Praeger.

DeVos, G. (1983). Ethnic identity and minority status: Some psycho-cultural considerations. In A. Jacobson-Widding (Ed.), *Identity: Personal and socio-cultural* (pp. 90–113). Upsala: Almquist & Wiksell Tryckeri AB.

DeVos, G. (1990). Conflict and accommodation in ethnic interaction. In G. DeVos & M. M. Suárez-Orozco (Eds.) *Status inequality: The self in culture* (pp. 204–245). Newbury Park, CA: Sage.

DeVos, G. (1992). *Social cohesion and alienation: Minorities in the United States and Japan.* San Francisco: Westview.

DeVos, G., & Romanucci-Ross, (Eds.) (1982). *Ethnic identity: Cultural continuities and change* (2nd. ed.). Chicago, IL: The University of Chicago Press. (First edition, 1975, by The Wenner-Gren Foundation for Anthropological Research, Inc.).

DeVos, G., & Suárez-Orozco, M. M. (1990). *Status inequality: The self in culture.* Newbury, CA: Sage.

DeVos, G., & Wagatsuma, H. (1966). *Japan's invisible race: Caste in culture and personality.* Berkeley, CA: University of California Press.

Ebel, R. L. (1974). And still the dryads linger. *American Psychologist, 29,* 485–492.

Ferguson, P. M., Ferguson, D. L., & Jones, D. (1988). Generations of hope: Parental perspectives on the transitions of their children with severe disabilities from school to adult life. *Journal of The Association for Persons with Severe Handicaps, 13,* 177–187.

Fine, M., & Asch, A. (1988). Disability beyond stigma: Social interaction, discrimination, and activism. *Journal of Social Issues, 44,* 3–21.

Foley, D. (1991). Reconsidering anthropological explanations of ethnic school failure. *Anthropology and Education Quarterly, 22*(1), 60–86.

Gibson, M. (1987). The school performance of immigrant minorities: A comparative view. *Anthropology and Education Quarterly, 18,* 262–275.

208 / The Interpersonal and Attitudinal Impact of Disability

Gibson, M., & Ogbu J. (Eds.) (1991). *Minority status and schooling: A comparative study of immigrant and involuntary minorities.* New York & London: Garland.

Goffman, E. (1963). *Stigma: Notes on the management of spoiled identity.* New York: Simon & Schuster.

Gove, W. R. (1976). Social reaction theory and disability. In G. L. Albrecht (Ed.), *The sociology of physical disability and rehabilitation,* (pp. 57–71). Pittsburgh: University of Pittsburgh Press.

Hahn, H. (1985). Changing perception of disability and the future of rehabilitation. In L. G. Perlman & G. F. Austin (Eds.), *Social influences in rehabilitation planning: Blueprint for the 21st century,* (pp. 53–64). A report of the Ninth Mary E. Switzer Memorial Seminar. Alexandria, VA: National Rehabilitation Association.

Hahn, H. (1989). The politics of special education. In D. K. Lipsky & A. Gartner (Eds.), *Beyond separate education: Quality education for all* (pp. 225–241). Baltimore: Paul H. Brookes.

Illich, I. (1977). Disabling professions. In I. Illich, I. K. Zola, J. McKnight, J. Caplan, H. Shaiken, *Disabling professions* (pp. 11–39). London: Marion Boyars.

Jenkins, W., Patterson, J. B., & Szymanski, E. M. (1992). Philosophical, historic, and legislative aspects of the rehabilitation counseling profession. In R. M. Parker & E. M. Szymanski (Eds.), *Rehabilitation counseling: Basics and beyond* (2nd ed., pp. 1–41). Austin: PRO-ED.

Kozol, J. (1991). *Savage inequalities: Children in America's schools.* New York: Crown.

Lipsky, D. K., & Gartner, A. (Eds.), (1989). *Beyond separate education: Quality education for all.* Baltimore: Paul H. Brookes.

Mandeville, K., & Brabham, R. (1992). The federal-state vocational rehabilitation program. In R. M. Parker & E. M. Szymanski (Eds.), *Rehabilitation counseling: Basics and beyond* (2nd ed., pp. 43–71). Austin, TX: Pro-Ed.

Matute-Bianchi, M. E. (1991). Situational ethnicity and patterns of school performance among immigrant and nonimmigrant Mexican-descent students. In M. Gibson, and J. Ogbu (Eds.), *Minority status and schooling: A comparative study of immigrant and involuntary minorities* (pp. 205–247). New York: Garland.

McBurney Disability Resource Center (1993, January). Memorandum on alternative-testing service changes. Madison, WI: University of Wisconsin-Madison, McBurney Disability Resource Center.

McKnight, J. (1977). Professionalized service and disabling help. In I. Illich, I. K. Zola, J. McKnight, J. Caplan, H. Shaiken, *Disabling professions* (pp. 69–91). London: Marion Boyars.

Mehan, H., Hertwick, A., & Meihls, J. L. (1986). *Handicapping the handicapped: Decision making in students' educational careers.* Stanford: Stanford University Press.

Nisbert, J., Covert, S., & Schuh, M. (1992). Family involvement in the transition from school to adult life. In F. R. Rusch, L. DeStefano, J. Chadsey-Rusch, L. A. Phelps, & E. M. Szymanski (Eds.), *Transition from school to adult life: Models, linkages, and policy* (pp. 407–424). Sycamore, IL: Sycamore.

Nosek, M. A. (1992). Independent living. In R. M. Parker & E. M. Szymanski (Eds.), *Rehabilitation counseling: Basics and beyond* (2nd ed.) (pp. 103–133). Austin, TX: PRO-ED.

Ogbu, J. (1974). *The next generation: An ethnography of education in an urban neighborhood.* New York: Academic Press.

Ogbu, J. (1978). *Minority education and caste: The American system in cross-cultural perspective.* New York: Academic Press.

Ogbu, J. (1987). Variability in minority school performance: A problem in search of an explanation. *Anthropology and Education Quarterly, 18,* 312–334.

Ogbu, J. (1989). The individual in collective adaptation: A framework for focusing on academic underperformance and dropping out among involuntary minorities. In L. Weis, E. Farrar, & H. Petrie (Eds.), *Dropouts from school: Issues, dilemmas, and solutions* (pp. 181–204). Albany, NY: State University of New York Press.

Ogbu, J. (1991a). Immigrant and involuntary minorities in comparative perspective. In Gibson & Ogbu, (Eds.), *Minority status and schooling: A comparative study of immigrant and involuntary minorities* (pp. 3–33). New York: Garland.

Ogbu, J. (1991b). Low school performance as an adaptation: The case of blacks in Stockton, California. In Gibson & Ogbu, (Eds.), *Minority status and schooling: A comparative study of immigrant and involuntary minorities* (pp. 249–285). New York: Garland.

Ogbu, J. (1992). Understanding cultural diversity. *Educational Researcher, 21*(8), 5–24.

Ogbu, J., & Matute-Bianchi, M. E. (1986). Understanding sociocultural factors: Knowledge, identity and school adjustment. In *Beyond language: Social and cultural factors in schooling language minority students* (pp. 73–142). Sacramento, CA: Bilingual Education Office, California State Department of Education.

Rehabilitation Act Amendments (1992).

Roosens, E. (1989). Creating Ethnicity: The process of ethnogenesis. In H. B. Bernard (Series Editor) *Frontiers of Anthropology, Volume 5.* Newbury Park, CA: Sage.

Roth, W. (1985). The politics of disability: Future trends as shaped by current realities. In L. G. Perlman & G. F. Austin (Eds.), *Social influences in rehabilitation planning: Blueprint for the 21st century,* (pp. 41–48). A report of the Ninth Mary E. Switzer Memorial Seminar. Alexandria, VA: National Rehabilitation Association.

Rubenfeld, P. (1988). The rehabilitation counselor and the disabled client: Is a partnership of equals possible? In S. E. Rubin & N. M. Rubin (Eds.), *Contemporary challenges to the rehabilitation counseling profession* (pp. 31–44). Baltimore: Brookes.

Rubin, S. E., & Roessler, R. T. (1987). *Foundations of the vocational rehabilitation process* (3rd ed.). Austin, TX: Pro-Ed.

Salifos-Rothschild, C. (1976). Disabled persons' self-definitions and their implications for rehabilitation. In G. L. Albrecht, *The sociology of physical disability and rehabilitation* (pp. 39–56). Pittsburgh: University of Pittsburgh Press.

Scotch, R. K. (1988). Disability as the basis for a social movement: Advocacy and the politics of definition. *Journal of Social issues, 44,* 159–2172.

Scott, R. A. (1969). *The making of blind men: A study of adult socialization.* New York: Russell Sage Foundation.

Shonkoff, J. P. (1983). The limitations of normative assessments of high-risk infants. *Topics in Early Childhood Special Education, 3*(1) 29–43.

Skrtic, T. M. (1991). *Behind special education: A critical analysis of professional culture and school organization.* Denver: Love.

Spindler, G. (1971). *Dreamers without power: The Menomini Indians* (with L. Spindler). New York: Holt, Rinehart and Winston. Republished by Waveland Press in 1984.

Spindler, G. (Ed.) (1955). *Education and Anthropology.* Stanford, CA: Stanford University Press.

Spindler, G. (Ed.) (1978). *The making of psychological anthropology.* Berkeley, CA: University of California Press.

Spindler, G., & Spindler, L. (1987). Teaching and learning how to do the ethnography of education. In G. Spindler & L. Spindler (Eds.), *Interpretive ethnograpy of education at home and abroad* (pp. 17–33). New Jersey: Lawrence Erlbaum.

Spindler, G., & Spindler, L., with Trueba, H., & Williams, M. (1990). *The American cultural dialogue and its transmission.* London: Falmer.

Storck, I. F., & Thompson-Hoffman, S. (1991). Demographic characteristics of the disabled population. In S. Thompson-Hoffman & I. F. Storck (Eds.), *Disability in the United States: A portrait from national data* (pp. 15–33). New York: Springer.

Stubbins, J. (1988). The politics of disability. In H. E. Yuker (Ed.), *Attitudes toward persons with disabilities* (pp. 22–32). New York, NY: Springer.

Stubbins, J. (1991). The interdisciplinary status of rehabilitation psychology. In R. P. Marinelli & A. E. Dell Orto (Eds.), *The psychological and social impact of disability* (3rd ed., pp. 9–17). New York: Springer.

Suárez-Orozco, M. M. (1987). Towards a psychosocial understanding of Hispanic adaptation to American schooling. In H. Trueba (Ed.), *Success or failure: Linguistic minority children at home and in school* (pp. 156–168). NY: Harper & Row.

Suárez-Orozco, M. M. (1991b). Immigrant adaptation to schooling: A Hispanic case. In M. Gibson, & J. Ogbu (Eds.), *Minority status and schooling: A comparative study of immigrant and involuntary minorities* (pp. 37–261). New York: Garland.

Suárez-Orozco, M. M. (1993). Three generations in the reshaping of psychological anthropology. Unpublished Manuscript. Center for Advanced Study in the Behavioral Sciences. Stanford University, Stanford, CA.

Suárez-Orozco, M. M. (Ed.). (1991a). Migration, minority status, and education: European dilemmas and responses in the 1990s, *Anthropology and Education Quarterly, 22*(2). (Entire Theme Issue).

Suárez-Orozco, M. M., & Suárez-Orozco, C. (1991). The cultural psychology of Hispanic immigrants: Implications for education research. Paper presented at the Cultural Diversity Working Conference, Teacher Context Center, Stanford University, October 4–6, 1991.

Szymanski, E. (1985). Rehabilitation counseling: A profession with a vision, an identity, and a future. *Rehabilitation Counseling Bulletin, 29,* 2–5.

Szymanski, E. M. (1994). Transition: Life-span, life-space considerations for empowerment. *Exceptional Children, 60,* 402–410.

Szymanski, E. M., Hanley-Maxwell, C., & Asselin, S. (1992). The vocational rehabilitation, special education, vocational education interface. In F. R. Rusch, L. DeStefano, J. Chadsey-Rusch, L. A. Phelps, & E. M. Szymanski (Eds.), *Transition from school to adult life: Models, linkages, and policy* (pp. 153–171). Sycamore, IL: Sycamore.

Szymanski, E. M., Rubin, S. E., & Rubin, N. M. (1988). Contemporary challenges: An introduction. In S. E. Rubin & N. M. Rubin, (Eds.), *Contemporary challenges to the rehabilitation counseling profession* (p. 1–14). Baltimore: Brookes.

Taylor, S. J., & Bogdan, R. (1984). An introduction to qualitative research methods. New York: Wiley.

Trueba, H. T. (1988a). English literacy acquisition: From cultural trauma to learning disabilities in minority students. *Journal of Linguistics and Education, 1,* 125–152.

Trueba, H. T. (1988b). Culturally-based explanations of minority students' academic achievement, *Anthropology and Education Quarterly, 19,* 270–287.

Trueba, H. T. (1991). Comments on Foley's "Reconsidering anthropological explanations . . ." *Anthropology and Education Quarterly, 22,* 87–94.

Trueba, H. T. (1991). Linkages of macro-micro analytical levels. *Journal of Psychohistory, 18,* 457–468.

Trueba, H. T. (1993a). Castification in multicultural America. In H. T. Trueba, C. Rodriguez, Y. Zou, & J. Cintron, *Healing multicultural America: Mexican immigrants rise to power in rural California* (pp. 29–51). Philadelphia: Falmer.

Trueba, H. T. (1993b). Ethnicity in school and society: Educational anthropology struggles between determinism and deconstructionism. Unpublished manuscript. School of Education, University of Wisconsin-Madison.

Trueba, H. T., Jacobs, L., & Kirton, E. (1990). *Cultural conflict and adaptation: The case of the Hmong children in American society.* London, England: Falmer.

Trueba, H. T., Rodriguez, C., Zou, Y., & Cintron, J. (1993). *Healing multicultural America: Mexican immigrants rise to power in rural California.* London, England: Falmer.

Trueba, H. T., Spindler, G., & Spindler, L. (Eds.). (1989). *What do anthropologists have to say about dropouts?* London, England: Falmer.

Trueba, H., Cheng, L., & Ima, K. (1993). *Myth or reality: Adaptive strategies of Asian Americans in California.* London, England: Falmer.

Wagatsuma, H., & DeVos, G. (1984). *Heritage of endurance: Family patterns and delinquency formation in urban Japan.* Berkeley, CA: University of California Press.

Wertsch, J. V. (1991). *Voices of the mind: Sociocultural approaches to mediated action.* Cambridge, MA: Harvard University Press.

Wright, B. A. (1983). *Physical disability—A psychosocial approach* (2nd ed.). New York: Harper & Row.

Wright, T. J., & Leung, P. (1993). *Meeting the unique needs of minorities with disabilities: A report to the President and the Congress.* Washington, DC: National Council on Disability.

15

People with Disabilities as Victims: Changing an Ill-Advised Paradigm

Ruth Torkelson Lynch and Kenneth R. Thomas

The concept of a person with a disability as "victim" is imbedded in the public press and everyday conversations of the general public. Other words synonymous or related to victim have also been associated with disability, such as casualty, sufferer, needed martyr, patient, and invalid (Landau, 1977). The emotionally-laden campaigns directed toward receiving donations for specific disability groups can be viewed as prime examples of promoting the victim concept. These fund-raising campaigns have been successful in raising millions of dollars for research and services, but at what cost to individuals with the particular disability targeted? Aziz (1992) reported that the 1992 Muscular Dystrophy Telethon, which raised $46 million, was the site of vocal protest for its use of a "pity" approach as a fund-raising tactic to solicit money from people. An associated concern of the protest was about what is done with the money once the Muscular Dystrophy Association gets it. The Muscular Dystrophy protestors, organized by a group called Barrier Busters, Inc., issued a press release charging the Telethon with promoting destructive and untrue stereotypes of people with severe physical disabilities as child-like, non-contributing members of society whose only hope is to be cured. In addition, the press release went on to state that the Telethon hurts all people with severe physical disabilities, including those who do not have muscular dystrophy, because the same pitiable stigma follows them. The search for sympathy for "victims" of disease and disability is big business. However, the message promoted does not emphasize a potential for independence or the individuality of each person.

In broadcast and print media, communication about people with disabilities has often highlighted either their helplessness or their heroism (National Institute on Disability and Rehabilitation Research, 1991). In this way, people with disabilities are characterized either as victims, or as inspirational figures

From *Journal of Rehabilitation, 60*(1) (1994), 8–11. Reprinted with permission.

who overcame their disability by some miracle. When these images are prevalent in the media and the press, it is difficult to bring public attention to the real issues facing people with disabilities. Most traditional media portrayals do not cover issues such as discrimination; societal attitudes; and physical, social and economic barriers. Instead, media portrayals have emphasized heartwarming stories of people who overcame their disabilities while being constantly good-humored, patient and courageous. Other portrayals have characterized the "sad victims, confined to beds or wheelchairs, dependent on the goodwill of others for every accomplishment in their lives, eliciting pity, charity, or both" (National Institute on Disability and Rehabilitation Research, 1991, p. 2). There have been several efforts to change media coverage through disability awareness programs as well as through written guidelines for reporting and writing about people with disabilities (Research and Training Center on Independent Living, 1987).

Almost more disconcerting than the portrayals by the media, however, is the prevalence of the "victim" concept in perceptions and communications by professionals: (a) Mr. Jones *suffered* a spinal cord injury in a motor vehicle accident.", (b) " This individual was the *victim* of a work-related injury.", (c) "Mr. Jones is *afflicted* with muscular dystrophy.", and (d) "Ms. Smith is *crippled* by post-polio disability." Rehabilitation professionals have, by use of such phrases, modeled and reinforced the victim concept. Although this process may be completely unintentional by the professional, the use of victim-laden terminology contributes to the perpetuation of this phenomenon. In order to reject the concept of victim, the more appropriate conceptualization and terminology would be the following: (a) "Mr. Smith sustained a spinal cord injury in a motor vehicle accident.", (b) "This individual experienced a work-related injury.", (c) "Mr. Jones has muscular dystrophy." and (d) "Ms. Smith is experiencing the effects of post-polio disability."

THE VICTIM CONCEPT IN ATTITUDES TOWARD PERSONS WITH DISABILITY

Attitudes towards people with disabilities are largely the result of an interactive process (Britton & Thomas, 1972). In this framework, persons with disabilities are not, as society so often perceives them, the passive recipients of negative or even positive attitudes. Instead, individuals with disabilities can affect the attitudes and reactions of others by their own behaviors. Examples of situations in which the person with a disability can affect the quality of interactions with others include the nature and frequency of requests for assistance or the demonstration of independent or dependent performance of life activities.

In a later work that focused on the contributions of sociology to the practice of rehabilitation counseling, Britton and Thomas (1976) commented on the relationship between the concept of deviance and Merton's (1957) self-fulfilling prophecy construct. Specifically, borrowing from Erikson (1962), Parsons (1956), and Garfinkel (1956), it was observed that the criminal trial, the psychiatric case conference, the verdict, the diagnosis, and the act of social placement into the role of inmate, patient, or rehabilitation client are all dramatic means of affirming deviance or "being different from normal." Moreover, this process can be viewed as decisive and often irreversible because of the few public rituals and rehabilitation interventions performed to reinstate individuals who have been affirmed as deviant into their original or "normal" roles. The inmate leaves the prison, the patient with a mental illness leaves the hospital, and the client with a disability leaves a rehabilitation agency with less support and structure than necessary to function effectively. Indeed, the community frequently places the former inmate, mental patient and rehabilitation client on some sort of probation, suspicious that their behavior will again become aberrant. Britton and Thomas (1976) proposed that Merton's self-fulfilling prophecy construct may explain instances of recidivism and poor outcomes among some individuals who have participated in rehabilitation programs. If a counselor has an attitude based on stereotypes that project a poor prognosis, this attitude can be conveyed to clients in terms of actions or inaction. In such a scenario, the rehabilitation process has been thwarted by a perception of the client as a victim, who is now different, and who is unlikely to break from the role of being different.

VICTIMIZATION IN AN ENVIRONMENTAL CONTEXT

The concept of victim is entwined with the concept of environment-person inter-action and implies helplessness, fate, and being at the mercy of the environment. Fortunately, much attention in the rehabilitation literature has been directed recently toward describing the inter-relationships between an individual's behavior and the environment (Parker, Szymanski, & Hanley-Maxwell, 1989; Szymanski, Dunn, & Parker, 1989; Szymanski & Parker, 1989). Although discussed primarily within the context of supported employment services, these observations have implications across a broad range of topics important to rehabilitation profession-als and clients. As suggested earlier by several authors (Barker, Wright, Meyerson, & Gonick, 1953; Glasser & Strauss, 1964; Goffman, 1967; Kleck, 1968; Kleck, Ono & Hastorf, 1966; Lemert, 1962; Richardson, 1969; Siegel, 1963), the behav-ior of people with disabilities affects not only the reactions of others toward them, but the reactions of others also affect their own behavior.

Clogston (1990) outlined the characteristics of models used to portray dis-ability. These characteristics can provide a framework for looking at environ-ments that promote a viewpoint of the client as a positive, active change agent or as a victim of the environment/system. A traditional medical model empha-sizes disability as illness and the person with a disability is portrayed as passive and dependent on health professionals and other well-meaning people. The tra-ditional social pathology model portrays the person with a disability as a disad-vantaged client who looks to the government or to society for economic support.

That support is considered a gift and not a right. Progressive models, however, portray people with disabilities as participating in and contributing to society. Society's inability to adapt its physical, social, or occupational environment and its attitude to those who are different is highlighted in these two models. The minority/civil rights model portrays people with disabilities as a minority group with clear rights and legitimate political grievances. The cultural pluralism model depicts a person with a disability as a multifaceted individual whose disability is just one personal trait among many personal traits.

Hahn (1991) also highlighted the importance of environment using a "minority group" model as a paradigm for examining disability. A "functional limitations" paradigm is based on both a medical interpretation that stresses physical inabilities or limitations and an economic view that emphasizes vocational restrictions. The "minority group" approach, however, is based on a sociopolitical definition that views disability as the product of the interaction between individuals and the environment. Rather than concentrating on the origin of disability within the individual (i.e., a victim model), models of behavior/environment interaction (e.g., an ecological model, a "minority group" model) utilizes and challenges the environment to assist the individual with a disability to function as effectively and naturally as possible.

Rehabilitation professionals need to be cognizant that the structure of a system or environment itself can promote the concept of the individual with a disability as singled out, different, and needing specific assistance. Public school systems, for example, require that students with special needs have to be identified and categorized in order to receive special educational services. Rehabilitation clients in the state-federal system must have a documented handicap to employment to receive services. If services are needed to maintain employment or new circumstances arise in the future, a new documentation procedure is necessary. Models have been proposed (Thomas, 1995; Walker, 1992), which would eliminate separate eligibility and identification of individuals for various human services. Instead, there would be a broader human service and education umbrella, which would provide a wide array of services through one eligibility process. This system could reduce the stigma and separation of individuals with disabilities who currently receive services from separate agencies because of disability. Since programs and policies themselves can perpetuate the "victim" model, rehabilitation professionals would be well-advised to keep these issues in mind when developing programs and influencing policy.

ELIMINATION OF THE VICTIM CONCEPT

Empowerment is a term that has popular appeal. The process of empowerment involves giving power or authority to individuals or systems. In the context of rehabilitation service delivery, an empowerment approach should facilitate and maximize opportunities for individuals with disabilities to have control and authority over their own lives (Emener, 1991). The empowerment model is incompatible with a victim model because empowerment focuses on providing the client with skills and encouragement to be an agent of self-change rather than a victim of circumstance with dependence on others. According to the empowerment model outlined by Emener (1991), empowerment is critical not only for rehabilitation clients but also for rehabilitation systems, rehabilitation professionals, and families of people with disabilities. The empowerment approach regarding individuals with disabilities assumes that people strive to grow and change in positive directions, empowerment is a mind set, and clients need to empower themselves. Regardless of how empowered the rehabilitation system and rehabilitation professionals are, unless this same expectation and *responsibility* is assigned to the client by the system and the professionals, the glass is still only half full. Clients will be likely to succeed when they expect and *are expected* to succeed.

In order for professional helping relationships to be devoid of victimization, a certain sense of objectivity, reality, and challenge is required. Instead of always doing things for the client, the rehabilitation provider would ideally often play more of a "behind-the-scenes" role which could include coaching, teaching, problem-solving and consulting with the client. That is, there are occasions when the counselor may need to challenge clients to proceed on their own with only background support and encouragement by the counselor. For example, clients are often able to make job contacts and inquiries into educational programs on their own rather than being led through the process by the counselor. The ultimate accomplishments are then the responsibility of the client and are visibly associated as a product of the client's efforts. The client is no longer a victim who is at the mercy of the environment and incapable of effecting change.

REHABILITATION EDUCATION

In order to eliminate the perpetuation of the victim model, students in professional preparation programs need to recognize the relationship between their own attitudes and their ability to provide beneficial service to individuals with disabilities. Students who enter rehabilitation professions want to "help people." Helping people is an admirable goal but it can easily be translated into "doing for others" rather than building skills and confidence in people to help themselves. Most students are also very sensitive to tragedies and perceived injustices which have affected their clients. In fact, it is likely and desirable for a human service professional to experience some sense of emotional pain themselves at the realities of client experiences. However, when "helping others" is expressed in practice as "doing for others" and personal emotions resemble "pity", then the client is placed in the context of victim. It is essential that rehabilitation educators assess and address these tendencies.

Rehabilitation education can also be influential in eliminating the victim model by focusing on client assets and strengths. This focus requires careful vigilance to patterns of communication (oral and written), to the emphasis of class discussions, and to the format of curriculum topics. As an example, there is a strong tendency in case study discussions to focus on the limitations and needs of the client and neglect strengths. In response, rehabilitation plans may end up emphasizing what can be done to eliminate or accommodate for deficits rather than on planning how to capitalize on assets. Since professional rehabilitation preparation is often focused on the development of student competencies, frank discussion of what expectations and responsibilities ultimately reside with the client may be unintentionally neglected. If rehabilitation coursework and clinical experiences emphasize client responsibility and empowerment and professional/client partnerships, there is a greater likelihood that the victim frame of reference will fade away.

REHABILITATION RESEARCH

Social policy has tended to isolate individuals with disabilities as different and has emphasized service provision which expects only the individual to change or adapt. In addition to personal variables, however, it is well recognized that environmental variables and social policy also affect the ease at which people with disabilities achieve their goals. It is important for researchers to carefully consider both person and environmental/social policy variables when examining outcomes. Otherwise, rehabilitation research tends to perpetuate the concept that people with disabilities are "victims of circumstance" or "victims of their own characteristics." Rehabilitation research can be more effective for practice when it emphasizes how people with disabilities have effectively utilized personal characteristics *and* the environment to achieve a desired outcome.

REHABILITATION PRACTICE

As illustrated earlier, rehabilitation professionals can make some simple changes in communication patterns to eliminate the concept of people with disabilities as victims. Rehabilitation professionals can have an impact merely by limiting/eliminating their use of "victimizing" language in casenoting and in verbal discussions. Rehabilitation professionals can, by their own actions, de-emphasize differences between people with and without disabilities by developing programs that are less "disability-specific." In day to day practice, rehabilitation professionals can emphasize client self-determination by placing increased responsibility on the client for action and results. This shift in perspective highlights the importance of the professional as a "partner," a resource person, an active participant in problem solving, and an advocate for social policy issues. It is imperative that the rehabilitation professional be attuned to and willing to tackle the true barriers posed by attitudes and environments rather than attributing "success" or "failure" to a client as a victim of these circumstances.

SUMMARY

Rehabilitation professionals must instill in their clients self-confidence and an expectation of success. Just as self-confidence building is essential to effective teaching, parenting, and athletic coaching, it is essential for rehabilitation professional to have respect, confidence and expectations of success for their clients. The portrayal of clients as victims, even if successful in eliciting sympathetic or financial support, is an ill-advised rehabilitation paradigm.

REFERENCES

Aziz, P. (1992). MDA Telethon and Jerry Lewis' tactics questioned again. *Moving Forward, 8*(5), 1, 20, 35.

Barker, R.G., Wright, B.A., Meyerson, L., & Gonick, M.R. (1953). *Adjustment to physical handicap: A survey of the social psychology of physique and disability* (2nd ed.). New York: Social Science Research Council.

Britton, J.O. & Thomas, K.R. (1972). Modifying attitudes toward the disabled: An interactive approach. *American Archives of Rehabilitation Therapy, 20,* 112–114.

Britton, J.O. & Thomas, K.R. (1976). Rehabilitation counseling practice: Some sociological insights. *Journal of Applied Rehabilitation Counseling, 7*(1), 34–39.

Clogston, J. (1990). Disability coverage in 16 newspapers. In *Targeting key adopters in the media for disability issues education* (Grant No. H133C90043). Washington, D.C.: National Institute on Disability and Rehabilitation Research.

Dowd, E.T. & Emener, W.G. (1978). Lifeboat counseling: The issue of survival decisions. *Journal of Rehabilitation, 44*(3), 34–36.

Emener, W.G. (1991). An empowerment philosophy for rehabilitation in the 20th century. *Journal of Rehabilitation, 57*(4), 7–12.

Erikson, K. (1962). Notes on the sociology of deviance. *Social Problems, 9,* 307–314.

Garfinkel, H. (1956). Conditions of successful degradation ceremonies. *American Journal of Sociology, 61,* 420–424.

Glasser, B. & Strauss, A. (1964). Awareness contexts and social interaction. *American Sociological Review, 29,* 669–679.

Goffman, E. (1967). *Interaction ritual: Essays on face-to-face behavior.* Garden City, NY: Doubleday.

Hahn, H. (1991). Alternative views of empowerment: Social services and civil rights. *Journal of Rehabilitation, 57*(4), 17–19.

Kleck, R. (1968). Physical stigma and non-verbal cues emitted in face-to-face interaction. *Human Relations, 21,* 19–28.

Kleck, R., Ono, H., & Hastorf, A. (1966). The effects of physical deviance upon face-to-face interaction. *Human Relations, 19,* 425–436.

Landau, S.I. (Ed.). (1977). *The Doubleday Roget's Thesaurus in Dictionary Form.* Garden City, New York: Doubleday.

Lemert, E. (1962). Paranoic and dynamics of exclusion. *Sociometry, 25,* 2–20.

Merton, R.K. (1957). *Social theory and social structure.* Glencoe, IL: The Free Press.

National Institute on Disability and Rehabilitation Research. (1991). Communications about disability *Rehab Brief, 13*(12).

Parker, R.M., Szymanski, E.M., & Hanley-Maxwell, C. (1989). Ecological assessment in supported employment. *Journal of Applied Rehabilitation Counseling, 20*(3), 26–33.

Parsons, T. (1956). *The social system.* Glencoe, IL: The Free Press.

Research and Training Center on Independent Living. (1987). *Guidelines for reporting and writing about people with disabilities.* Lawrence, Kansas: Author.

Richardson, S.A. (1969). The effect of physical disability on the socialization of a child. In D. Goslin (Ed.), *Handbook of socialization theory and research* (pp. 1047–1064). Chicago, IL: Rand McNally.

Siegel, G.M. (1963). Adult verbal behavior with retarded children labeled as "high" or "low" in verbal ability. *American Journal of Mental Deficiency, 68,* 417–424.

Szymanski, E.M., Dunn, C., & Parker, R.M. (1989). Rehabilitation of persons with learning disabilities: An ecological framework. *Rehabilitation Counseling Bulletin, 33*(1), 38–53.

Szymanski, E.M., & Parker, R.M. (1989). Supported employment in rehabilitation counseling: Issues and practices. *Journal of Applied Rehabilitation Counseling, 20*(3), 65–72.

Thomas, K.R. (1995). *Attitudes toward disability: A phylogenetic and psychoanalytic perspective.* In J. Siller, K.R. Thomas, and Associates, Essays and Research on Disability. Athens, GA: Elliott and Fitzpatrick.

Walker, M. (1992). *Study circle guide—Reauthorization of the Rehabilitation Act: What should our goals be?* Alexandria, VA: American Rehabilitation Counseling Association.

16

Loss, Loneliness, and the Desire for Love: Perspectives on the Social Lives of People with Schizophrenia

Larry Davidson and David Stayner

> *So, after all, we have not failed to make use*
> *of the spaces, these generous spaces,*
> *these, our spaces. (How terribly big they*
> *must be, when, with thousands of years of*
> *our feeling, they're not over-crowded)*
>
> —Rainer Maria Rilke,
> *The Duino Elegies, Number VII*

INTRODUCTION

The following report differs somewhat from the usual journal article in its approach to the question: What factors influence the presentation of severe psychiatric disability? Numerous studies in this and other journals approach this question by searching for the objective factors that externally shape the production, exacerbation, and maintenance of the signs and symptoms of psychiatric disorder. In this report, however, we will focus on subjective factors that internally shape how individuals view the nature and consequences of one form of psychiatric disability—in this case, schizophrenia. Rather than examine the relation of genetic, neurobiological, or environmental factors to the incidence and prevalence of schizophrenic symptomatology, we will explore how the sociocultural and psychological "spaces" of experience—the interior spaces described

From *Psychiatric Rehabilitation Journal, 20*(3) (Winter 1997), 3–12. Reprinted with permission.

poetically by Rilke in the passage above—influence the ways in which schizophrenia *appears* in a person's relationships to him- or herself and to others.

These sociocultural and psychological spaces are the personal and professional perspectives, based on a combination of historical, social, cultural, political and life-historical factors, that shape the perceptions and attitudes of persons or groups encountering schizophrenia and its sequelae (McHugh & Slavney, 1983; Schutz, 1962; Schwartz & Wiggins, 1988). The perspectives in question include the clinical perspective of mental health providers and investigators who work with individuals with schizophrenia, the family perspective of those who have a loved one with this disorder, and the fist-person perspective of the individual with schizophrenia. In this article, we will examine the ways in which the social lives of people with schizophrenia appear within each of these perspectives, and how aspects of each of these three sociocultural and psychological spaces may be brought together to provide a three-dimensional view of this complex phenomenon (Miller, 1994).

We draw our data for this exercise from a larger study on the phenomenology of social functioning in people with schizophrenia. The methodology and overall findings of this study have already been presented elsewhere (Davidson, Stayner & Haglund, 1998). For this report, we will focus specifically on the core images that best capture the essence of a particular perspective on schizophrenia, and we will elaborate on these images through the use of empirical findings from the clinical literature and illustrative subjective accounts from the family and patient literatures. While each perspective has a validity and importance in its own right, we conclude by arguing that the first-person perspective provides the only direct access to the interior spaces of the person with the disorder; spaces that may be inaccessible to the objective approaches of clinical instigators, but that must be incorporated into our science if we are to do justice to the complexity of the person who is trying to recover (Strauss, 1994). Within this broader view of science, access to the interior spaces of the person with the disorder places the first-person perspective in a priority and privileged position, providing a necessary grounding that can enrich and deepen the other two perspectives.

THE CLINICAL PERSPECTIVE

> Delusions, hallucinations, and disorganized speech tend to occur early in the illness. As it progresses, these symptoms sometimes "burn out." The patient is then left only with prominent negative or defect symptoms. Looking at things superficially, one might think that a person is better off no longer hearing voices or feeling persecuted. . . . But the "burned-out" schizophrenic is an empty shell—[s/he] cannot think, feel, or act. . . . She or he has lost the capacity both to suffer and to hope—and at present, medicine has no good remedy to offer for this loss. (Andreasen, 1984, pp. 62–3)

As is evident in this passage, the clinical perspective of many professionals views the disease process of schizophrenia as transforming the person into an "empty shell" of who she or he was prior to the onset of the disorder. With the "burning out" of the more flagrant positive symptoms, nothing remains behind the blunted and dull facade of the person. Gone are the thoughts, feelings, and intentions that we most often and most personally identify with who we are as individuals. Gone is the capacity both to suffer and to hope; a capacity we consider to be basic to our nature as human beings. In these ways, the person *as a person*—as a feeling, thinking, and intending subject—is thought no longer to be home. The person having become victim to the illness, all that remains is an empty husk that can be bandied about by the winds and tides of the eternal environment, and which otherwise remains passive, withdrawn and inert.

The implications of such an image for the social functioning of people with schizophrenia are obvious. Empty shells would not be expected to have much of a social life. And, in fact, so well accepted is this expectation of a diminished capacity for socialization in people with schizophrenia that it is included as a diagnostic criterion for schizophrenia in the *DSM-IV* (American Psychiatric Association, 1994). There is a wealth of clinical research literature to support this view, with a multitude of studies demonstrating the constricted nature of the social network of people with schizophrenia and their considerable limitations in social interactions with others. In these studies, people with schizophrenia typically are described as withdrawn and socially isolated, initiating few social contacts, reporting having no friends or only superficial acquaintances, relying heavily on family members for what contacts they do have, and receiving significantly more support from these relationships than they are able to give back (Breier, Schreiber, Dyer & Pickar, 1991; Cohen & Sokolovsky, 1978; Gilliland & Sommer, 1961; Hirschberg, 1985; Rosen et al., 1980; Schooler & Spohn, 1960; Sylph, Ross & Kedwarth, 1977; Tolsdorf, 1976; Wallace, 1984. For a review, see Davidson et al., 1998). While the shell may not be totally empty in all of these instances, it has been a consistent finding in the clinical literature that the person with schizophrenia is more often isolated than not, and more often seen as being cared about and for by family than being caring toward others.

In addition to being a consequence of the burnout of the positive symptoms of hallucinations, delusions, and thought disorder, social isolation in schizophrenia has been associated with a number of other factors. These include indirect manifestations of the disorder such as alienating behaviors and appearance that provoke stigmatizing responses from others, a pervasive lack of basic social skills and judgment, and undesirable side effects of treatments for the disorder ranging from medication side effects to the effects of institutionalization (Davidson et al., 1998). As a result of this myriad of factors, people with schizophrenia are not only considered incapable of approaching and initiating social contacts with others, but they also are seen as more likely to be avoided and shunned by others, particularly by those people who did not know them or care about them before they became disabled. To strangers, the prominent negative symptoms reflected in the empty shell image do not offer much promise for a meaningful sense of social connection; it is easiest just to pass by. For family members and other loved ones and friends who already know the person, the situation is more complicated. It is to this situation that we now turn.

THE FAMILY PERSPECTIVE

> The anguish is that this demon, schizophrenia, having completely deranged a brain and ravaged a life, has now released an empty shell of a person, as though shaking it like a rag doll and throwing it to the ground. (Smith, 1991, p. 690)

At first glance, this passage echoes the quotation chosen to represent the clinical perspective described above, in that both authors—in the first instance a psychiatrist, in the second, the mother of a young woman with schizophrenia—describe the disorder as wreaking havoc on the person's life and releasing, in the wake of this storm, an "empty shell of a person." And in fact, family accounts of schizophrenia are most often pervaded by a profound sense of loss of the person with the disorder, and of a growing chasm between who this person was before getting sick, including his or her goals and dreams for the future, and who he or she has since become. Similar to clinical investigators, family members describe their loved ones having grave difficulties in relating, which they attribute to the illness. The mother quoted above, for example, writes that "sustaining or contributing to a relationship of any kind [has become] beyond the realm of possibility" for her daughter (Smith, 1991, p. 690). As a consequence of this social disability, family members feel at an increasing emotional distance from their loved one, and in this way appear to confirm the empty shell image offered by the clinical perspective outlined above.

Family accounts differ from clinical accounts, however, in at least one important respect. Despite the social disability, withdrawal and isolation, and apparent emotional vacancy that they attribute to the rages of the illness, family members appear to hold onto a conviction that their loved one somehow remains, somewhere inside of the shell, even if concealed or buried within the negative symptoms of the disorder. This conviction in the lingering of the person they knew prior to the onset of the disorder can take on a variety of forms. Some family members, for example, describe the heightened vulnerability, hypersensitivity, and fear that they sense their loved ones experiencing behind the clouds of the disorder. Rather than viewing their brother or daughter as incapable of feeling, they view him or her as overwhelmed by feelings that are too much for his or her internal resources to manage. The sister of one young man with schizophrenia describes her brother as having a "sixth emotional sense" through which he comes to see the world as "through a magnifying glass"; a capacity that can leave him transfixed by paralyzing fear and anxiety. In a significant and provocative move beyond the empty shell image to one that we feel better captures the insight, sensitivity, and pathos of the family perspective, she describes his eyes as "vacant and haunted with the naked look of a frightened animal frozen by the beam of approaching headlights" (Brodoff, 1988, pp. 114–5). In a similar vein, a mother describes her son's blunted feelings as a way to "shield himself from the intensity of his emotions" (Bouricius, 1989, p. 207).

In addition to sensing the presence of extreme and overwhelming feelings behind the clouds of the disorder, family members also feel that they are able to understand some of the bizarre behaviors and speech of their loved ones and are aware of the fact that their loved ones are experiencing their own sense of profound loss of the lives and dreams they had prior to becoming disabled. They write often and eloquently of the failures of a mental health system that they feel ignores the person with the disorder by focusing almost exclusively on the treatment of the illness at the expense of attending to the basic human needs that people continue to experience either despite or because of their disorder. Being acutely aware of the presence and importance of these unmet needs, family members go to great lengths to lobby and advocate to change the mental health system and its treatment of people with schizophrenia. Concerned that mental health providers can be misled by the appearance of emotional vacancy in people with schizophrenia to assume that these people no longer have feelings at all (which is, in fact, a core assumption of the clinical perspective, as we have just seen), a mother of a young man with schizophrenia offers another telling image for the social facade of her son, comparing him to a poker player who experiences emotions he cannot or will not reveal. Insisting that her son is not in fact an empty shell, she asks that "those who work with him will make every effort to find the emotions that may be hidden behind an expressionless face" (Bouricius, 19889, p. 207).

On a more positive but equally painful note, family members also describe the thrill they experience during occasional periods of improvement in their loved one's condition, when they see once more the real person break through the illness (Moorman, 1988; Smith, 1991). It is perhaps this experience more than any other which distinguishes the family perspective from that of the clinician, and which captures the dynamic tension inherent in family accounts of life with a person with schizophrenia. This tension is between the need, on the one hand, of family members to distance themselves from the person with schizophrenia and all of the havoc and chaos it creates, to accept that their relationship with this person has been irrevocably changed as a result of the disorder, and, on the other hand, the lingering desire and hope for the return of the person who has been lost to the illness. Family members look expectantly to the newest medication or the next treatment, hoping that this will be "the one" to bring about a cure; and they find their hopes bolstered when they see incremental improvements in their loved one's condition (Moorman, 1988; Najarian, 1995). Yet just as often, family members experience repeated setbacks and disappointments, and see the person disappear yet again behind the illness. Pulled back and forth between their need to accept the reality of the illness and protect themselves from its effects and their tireless hunger for the return of the person they have lost to the disorder, families describe a heartrending tension that is all the more difficult to tolerate because it appears to be unending and unresolvable. Unlike grief over a loss, which can eventually lead to acceptance, this partial loss and partial hope for the return of the person suspends the family member in a no-man's land from which there appears to be no way out. As a sister of a man with schizophrenia writes:

> Although grieving for someone who has died is painful, some sense of peace and acceptance is ultimately possible. However, mourning for a loved one who is alive— in your very presence and yet in vital ways inaccessible to you—has a lonely, unreal quality that is extraordinarily painful. (Brodoff, 1988, p. 116)

THE FIRST-PERSON PERSPECTIVE

> If I am to survive this maelstrom called schizophrenia, I must continuously try to gain the comprehension I need to withstand each plunge into darkness and find a way to share as much as I can in a way that will make me feel the least alone. (Ruocchio, 1991, p. 358)

Family accounts paint an image of the person with schizophrenia as a frightened animal or calculating poker player, in either case with the person hiding his or her feelings and thoughts behind a haunted and expressionless face. If family members are engaged in a painful and prolonged waiting game, hoping against hope for the person to reemerge from behind this vacant facade, the person with schizophrenia may be involved at the same time in a struggle to resurface from the depths and darkness of the disorder in an attempt to reconnect with others, as well as with him- or herself. First-person accounts of schizophrenia are pervaded by the themes of loss of interpersonal relationships, loneliness, and social isolation, and the desire for, and attempt to establish, social connections. People describe the illness as robbing them of access to themselves as well as to others, and as leading to profound feelings of alienation and estrangement coupled with painful yearnings for comfort, companionship, and caring. While perhaps appearing wooden and vacant to others, and perhaps also feeling at an extreme emotional distance even from themselves, people with schizophrenia continue to describe a fervent wish for love and relationships that contrasts starkly with the empty shell image descried above. The diary of one young man with schizophrenia who was rated independently by five clinicians as having negative symptoms, for example, includes such statements as: "I am a lonely nothing. . . . My afflictions fill the place that was meant for sharing love. . . . I have a dreadful fear of not loving. . . . I want to love" (Bouricius, 1989, pp. 202–5). The desires and needs of many such individuals are captured well in an eloquent plea by Esso Leete, a national spokesperson for the mental health consumer/survivor movement in the United States and herself diagnosed with schizophrenia:

> What makes life valuable for those of us with mental illness? . . . Exactly what is necessary for other people. We need to feel wanted, accepted and loved. . . . We need support from friends and family. . . . We need to feel a part of the human race, to have friends. We need to give and receive love. (Leete, 1993, p. 127)

If people with schizophrenia continue to desire love and connections so strongly, then why do they describe feeling at such an emotional distance from themselves and others? To what do they attribute their experiences of loss, isolation, and loneliness, at times to the point of despair? First-person accounts make mention of a number of obstacles and barriers to relating that people with schizophrenia see as keeping them at a painful distance from others. We will review some of these briefly before moving on to propose an image that captures the social situation entailed in these experiences from the inside, i.e., from the perspective of the person with the disorder.

Most often, people with schizophrenia describe a range of issues which they face that are not due inherently to the disorder itself, but that are related to it more indirectly. Such issues include stigma, rejection, poverty, and unemployment. Particularly early in the course of their illness, people with schizophrenia credit stigmatizing attitudes on the part of mental health providers and their loved ones as a primary cause of their experiences of rejection and loss. They also identify stigma as a main factor in their continuing difficulty in initiating new relationships once they have become a patient of the mental health system. Underlying all of the many examples of encountering stigma described in first-person accounts is the dehumanizing experience of being seen by others primarily, if not solely, as a mental patient—and, to that extent, no longer as an individual like themselves. In addition to the effects of stigma, people with schizophrenia may act in ways which inadvertently (or intentionally) keep others at a distance. Alienating behaviors associated with this disorder include talking out loud to hallucinated voices, acting in bizarre ways in response to delusional ideas, and demonstrating poor social judgment and personal hygiene. With the increased social distance that results from the combination of discrimination, alienation, and rejection, people with schizophrenia are left feeling less than human, needing even more persistence and courage to make another attempt at establishing a relationship in spite of these odds.

Attempts to socialize and develop new connections may be further undermined by the unemployment and poverty experienced by many people with schizophrenia. With the loss of work, people also lose one of the primary sources adults have for meeting people and establishing new connections. With the loss of expendable income, people also find their options for engaging in social and recreational activities severely restricted. Entitlements leave scarce money for leisure activities, and it is hard to feel like going out and being with others when you have no money in your pockets or purse. Both unemployment and poverty also can exert a significant negative impact on a person's confidence, self-esteem, and social status, making it more difficult for him or her to take the social risks required to form new relationships. As one consumer advocate describes:

> Many of us have to learn to cope with little money, or no money from time to time. It almost always has an effect upon our relationships. If we lose a job . . . it is difficult to maintain self-respect and relationships with those we love, no matter what kind of relationship it is. (Seckinger, 1994, p. 20)

Of those barriers to relating resulting directly from the disorder itself, hypersensitivity to stimulation and affect appears most often in first-person accounts. This hypersensitivity crosses sensory domains—it may be visual, auditory, tactile, or olfactory—and also may permeate the interpersonal sphere, imposing an additional emotional burden on relationships. Leete (1993) describes the impact of this enhanced sensitivity and intensity on both the perceptual and social levels:

> We mst learn to go through life experiencing our surroundings with a greater intensity than others do. Sounds are louder, lights brighter, colors more vibrant. These stimuli are distracting and confusing for us, and we are unable to filter their impact to lessen their effect. In addition, I believe we are more sensitive in an interpersonal sense as well. I have noticed that others like myself are easily able to pick up emotional nonverbal cues and feelings that may be "hidden." (p. 119)

Going through life experiencing "a greater intensity than others do" both perceptually and socially can pose a number of challenges in relating to others. Heightened sensitivity to sensory stimulation can lead people to become preoccupied with their immediate perceptual environment, at the expense of attending to co-occurring social demands and cues. People also may be overwhelmed by the constant bombardment of intense sensory impressions, leading them either to become numb or to shut down altogether. On the interpersonal level, a heightened sensitivity to subtle cues and "hidden" feelings may make it difficult for people to sort out what information is most relevant for social encounters and what messages can remain implicit. Experiencing others' emotions as if "through a magnifying glass," people also may feel that customary social responses do not do justice to the enormity of the encounters in which they are involved. As one person describes:

> I find emotions tremendously complex, and I am quite acutely aware of the many over- and undertones of things people say and the way they say them. . . . I have difficulty handling social situations that require me to be artificial or too careful. (Hatfield & Lefley, 1993, p. 63)

The increased intensity of affect experienced by people with schizophrenia seems to pose particular problems in relating when the affect in question has a negative valence. Emotions and experiences like anger, hostility, criticism, disapproval, and rejection may be especially difficult for them to tolerate, and may lead to an exaggerated tenuousness and precipitous breaks in relationships. As one person describes: The largest problem I face—I think the basic one—is the intensity and variety of my feelings, and my low threshold for handling other people's intense feelings, especially negative ones" (Hatfield & Lefley, 1993, p. 55). As a result of their confusion and low tolerance for affect, people with schizophrenia may find relationships difficult to manage and navigate, and gradually may withdraw from opportunities for relating due to their anticipation of future embarrassments and failures. As one person explains: "I began to be afraid of people, of my family and friends; not because of what they represented . . . but because of my own inability to cope with ordinary human contacts" (Hatfield & Lefley, 1993, p. 56).

Another barrier to relating inherent to schizophrenia results from impairments in attention, concentration, and communication experienced by people with this disorder. In addition to hypersensitivity, people often report difficulties in focusing their attention, filtering out distracting and irrelevant details, and being able to concentrate on objects or events that interest them. With their perceptions, thoughts, emotions, and intentions constantly being pulled in a variety of directions in response to the slightest breeze people may find it exceedingly difficult to pursue a single train of thought or sustain a simple dialogue for any extended period of time. While they may be acutely aware of the consequences of their "yielding to associative connections" (Freedman, 1974, p. 335) in this way, they also may feel powerless and helpless to change this condition, watching themselves passively and impotently from the sidelines as they stumble and fail repetitively in their attempts to sustain conversations with others. As one person describes:

> My thoughts get all jumbled up. I start thinking about something but I never get there. Instead I wander off in the wrong direction and get caught up with all sorts of things that might be connected with the things I want to say but in a way I can't explain. People listening to me get more lost than I do. (Torrey, 1983, p. 18)

In this case as well, people may restrict their social interactions and become increasingly withdrawn in anticipation of the tremendous energy, persistence, and repeated difficulties entailed in attempting to converse with others. In the following report, this person adds memory difficulties to the mix and describes how she has come to keep her verbal interactions with others to a minimum to spare herself the strain and disappointments involved in trying to sustain a dialogue:

> I can hear what they are saying all right, it's remembering what they have said in the next second that's difficult—it just goes out of my mind. . . . I am speaking but I'm not conscious of what I'm saying . . . so I don't know what I'm talking about. I've got a rigmarole in my mind now for checking what I say in advance so if somebody speaks to me I get on my guard straight away so that I can make ia sensible answer. I try to say something sensible and appropriate but it is a strain . . . and when the conversation is going on . . . I don't know what they are talking about or what I was talking about. I keep talk to a minimum to prevent these attacks coming on. (Chapman, 1966, p. 237)

Another exceptionally distressing aspect of the subjective experience of schizophrenia that interferes with social functioning is the loss of sense of self reported by people with the disorder. In addition to the experience of stigma and attentional impairments described above, people also report severe memory impairments that lead to a loss of any continuity between past, present, and future in terms both of day-to-day life and of personal identity. This combination of factors appears to leave people feeling that they are no longer an enduring subject or agent of their own sensations, ideas, and emotions, but that these subjective functions have been taken over by forces external to the person (Davidson, in press). With no abiding center, people become unsure of where they leave off and others begin, and become increasingly vulnerable and susceptible to the influence of others. Fears of engulfment then become another powerful motivator to avoid social contact (Ruocchio, 1991). With no abiding center, there also is no one left inside of the person to initiate and sustain contact with others (Deegan, 1993). In this vein, people with schizophrenia describe losing themselves to their illness, feeling that they are "giving in to death" and becoming separated from themselves by a "wall of glass" (Ruocchio, 1991). They describe the horror and powerlessness of becoming inaccessible to themselves as well as to others, and feeling pushed out to the margins of their own awareness where they can be only passive and distant spectators of the chaos that rages in their minds. Perceiving themselves to be at the mercy and whim of the storms of illness, people may have little choice but to act and appear to others as they themselves feel internally: like a "nobody nowhere" (Weingarten, 1994, p. 374).

Given the range of barriers to relating described above, it is no wonder that people with schizophrenia appear significantly compromised in their social functioning. If, as we suggest, they continue nonetheless to desire connections to others, we might expect that one way for them to cope with this state of affairs would be to share their internal struggle with others by articulating their experiences of the difficulties and obstacles they encounter. And, in fact, this is one important function served by the fist-person accounts from which we draw the data for this section. In relating their own stories through interviews and autobiographies, individuals with schizophrenia have already made efforts to communicate their dilemma and struggles to the larger community. The passage with which we opened this section also addresses this issue on the interpersonal level, describing the importance one woman with schizophrenia placed on being able to share a much of her experience as possible with her therapist so that she could feel "the least alone" (Ruocchio, 1991). People with schizophrenia may find it exceedingly difficult, however, to communicate to others *about* the difficulties they have in communicating, and this for some of the same reasons we have already described.

In addition to those issues already described, there are at least two more factors that undermine individuals' attempts to share their experiences of the disorder and its sequelae with others as a first step toward reentering the social sphere. First, the impact of the disorder may be so confusing and disorienting, at least initially (and, for some, for an extended period of time), that people often do not know where to begin in describing their situation to others, nor do they know what exactly to say about it. In addition, some aspects of the disorder itself, such as the heightened intensity of sensation, the fragmentation of thoughts brought about by yielding to associative connections, and the loss of self, may take place on such a basic and foundational level that they may border on ineffable, leaving the person without a language to capture these experiences. The woman quoted above as trying to find a way to share her experience with her therapist describes the painful process of trying to find words to express these deeply personal and deeply disturbing experiences this way:

My own inadequacy to use language to express what lies buried so deeply inside me, even when I am lucid, makes words a curse that blocks the proverbial light within the tunnel, and I am alone with my darkness. There are things that happen to me that I have never found words for, some lost now, some which I still search desperately to explain, as if time is running out and what I see and feel will be lost to the depths of chaos forever. With each uncommunicated experience the darkness grows. (Ruocchio, 1991, p. 358)

Even when people do find the words to capture their experiences, they are faced with the second challenge of finding a way to communicate their struggles so that others can hear, tolerate, and accept the despite the stigma of mental illness. As another person explains:

Aggravating matters more is the painful knowledge that you can't talk to anybody about these things. Not only are these things hard to talk about, but if you admit to having any of these kinds of problems you are likely to get puzzled looks or face immediate and often final rejection. Most people will put you in the category of "crazy" or "looney tunes" or "nutcase" or something similar. So to avoid this kind of abuse you are forced to hide or conceal your thoughts and feelings from others, and then ultimately from yourself, which only serves to worsen your situation. This is why persons with mental disorders are often passive, withdrawn, and avoid human contact. They are engaged in an inner struggle they can't express and which consumes them. . . . The invisibility of [this] struggle . . . and the isolation that results is what makes their situation so tragic. (Weingarten, 1994, p. 374)

As both of these last two passages suggest, failed attempts to share the burden of the illness with others leave the person feeling increasingly alienated and alone. With each such failure, the person's sense of darkness and chaos deepens, as does his or her rage and frustration over the inability to connect. Despair and hopelessness may move more and more to the foreground, at times overshadowing continuing desires for relationships. At these times, people may hide their feelings, thoughts, and desires even from themselves, risking becoming dead inside and appearing to others as the "nobody nowhere" they already feel. It is at these times that the empty shell image first offered by the clinical perspective may be the most accurate in capturing how the person with schizophrenia can appear to others. First-person accounts consistently document, however, that even at these extreme times an inner struggle continues to be waged within the person between, on the one hand, giving in to the illness and giving up, and, on the other hand, venturing out again and again into the social domain to risk yet another failed attempt to relate. While what the last author quoted above describes the invisibility of this inner struggle can mislead people into thinking that the war has already been lost and that the person is no longer home, this misperception only leads to increased isolation and loneliness for the person struggling to resurface and break through the illness. What is needed is a more accurate image of the interior space of the person with the disorder, which makes visible the struggle in which he or she is engaged and which thereby draws others to him or her as sympathetic allies in this fight.

Such an image is offered implicitly in the dairy of the young man quoted earlier, who had been rated independently by five clinicians as having pronounced negative symptoms. In one passage from his diary he describes a profound sense of paralysis and incapacity in social functioning that thwarts his earnest and ongoing efforts to give and receive love. He writes:

> I want to love. I envy those who can relate to each other. . . . When my heart burns away, will they pick up the ashes and say, "He loved too much but he never knew how to show it so his heart burned away and here are the ashes"? . . . My desire burns to sorrow and freezes to ice. My cries hide in my heart. (Bouricius, 1989, pp. 204–5)

The images of desires frozen to ice and cries hiding in the young man's heart bring to mind the panther in Rilke's (1907/1981) poem of that name. In this poem, the panther has become so accustomed to encountering only the bars of the cage in which it lives, rather than the world that lies beyond the cage, that it has since ceased even to attempt to muster a response to the impressions that continue to slip into its awareness through the bars. Like this caged panther, the will of people with schizophrenia can become so stunned and numbed by their repeated failures in trying to connect with others that they may at times suspend acting on their continued desires for relationships. While opportunities for relating may initially arouse interest, the impulse to act may reach the person's heart, as it does with the panther, only to die there very quickly thereafter. Both the existence and the death of these desires and impulses may be invisible to others, taking place perhaps behind a wooden and vacant expression; but it is still quite possible that "great will" stands poised there, waiting for a more promising opening or for the replenishment of sufficient strength to try again. We close this section with Rilke's complete poem, "The Panther," which we offer as an alternative to the empty shell, frightened animal, and poker player images to represent the first-person perspective on social functioning in schizophrenia:

The Panther

From seeing the bars, his seeing is so exhausted
that it no longer holds anything anymore.
To him the world is bars, a hundred thousand
bars, and behind the bars nothing.
The little swinging of that rhythmical easy stride
which circles down to the tiniest hub
is like a dance of energy around a point
in which a great will stands stunned and numb.
Only at times the curtains of the pupil rise
without a sound . . . then a shape enters,
slips through the tightened silence of the shoulders,
reaches the heart, and dies.
(*The New Poems,* 1907/1981, p. 139.)

DISCUSSION

> The professionals called it apathy and lack of motivation. They blamed it on our ill-
> ness. But they don't understand that giving up is a highly motivated and highly goal-
> directed behavior. For us giving up was a way of surviving. Giving up, refusing to
> hope, not trying, not caring: all of these were ways of trying to protect the last frag-
> ile traces of our spirit and our selfhood from undergoing another crushing. (Deegan,
> 1994, p. 19)

Each of the perspectives on social functioning in schizophrenia reviewed in
this report has a legitimacy and validity in its own right. It is important, in comprehending this complex phenomenon, to know that people with schizophrenia
may appear to third parties as empty shells in relation to them, and to know that
family members can perceive the lingering flame of a life behind this facade,
even if it remains for the most part beyond their reach. It is important to know
how restricted and limited the social lives of people with schizophrenia may be,
and to recognize the painful feelings of loss and mourning experienced by their
loved ones as a result. In these and other ways, the sociocultural and psychological spaces traversed by clinicians and family members in their relations to the
person with schizophrenia reflect important aspects of that person's situation and
plight. But it may be even more important in coming to a comprehensive understanding of this phenomenon to listen to the voice from behind the expressionless face, appreciate the obstacles the person is encountering in trying to
reemerge, and continue to believe in and bear witness to that person's integrity
and potential, even when things seem their bleakest.

The above passage from Patricia Deegan, another national spokesperson for
the mental health consumer/survivor movement in the United State and herself
diagnosed with schizophrenia, argues that even giving up and not caring are goal-
directed and intentional acts of a person who continues to fight to survive, to
"protect the last fragile traces" of his or her spirit, until a better day dawns and
offers more promise. Deegan suggests that even those people who, for the time
being, have lost the capacity to hope still retain a capacity to feel and to think,
and do in fact continue to suffer, at times to unspeakable depths of anguish and
despair. From a third-person point of view, it is understandable how a person's
inner struggles may remain invisible, and how others may come to assume that
there is no longer anyone home. Both family members and individuals with
schizophrenia attest, however, that the shell is in fact not empty; and first-person
accounts of what goes on inside of the shell are crucial in giving us access to the
interior spaces of the person with the disorder which we might otherwise fail to
make use of. We would suggest that it is only through a reclamation of these
spaces—and, in fact, in the process *of* reclaiming them—that we will be able to
figure out first, how to reconnect with, and then, second, how to assist the person
confined within the bars of his or her own disorder in reemerging and rejoining
the social sphere.

To return briefly to our introductory and more general comments regarding the influence of sociocultural and psychological spaces on the appearance of psychopathology, this exercise demonstrates the value of integrating various perspectives on aspects of human behavior, and also suggests at least one principle to guide such efforts. This principle, derived from the work of Edmund Husserl and the phenomenological tradition, holds that when studying human beings one should begin with the experiences of the subject under study. Objective approaches are useful and can produce valuable findings that could not be obtained by other means. Science also depends upon our ability to acquire a reflective, theoretical attitude toward data, and to move to a level of abstraction that goes beyond our day-to-day, common sense understanding in making sense of these data. But when the object of our science is human subjectivity, our reflections and theoretical abstractions must first be grounded in an empathic appreciation of the lives of our subjects from the perspective of their own life experience and intentionality (Davidson, 1994). As Husserl (1952/1989) wrote: "I can experience others [as subjects], but only through empathy. . . . No causal research, no matter how far-reaching, can improve the understanding which is ours when we have understood the motivation of a person" (pp. 210, 241). Only by continuing to treat our subjects *as subjects,* and by developing such empathic bridges to their experiences, will we be able to avoid the mistake of treating the shell as if it were empty, and in the process further alienating and isolating people who already are at the margins of the social world (Estroff, 1989). As scientists, a first crucial step toward facilitating the reintegration of people with schizophrenia is for us to *not fail* to make use of their own interior spaces and experiences in our science, but to seek out and solicit their stories and perspectives in addition to those of clinicians, clinical investigators, and family members (Davidson & Strauss, 1995; Strauss, 1989). In the end, it will be these stories that will enable us to discover the otherwise invisible ways that people with schizophrenia have of surviving, and that will teach us how to be most useful to them in their continuing efforts to replenish their strength and to reemerge from the chaos and storms of the illness.

REFERENCES

American Psychiatric Association (1994). *Diagnostic and Statistical Manual of Mental Disorders, fourth edition.* Washington, DC: APA Press.

Andreasen, N. C. (1984). *The broken brain: The biological revolution in psychiatry.* New York: Harper & Row.

Bouricius, J. K. (1989). Negative symptoms and emotions in schizophrenia. *Schizophrenia Bulletin, 15,* 201–8.

Breier, A., Schreiber, J.L., Dyer, J., & Pickar, D. (1991). National institute of mental health longitudinal study of chronic schizophrenia. *Archives of General Psychiatry, 48,* 239–246.

Brodoff, A.S. (1988). Schizophrenia through a sister's eyes: The burden of invisible baggage. *Schizophrenia Bulletin, 14,* 113–6.

Chapman, J. (1966). The early symptoms of schizophrenia. *British Journal of Psychiatry, 112,* 225–51.

Cohen, C.I., & Sokolovsky, J. (1978). Schizophrenia and social networks: Ex-patients in the inner city. *Schizophrenia Bulletin, 4,* 546–60.

Davidson, L. (1994). Phenomenological research in schizophrenia: From philosophical anthropology to empirical science. *Journal of Phenomenological Psychology, 25,* 104–30.

Davidson, L. (in press). Intentionality and identity in schizophrenia: A phenomenological perspective. *Duquesne Studies in Phenomenological Psychology, 5.*

Davidson, L., Stayner, D., & Haglund, K.E. (1998). Phenomenological perspectives on the social functioning of people with schizophrenia. In K. T. Mueser & N. Tarrier (Eds.), *Handbook of social functioning in schizophrenia.* Needham Heights, MA: Allyn & Bacon Publishers.

Davidson L., & Strauss, J.S. (1995). Beyond the biopsychosocial model: Integrating disorder, health and recovery, *Psychiatry, 58,* 43–55.

Deegan, P.E. (1993). Recovering our sense of value after being labeled mentally ill. *Journal of Psychosocial Nursing, 31,* 7–11.

Deegan. P.E. (1994). A letter to my friend who is giving up. *The Journal of the California Alliance for the Mentally Ill, 5,* 18–20.

Estroff, S.E. (1989). Self, identity, and subjective experiences of schizophrenia: In search of the subject. *Schizophrenia Bulletin, 15,* 189–96.

Freedman, B.J. (1974). The subjective experience of perceptual and cognitive disturbances in schizophrenia: A review of autobiographical accounts. *Archives of General Psychiatry, 30,* 333–40.

Gilliland, G.W., & Sommer, R. (1961). A sociometric study of admission wards in a mental hospital. *Psychiatry, 24,* 367–72.

Hatfield, A.B., & Lefley, H.P. (1993). *Surviving mental illness: Stress, coping and adaptation.* New York: The Guilford Press.

Hirschberg, W. (1985). Social isolation among schizophrenia outpatients. *Social Psychiatry, 20,* 171–8.

Husserl, E. (1989). *Ideas pertaining to a pure phenomenology and to a phenomenological philosophy, Second book: Studies in the phenomenology of constitution* (R. Rojcewicz & A. Schuwer, trans.). Boston: Kluwer Academic Publishers. (Original work published 1952.)

Leete, E. (1993). The interpersonal environment—A consumer's personal recollection. In A.B. Hatfield & H.P. Lefley (Eds.), *Surviving mental illness: Stress, coping and adaptation* (pp. 114–28). New York: The Guilford Press.

McHugh, P.R., & Slavney, P.R. (1983). *The perspectives of psychiatry.* Baltimore: Johns Hopkins University Press.

Miller, S.G. (1994). Borderline personality disorder from the patient's perspective. *Hospital and Community Psychiatry, 45,* 1215–9.

Moorman, M. (1988, September 11). A sister's need. *New York Times Magazine,* pp. 44ff.

Najarian, S.P. (1995). Family experience with positive client response to Clozapine. *Archives of Psychiatry Nursing, 9,* 11–21.

Rilke, M.R. (1939). *The duino elegies* (J.B. Leishman & S. Spender, trans.). New York: W.W. Norton & Company. (Original work published 1923.)

Rilke, M.R. (1981). The panther. In R. Bly (ed. & trans.), *Selected poems of Rainer Maria Rilke* (p. 139). New York: Harper & Row Publishers. (Original work published 1907.)

Rosen, A.J., Tureff, S.E, Daruna, J.H., Johnson, P.B., Lyons, J.S., & Davis, J.M. (1980). Pharmacotherapy of schizophrenia and affective disorder: Behavioral correlates of diagnostic and demographic variables. *Journal of Abnormal Psychology, 89,* 378–89.

Ruocchio, P.J. (1991). The schizophrenic inside. *Schizophrenia Bulletin, 17,* 357–9.

Schooler, C., & Spohn, H.E. (1960). Social interaction on a ward of chronic schizophrenics. *International Journal of Social Psychiatry, 6,* 115–9.

Schutz, A. (1962). *The problem of social reality. Collected papers, Volume 1* (M. Natanson, Ed.). Boston: Martinus Nijhoff.

Schwartz, M.A., & Wiggins, O.P. (1988). Perspectivism and the methods of psychiatry. *Comprehensive Psychiatry, 29,* 237–51.

Seckinger, S.S. (1994). Relationships: Is 1-900 all there is? *The Journal of the California Alliance for the mentally Ill, 5,* 19–20.

Smith, E. (1991). Living with schizophrenia. *Schizophrenia Bulletin, 17,* 689–691.

Strauss, J.S. (1989). Subjective experiences of schizophrenia: Toward a new dynamic psychiatry II. *Schizophrenia Bulletin, 15,* 179–87.

Strauss, J.S. (1994). The person with schizophrenia as a person II: Approaches to the subjective and complex. *British Journal of Psychiatry, 164,* 103–107.

Sylph, J.A., Ross, H.E., & Kedwarth, H.B. (1977). Social disability in chronic psychiatric patients. *American Journal of Psychiatry, 134,* 1391–1394.

Tolsdorf, C.C. (1976). Social networks, support, and coping· An exploratory study *Family Process, 15,* 407–417.

Torrey, E.F. (1983). *Surviving schizophrenia: A family manual.* New York: Harper & Row.

Wallace, C.J. (1984). Community and interpersonal functioning in the course of schizophrenic disorders. *Schizophrenia Bulletin, 10,* 233–257.

Weingarten, R. (1994). The ongoing processes of recovery. *Psychiatry, 57,* 369–375.

Part IV: *Study Questions and Disability Awareness Exercise*

1. Are the principles related to the acceptance of relationships between persons with mental retardation and other mental impairments, and persons who are temporarily able-bodied, transferable to other populations, such as persons with chronic mental illness, traumatic brain injury, and people with AIDS?
2. Your client, who has a facial disfigurement as a result of severe burns, presents concerns to you regarding the best ways for her to handle people who either exclude her from social contact or who intrude on her by "prying" into the causes of her disfigurement and its impact on her. How would you respond to her request for specific suggestions on how to cope with or change this situation?
3. What is the common ground between persons with disabilities and persons of ethnic and racial minorities?
4. Give an example of how constructs or definitions of disability relate to the perspective of the defining group.
5. Discuss how castification in a historic context may provide insight into future issues in rehabilitation and health care.
6. Can castification ever be empowering? If so, give an example.
7. How does the media promote the image of victim for some people with disabilities?
8. How can the media present empowering images of people with disabilities?
9. Can victimization ever be empowering for people with disabilities?
10. What argument would you present to the March of Dimes Muscular Dystrophy Association to convince them to change their "victim-based" marketing? What would you anticipate as their counter argument to you?
11. How does the concept of " empty shell" limit the expectations for recovery for people with schizophrenia?
12. Why does the family experience a sense of profound loss when living with a member with a psychiatric disability?
13. What is your reaction to the first person, family, and investigator accounts in the Davidson and Stayner article? Which one do you relate to most, and why?

DONOR OR RECIPIENT?

This experience focuses on complex issues arising for donors of organs for transplant. An intense situation may be created because the person requiring a kidney is someone who is emotionally close to you.

Goals

1. To explore reactions when a person has the opportunity to consider the donation of his or her kidney.
2. To present a situation that is complicated by the needs of a loved one or a non loved one.
3. To examine differing perspectives when the role of a person in need is reversed.

Procedure

1. Leader reads the following statement: "You have just received a phone call from the person you are closest to and love dearly. Stop and reflect on who this person would be in your life now. This person has just received word of having renal failure and is very distressed about his or her health. Due to medical complications the doctors feel that a kidney transplant is critical; without it, the person is in danger of dying."
2. Participants write a one-page statement of their reactions to this information.
3. Group members are selected at random to read their responses.
4. After all members have read their statements an open group discussion takes place.
5. During this discussion particular attention should be paid to the quality of the relationship.
6. The leader introduces the concept of significant others (e.g., if you would be hesitant to donate a kidney to this person, is there anyone whom you might consider as a donor?).
7. Having processed this, the leader moves to the role reversal stage in which the group members become the person in need.
8. The leader reads the following statement: "You have just been informed by your physician that you have renal failure, unless you receive a kidney within three months you are risking death."
9. The leader asks participants to write a paragraph on the initial reaction to this news.
10. Next the group leader asks the group to write down the name of a person they would ask to donate a kidney to them and to list five reasons why they might ask this particular person.
11. Two group members are selected to role-play the situation, asking the named person for his or her kidney.
12. What would your response be if a severely disabled family member volunteered to donate a kidney? Did not volunteer? Was in need of a kidney?
13. What if the person who wanted or could donate a kidney was someone you hated and considered an enemy?

Part V

Sexuality and Disability

The sexuality of persons with disabilities has traditionally been given little attention by professionals, although currently this is a major area of concern during treatment and rehabilitation. It has been suggested that this avoidance, in part, stems from taboos against the discussion of sex. Another reason for avoidance is the lack of education and information about sex and sexuality as they relate to people with disabilities. The chapters in Part V have been selected to create a perspective focusing on attitudinal and informational problems related to sexuality and disability.

Cole and Cole address sexuality, disability, and reproductive issues throughout the life span in chapter 18. Four perspectives are provided in their comprehensive article: 1) sexuality and developmental disability; 2) sexuality and acquired disability; 3) reproductive issues, and 4) sexuality and aging. They emphasize, throughout, that sexuality and fertility are natural experiences for persons with disabilities, as they are for persons without disabilities, and as such, should not be artificially separated from the spectrum of our lives.

In chapter 19, McAllan and Ditillo present practical information to assist rehabilitation practitioners in working more effectively with gay and lesbian clients with disabilities. These include 1) understanding and countering myths, 2) the reality of being gay or lesbian, 3) learning about ourselves and our biases, and 4) necessary skills and resources. The importance of rehabilitation practice embracing diversity to include all persons is emphasized.

Sexual abuse, a pervasive problem in our culture, does not exclude those with physical or mental disabilities. In fact, research has shown that persons with disabilities face an increased risk of abuse as compared to persons without disabilities. The purpose of chapter 20 is to increase the awareness of the issues surrounding the sexual abuse of persons with disabilities. Recommendations for counselor intervention are made and resources for additional information are provided.

In her sexual autobiography (chapter 21) Vash presents a candid portrayal of her sexual experience as a woman with an acquired disability. Using her personal-psychospiritual-theoretical model, she provides the reader with an analysis of this experience which proves beneficial in understanding the meaning of sexuality in her life, in that of others and in ourselves.

The overall theme of Part V is that a person has many issues to address during the life and the living process. Sexuality is a major factor that cannot be ignored and must be part of the treatment and rehabilitation process. As people with disabilities have become more socially liberated at the close of the 20th century, so too must they become more sexually liberated.

17

Sexuality, Disability, and Reproductive Issues Through the Lifespan

Sandra S. Cole and Theodore M. Cole

The decade of the 1990s presents an opportunity for America to reflect on the progress that has been made in services, attitudes, and opportunities for people with disabilities. In her book, *Sex, Society and the Disabled*, Robinault (1978) reminds us that Margaret Mead said, "The character of a culture is judged by the way it treats its disabled." In the United States we are now implementing the Americans with Disabilities Act (ADA), and Margaret Mead would be pleased to judge our culture by our commitment to the ADA.

Biology is the determinant of anatomic sex. It is not the determinant of behavioral sex, and the primate learns sexual behavior. More is needed than biology alone—education influences the final product of sexual health. However, in animals, sexual behavior is determined neurochemically. It is related to reproduction, which is its final intent. In humans, reproduction and sexual behavior are not synonymous. Men and women must learn not only about sexuality, but they must also learn about sexual relationships. Add to this the need to learn about love, and it becomes apparent that both the tasks and the rewards become complex. Beyond sexual love is the more generic love for humankind, a noncoital love involving personal interaction and charm.

Historically, disability in the Western world has a grisly past. In early cultures, an imperfect child was usually killed. In the Middle Ages, such a child was tolerated but was the object of ridicule or fear. Court jesters were sometimes the adult products of birth defects. By the time of the Renaissance, many people with disabilities could look forward to living out their adult lives in asylums.

It was not until the 18th century that the first "modern care" for people with disabilities was begun, in Switzerland. In the 19th century, the first glimmers of education and scientific inquiry into physical disabilities and mental retardation were seen.

From *Sexuality and Disability, 11*(3) (1993), 189–205. Reprinted with permission.

By the middle of the 20th century, what has come to be known as modern rehabilitation first appeared. It was the by-product of a society sympathetic toward survivors of military encounters. Now at the close of the 20th century, we are just beginning to demonstrate our concerns for personhood, body image, and human sexuality as a part of rehabilitation (Robinault, 1978).

AN OVERVIEW

Sexuality and reproductive issues encountered by people with physical disabilities during early childhood, adolescence, and early reproductive years are likely to be different from those that people without disabilities experience. Earlier years (infancy) and later years (adult reproductive years) have many similarities for both groups.

It is most convenient to think about these issues from four points of view: 1) sexuality and developmental disabilities, 2) sexuality and acquired disabilities, 3) reproductive issues, and 4) issues pertaining to the aging process.

Early onset disabilities are likely to affect sexual development in terms of gender roles, the language of sex, privacy, self-exploration, sex education, and personal learning. Socialization experiences in early childhood give direction and meaning to adult sexuality. Examples of medical correlates include musculoskeletal disabilities and neurogenic impairments that can affect fertility and sexual options (Hanks & Poplin, 1981).

Disabilities that are acquired after sexual maturity may affect these same areas, but in different ways. Gender roles may become blurred, past sexual patterns of activity may impede creativity needed after disability, and medical experiences may have a desexualizing effect upon self-esteem and libido. Birth control, sexually transmitted diseases, pregnancy, reproduction, and parenting present similar concerns for early onset and adult onset disabilities.

Individuals with and without disabilities have the same rights to information, services, and to health service providers with adequate knowledge, sensitivity, and experience in areas of sexual development. Self-empowerment, life skills, parenting, and medical concerns are common to everyone, but these are issues that may need special attention in individuals with physical disabilities. As individuals mature, new problems may be added to underlying disability issues: for example, further confusion of gender role, stigma, need for more adaptive equipment, societal expectations of the aging adult, and the anticipated transition from health to illness (Frank, 1988; Goffman, 1963).

DEVELOPMENTAL ISSUES

Gender

As children grow, a tremendous focus of energy and instruction, both from the individual and society, is on the careful preparation and development of the gender role of female or male. Much of the childhood experience lays the foundation for the masculinity and femininity of personalities and relationships with others. It must be recognized that the presence of a physical disability influences and in some ways may limit the development of psychosexual/social maturity.

It is reasonable to assume that parents, in anticipation of the birth of a child, have fantasies and dreams of what their "perfect little child" will be as a man or a woman. Needless to say, parents are generally not prepared for the birth of a child with a disability, and, although they can learn to understand and work with the presence of a disability, many of their dreams, plans, and preparations for the child and for the family will be altered (Darling, 1988; Shapiro, 1983).

Privacy

In the early years when children first demonstrate independence and curiosity, including curiosity about themselves and their sexual bodies, the child with a disability probably experiences some alteration in natural opportunities for privacy. He or she may be more closely observed or supervised by family or caregivers and therefore less able to be spontaneous and private with sexual curiosity than a typically developing child. This lack of privacy can affect a child's perception of his or her body, its function, and personal boundaries regarding appropriate or inappropriate touch. Most learning in children is done spontaneously and includes a great deal of physical involvement with other children, adults, and with the environment—physical involvement being a catalyst to learning. Spontaneity is dramatically affected and can be severely limited by the presence of a disability (e.g., affecting vision, mobility, speech and/or hearing) (Cole & Cole, 1990).

During these years, children are simultaneously gaining language skills: first, recognizing language; second, gaining cognition; and third, developing individual skills to communicate with parents, family, and the environment. During these early years, children are also obtaining the "language of sex," learning terms and phrases for body parts and behaviors, and striving to gain an understanding of word usage in expressing thoughts and feelings about sex and sexuality. Their efforts sometimes range from embarrassing and silly to dramatic. This phase is a time for adults and parents to provide children with accurate language for body parts and their functions, appropriate and accurate sex education, in addition to their usual private and personal words, names, and sexual expressions used within the family.

It is helpful for all children, including the child with a disability, to know correct words, their usage, and to be able to express him- or herself appropriately regarding sexual matters. This knowledge and ability increases the child's self-confidence and self-esteem and can be a contributing factor in prevention of sexual abuse, molestation, or exploitation. Increased knowledge, awareness, and language confidence can help the child to recognize inappropriate behavior, abuse, or violence that may be imposed on him or her, since persons with disabilities are particularly vulnerable to sexual perpetrators (Cole, 1986; Sobsey & Varnhagen, 1988).

Many common expletives in adult language make reference to sexual activities. A child very likely will have heard such "swearing" and, most naturally, tries to repeat those words to emulate adult behavior, even if the words are not understood. This spontaneous behavior of children frequently generates a startled reaction from adults and can sometimes result in an immediate opportunity to provide sex education, helping the child to distinguish appropriate and inappropriate language and social situations. (Unfortunately, occasionally the response from an adult is to admonish and punish the child.) A child with a disability may be quite insulated from having these spontaneous experiences. For children with disabilities, particularly those who have limited mobility, it is entirely possible that a part of their development may be influenced by isolation or limited access to peers, and that they may not have had many opportunities to explore and learn about life and its events with their peers. As children with disabilities get older, these life experience omissions become more evident and they may experience social handicaps because of their lack of awareness or understanding of society and the behaviors of the adult world. Since most information about sex is learned quietly, covertly, and is greatly and dramatically influenced by peers and the media, children with disabilities may experience distinct limitations in knowledge and communication about sex education and sexual behavior (Robinault, 1978).

Touch

Touch is a major element in human development and has a powerful effect on all individuals. Infants and children first learn feelings of security, intimacy, and bonding through touch. Love and affection are expressed through touch and language. Children with physical disabilities have additional touch experiences that relate to medical care procedures or to assistance with activities of daily living (ADL).

Children with physical disabilities may require specific assistance with movement or positioning and may require apparatus or equipment to facilitate ambulation and mobility. As a result, they may experience a profound difference between being handled for management and health care purposes and being touched and held for tender and loving purposes. Many children with disabilities experience far more "handling" than tender loving caresses. Similarly, having a disability that requires medical attention presents the possibility of more public nudity than that experienced by a typical child. Having one's body examined and impersonally handled by health care providers often involves this type of physical exposure, and this type of touch most often is not negotiated with the child by health care providers. It is a common experience for individuals with disabilities to have medical procedures, examinations, and inquiries made by health care providers who touch their bodies for purposes of examination but who neglect to be sensitive to this intrusion. Any effort to acknowledge and negotiate personal boundaries of touch is generally overlooked, and the implications of being touched by strangers usually are left unresolved. Obviously, vulnerability to exploitation, misinterpretation, or misinformation is increased with these situations.

Such behavior is common, although inappropriate, in the health care professions. For example, a child with an orthopedic condition may have experienced many examinations that take place with five or more members of a health care team in attendance. In addition, the procedures may be videotaped and the child may be wearing only underpants during the examination. Vulnerability during pubescent years when children are naturally modest, particularly as they experience genital development, is heightened. Perhaps one of the most important lessons for professionals in health care to learn is to respect their individuality, personal dignity, and privacy of patients, something that is not often demonstrated in public examinations in amphitheaters or lecture halls.

When boundaries of appropriate touch are not clear, a child with a disability may not learn to distinguish between appropriate and inappropriate touch and may not have a healthy understanding of the subtleties between public and private nudity and public and private sexual behavior. For some children, especially in institutions, inappropriate touch may have been the only form of affection they have received, and, therefore, their ability to distinguish appropriateness has been impaired. It is well known that health care providers are not infrequently the abusers of persons with disabilities (Griffith, Cole, & Cole, 1990; Sobsey & Varnhagen, 1988).

These issues add to the well-established societal fact that adults handle and interact differently with male and female children (Allgeier & Allgeier, 1991). Adults tend to be more aggressive and physically firm in the way boys are handled in daily activities. Girls are more frequently stroked and caressed, spoken to softly, and handled gently. With all children, society begins to shape the gender roles of masculine and feminine from infancy. A child with a disability may experience additional limitations by being unable to participate fully in his or her expected and implied gender role (Gordon, 1975).

Self-Exploration

In early childhood, self-exploration of genitals is a natural activity. Male genitals are exposed, available, conspicuous, and of great interest to the little boy. Female genitals are hidden, less conspicuous, and much more mysterious and difficult to access for the little girl. For boys who are easily able to handle their own genitals, there is a direct opportunity to touch and stimulate their penises. Girls experience a more diffuse and sensual kind of touch in sexual expression, through caressing and stroking, as their genitals are hidden and more obscure. These distinguishing sexual aspects of masculinity and femininity are carried into adult sexual roles, each role having been developed and refined through puberty and adolescence. Some children with disabilities may have difficulty reaching and touching their own genitals. They also may lack the ability to experience touch

246 / Sexuality and Disability

sensation in their genitals. They may not directly experience their whole bodies, particularly if there is sensory loss and no feeling in some parts of their bodies. The spontaneous, curious, and innocent ways in which children learn about their bodies through touch may be less prevalent in the child with a disability than in typical peers, either through personal sensory limitations or through limitations such as lack of privacy, the need for assistance, and being discouraged in these activities by adults or by an environment controlled by adults (i.e., an institution).

The situations that have been described indicate the specific need for accurate and comprehensive sex education and gender role preparation for children with disabilities. Society must be more diligent in providing opportunities for children with early onset disabilities to acquire knowledge about themselves as sexual individuals, about sexual mores in the culture, and about the informal world of sex that their nondisabled peers more easily access. Toward that end, parents and educational systems are encouraged to provide structured sex education and to help children with disabilities to obtain accurate information about sexual health and to form positive role models for themselves.

Adolescence

During adolescence, the most common means of learning about sex is through private, informal, and perhaps secret opportunities alone or with others to rehearse the roles of a sexual man or woman. The need for opportunities for sexual rehearsal cannot be overemphasized, as it is during these occasions that adolescents begin to sort out the many mixed messages they have learned about sex and sexuality (Money, 1986). There are dramatic changes in their bodies as secondary sex characteristics begin to develop. It is a time for practicing and refining one's masculinity or femininity, and, similarly, it is during this time that the young adolescent boy and girl will begin to talk only with peers about matters of sexual development, behavior, and desires. They will practice relating to peers and to the opposite gender in sexual ways and will enter into the dramatic, sensuous, and momentous experiences of rehearsing their adult roles (Gordon & Gordon, 1983).

As many adults recall, some of the most significant memories of adolescent sexual development were of those events that occurred privately and unobserved. These opportunities of spontaneous learning may not be available to adolescents with disabilities, who often lack easy accessibility to other adolescents. Dynamics change considerably if, as a teen, one has to be catheterized, transferred into an electric wheelchair, assisted into a van, and delivered to a friend's home or public event where further assistance is needed to get into the building. At the end of the event, all of the maintenance activities are repeated in reverse. Spontaneity and social experiences and risk-taking are inhibited in these circumstances. Women who experience a disability before adolescence report their first social and sexual experiences later than their peers for these reasons (Rousso, 1988).

Society has a tendency to reinforce the dependency of children and young adults with disabilities. They are frequently infantilized in their relationships and communications with adults. A child may quickly learn that he or she is perceived and treated as helpless or less able, and this may actually facilitate the development of a "helpless individual" or "learned helplessness" (Romeis, 1990).

The pubescent child with a disability can be at risk for stigmatization by an insensitive, uncaring, and ignorant able-bodied society. At a time when conspicuousness and vulnerability is at its peak in boys and girls, the presence of a disability can further compound the difficulty of natural sexual and social development. The young person may have had so little opportunity to spontaneously interact with peers that he or she may not have the ability to develop the social skills of adolescence so necessary to carry out the culturally expected roles of male and female.

Perfection/Body Image

Society places enormous positive value and emphasis on having a perfect body. This message is taught and reinforced in the early years by the presence of role models with perfect bodies and by the lack of role models with disabilities. Advertising and media rarely show a person with a disability. By the time a child acquires language, he or she has already learned that to be disabled is to be different, imperfect, and perhaps unacceptable (Fine & Asch, 1985). To be imperfect is to be asexual and anonymous or overlooked in the sexual spectrum of adult life. The continuing emphasis on the healthy and physically fit adult (who must also achieve a perfect body) is a concrete message learned repeatedly from early childhood through media and advertising. This is often a further assault on the vulnerability of self-esteem for all people without perfect bodies, increasingly reinforced for persons with disabilities (Bogdan, Biklen, Shapiro, & Spelkoman, 1990; Brolley & Anderson, 1990; Ruffner, 1984).

Social Opportunities

Social opportunities for adolescents to interact with peers assist young adults to gain self-esteem. Clothing and fashion, music and the media, community activities, social events, and school experiences are major contributors to gender development at this age. The technical aspects of having physical access to settings where social events occur are often taken for granted by the nondisabled population. These years are times for intense peer interaction, communication, and learning by watching, doing, and rehearsing. Parental influence and values are challenged during these years and often are replaced by peer and media influence. Each adolescent matures at a different rate, but, all in all, these years are extremely full of sexual and sensual overtones, messages, and activities for those who can access them.

The sexual messages in the media about perfection and the artificiality of adult life as presented on television and in magazines tend to be one-dimensional and value-laden and provide few opportunities for the adolescent to discuss and clarify such values and their implications. These aspects of sexual socialization strongly shape and influence the emerging adult (Blackwell-Stratton, Breslin, Mayerson, & Bailey, 1988). It is entirely possible that the adolescent with a disability may have to be a spectator on the sidelines rather than a participant in exciting and demanding experiences of social-sexual development.

Socialization opportunities are essential to growth and development. If the process is healthy, essential self-esteem is achieved through daily activities, social events, and by wearing particular clothing and observing contemporary fashions. It is assumed that the child has access to settings in which these events occur. For most children, the setting does not limit them to the role of spectator but allows active participation and peer interaction. The child with a physical disability may have a more passive than active role, and learning may result more from reading and watching than from doing and experiencing.

Medical Issues

More and more, medical care includes educating the individual and the family about physical, emotional, and behavioral aspects of the disability. Even so, education is frequently presented from the perspective of the health practitioner and may be more technical than useful to the individual and family (Biklen, 1988).

Issues that should be included in patient education are mobility limitations, weakness and fatigue, management of spasticity, and adaptation to somatosensory and perceptual dysfunctions (e.g., loss of vision, hearing, smell, or touch). This material is always best presented in a nonjudgmental fashion, while the educator helps to broaden the individual's and family's concept of human diversity. (Cole & Cole, 1990).

In terms of sexuality, it is advisable to avoid a narrowly defined concept of sexuality (e.g., coitus and reproductive physiology). It is useful to include information that helps the adolescent or adult prepare for sexual fantasies and activities. Avoiding unwanted pregnancy and sexually transmitted diseases would be high on the list of desirable topics to be taught. It is all too possible that an individual with a physical disability may have alterations of body functions that interfere with the timely and accurate recognition of symptoms of sexually transmitted diseases.

Inherent in this more modern approach to health care is the assumption that the physician and other health professionals are educated and knowledgeable, both about human sexuality and the individual and the specific disability (Sandowski, 1989). It is pleasing to see that some medical examination rooms incorporate examining techniques and equipment that are user-friendly to the "disabled customer." The paraplegic woman will readily attest to the awkward, if not embarrassing, experience of being subjected to a pelvic examination that is carried out on a traditional and inaccessible examining table—too high for trans-fers, too narrow for safety, and with stirrups that require leg positions that may be impossible. (Ferreyra & Hughes, 1982).

ISSUES CONCERNING ACQUIRED DISABILITIES

Disabilities acquired in early adulthood after maturation may most specifically affect the established and well-developed sense of masculine and feminine iden-tity of the individual. In fact, the elaborate preparations for masculine and femi-nine roles of individuals are interrupted by the onset of the disability. Life plans, goals, dreams, and ideals are significantly challenged and perhaps changed by the onset of disability. The individual will most likely experience grieving, not only for specific body changes and losses, but also regarding the trauma of having one's private dreams altered, including one's sexual identification as a man or woman.

Stable and Progressive Disabilities

A disability acquired as an adult may be characterized as stable (e.g., a spinal cord injury) or progressive (e.g., multiple sclerosis). There are differences between these types of disabilities. Although the trauma of an acquired disability is unde-niable, once the disability is stabilized, an individual can proceed with organizing his or her life and achieving some semblance of control, with adaptation.

It is more complicated, however, to experience a progressive disability, because it is hard to predict the course medically and physically. It is therefore difficult to be confident about being in charge or in control of daily living, spon-taneity, and planning for the future. When individuals are in the stages of dating or planning a family, these uncertainties may complicate the usual challenges of relationships and family living.

Through the rich use of memory and the creative use of fantasy, much plea-sure can be retained from previous sexual experiences of individuals who have acquired disabilities in adult life. Sensuality can be enhanced through memory and retained throughout various sexual pleasures and activities, even with phys-ical changes or limitations. With some disabilities, intimate behaviors and pre-ferred sexual positions may have to be changed or adapted. However, severe physical losses (e.g., for a male with spinal cord injury) often cause distinct and serious concerns about fertility and the ability to be a parent, in addition to gen-eral and obvious concerns about erectile dysfunction and being accepted by soci-ety as a "real" man or woman (Mooney, Cole, & Chiligren, 1975; Neistadt & Freda, 1987; Rabin, 1980; Sha'ked, 1981).

Partners of persons with disabilities may experience the dual roles of per-sonal care assistants and of intimate partners. These challenges can create feel-ings of conflict for both the partner and the person with the disability and may contribute to stress in the relationship. Efforts must be taken by the health care worker to be sensitive to these situational dilemmas and to assist in creative problem-solving recommendations (Griffith et al., 1990).

Persons socialized in contemporary American culture are surrounded by traditional societal messages about parenting and disability (Hahn, 1981). It is imperative that health care practitioners avoid falling into the trap of stereotypical responses of pity, avoidance, infantilization, and excessive attention to persons with disabilities. Independence, personal esteem, positive body image, and positive sex messages should be emphasized. Silence from the medical community concerning disability, sexuality, and reproductive issues relays the stronger message of rejection and repression and gives the impression that parenting is not to be considered. This approach is not helpful.

GENERAL MEDICAL CARE

Men and women with acquired disabilities frequently avoid general medical care. The reason commonly given is that they believe that physicians providing general health care are not sensitive to the specific urologic and gynecologic needs and conditions of a person with a disability. Women who have disabilities often find that their gynecologist is not trained in alternative methods of conducting a pelvic examination on women with a variety of physical limitations. Many health care facilities and offices are not even accessible for the individual with a disability.

Among the general population, it is well established that sexual exploitation occurs in one out of three females and one out of seven males before they reach adulthood (Finklehor, 1979). The statistics are even more grave among those with disabilities (Mullan & Cole, 1991; Sobsey & Varnhagen, 1988). Early research has indicated that men and women with disabilities are more frequently sexually exploited than nondisabled persons and that it is almost always done by someone known to the individual. As is the case with all sexual exploitation, the psychological effect can be traumatic, and, when the trauma experienced is compounded by a disability and a lack of sex education or healthy sexual experiences, we can only assume that understanding and concerns about sexuality and confidence about one's sexual self-esteem are dramatically affected.

Certainly, there is great recognition that particular medical attention should be paid to persons with disabilities, not only to be observant to clues or indications of sexual abuse, but also for opportunities to provide information about birth control and the prevention of sexually transmitted diseases.

Consistent with the general lack of sex education available to people with disabilities, there is also an equal lack of knowledge regarding specific reproductive technology and birth control options. The sensitive clinician provides pertinent and accurate education and information (Neistadt & Freda, 1987). Such a clinician increases sexual knowledge, personal skills, and self-confidence regarding sexual health.

Sexually Transmitted Diseases

An important consideration in adolescent and adult sexual experiences is the threat to health and fertility from acquiring sexually transmitted diseases (STDs). Accurate and explicit information regarding the prevention of STDs, including AIDS, must be available to all children and adults in our society.

Of particular concern are persons with disabilities, who may lack basic sex information and education that makes them more vulnerable for acquiring these diseases. Specific recommendations for STDs and pregnancy prevention must include the use of latex dental dams and of condoms that contain nonoxynol-9. Information about the identification of symptoms and management of various STDs should be as available to individuals with disabilities as it is to others. This requires deliberate efforts by health practitioners.

Options

Just as artificiality and awkwardness are recognized by nondisabled individuals as an occasional accompaniment to sexual activities, they are also recognized by persons with disabilities. The difference is more one of quantity than quality. However, technology can be helpful for all people. A sizable portion of the nondisabled population has found that sexual diversity and adaptation can be welcome in the bedroom. So, too, people with disabilities can find that technology can be of assistance in sexual activities as it is with other activities of daily living. Surgery has contributed to the advances in technology affecting sexuality (e.g., breast enhancement, penile prosthesis). The rehabilitation practitioner or other professional should supplement the technology with information to facilitate its use. Insights into sexual kinesiology or "the athletics of sex" can be a helpful as the technology itself. Thus, the practitioner assists the person with a disability in coping with pain, fatigue, or spasticity as they affect sexual activity.

Ten percent of the population in the United States has a homosexual orientation (Kinsey & Pomeroy, 1948; Reinisch, 1990). This should be kept in mind, so that the information and technology provided dose not burden the recipient with the need for "gender translation." All medical care should be extended nonjudgmentally (Moses & Hawkins, 1982).

Physical disabilities that produce sexual dysfunctions or concerns are seen in everyday medical practice. Most practitioners encounter a patient every day with neurotrauma, skeletal disease, cardiopulmonary disabilities, metabolic diseases, dermatologic disorders, pain, malignancy, or sensory disturbances, any one of which can and usually does affect sexuality in major or minor ways.

SPECIFIC REPRODUCTIVE ISSUES AND OPTIONS

Basic reproductive concerns for men and women in the general population are also of concern for the person with a disability and, in addition, specific topics require particular attention.

Family Planning

Medical advice may facilitate pregnancy and the activities of preparing for pregnancy. Spontaneity of intimacy must also be considered. A woman who is beginning intimacy with a disabled man may wish to consider the gender role into which she has been socialized. She may be well advised to be assertive and playful and to take greater initiative. If her partner is paralyzed and cannot initiate physical activities, it may no longer be sufficient for her simply to "not say no."

In the areas of family planning, there must be more linkages between those who provide these services and the rehabilitation professionals who understand and work with the problems imposed by physical disabilities. So, too, medical information needs to be tailored to a more diverse population that includes people with physical disabilities. Research in this area is not abundant. Information for the public is not generally available, and many practitioners are unprepared to think about issues of fertility, conception, pregnancy, delivery, or even the monthly occurrence of menstruation for women with physical disabilities (Miller & Morgan, 1980; Neistadt & Freda, 1987).

In discussing reproductive options and potentials with an individual with a disability, one must assess whether the disability influences fertility and fertility options (Neistadt & Freda, 1987). Evaluations must include whether genital sensation and genital function are affected. An example would be a male with a spinal cord injury who is unable to ejaculate. This is a case in which a urologist, specially trained in electroejaculation procedures, would be instrumental in assisting with the evacuation and obtaining of sperm for insemination.

Some birth control methods may be contraindicated for women with specific disabilities. For example, a woman with spinal cord injury who is unable to feel sensation in her genital area and has diminished hand function from quadriplegia would not be a candidate to insert and use a diaphragm. There may also be unrecognized and ongoing medical conditions that affect fertility, such as irregular menses and chronic infection. What reproductive choices might be available for a woman with a disability? She would need to be evaluated to determine if she could physically carry a fetus to full term once she conceived. If this is contraindicated, it may be important to consider other alternatives for reproduction, perhaps using a female surrogate. Evaluating and recommending the type of delivery suited for a woman with a disability is extremely important for the safety of both mother and child. Many obstetricians are not trained to specialize in pregnancies of women with physical disabilities and should consult physiatrists who can assist in consultation and health care of the patient. The presence of sexually transmitted diseases would need to be identified, as would be necessary for any pregnancy.

Additional Considerations

There are several other considerations related to the ability to reproduce that are not routinely considered but potentially could have a tremendous impact on an individual with a disability and his or her partner.

People with disabilities frequently live on fixed incomes or are medically subsidized in some way. Therefore, money and finances may be limited or strained, which creates limitations on one's ability to socialize, establish relationships, and find partners (Hanks & Poplin, 1981). Does the individual with a disability have life skills that include the ability to parent? Does the possibility exist of someone assisting with parenting tasks? In addition, does the individual with the disability require a personal care assistant or someone to assist with general daily living tasks? What is the person's level of independence? What kinds of reasonable accommodations can be provided?

Social skills, body image, self-esteem, and personal integrity are central to one's ability to enjoy life and to participate in the development of relationships, intimate behavior, and preparation for pregnancy, birthing, and parenting. (DeLoach & Greer, 1981).

When medically evaluating individuals for fertility, the potential for substance abuse, the use or abuse of medications and, as mentioned earlier, a routine evaluation for determination of sexually transmitted diseases or other genital disorders must also be assessed. What previous investigation has been done in the form of tests, procedures, and assessment of sexual activities regarding reproduction? Does the individual understand his or her exact situation and options from a medical perspective? If so, then the individual deserves commendation for determination to learn and challenge a rather passive medical system until there are more answers and solutions.

AGING

As we age as sexual individuals, we continue to function in our male and female roles, which have been established since adolescence. We experience normal changes of aging, which can include physical disabilities. These changes affect the flexibility and ease with which we are able to conduct our daily lives. Additions such as wheelchairs, new and unfamiliar devices, apparatus, or equipment, which support the body, increase mobility, or enhance and make safe daily living tasks, can be cumbersome and awkward. Changes such as these can be overwhelming to the individual and his or her sense of self-confidence, dignity, and self-esteem.

We are sexual until our death. However, the gender roles we have carefully created for ourselves can be eroded during the aging process by the realization and personal experience of being slow, being viewed as less important, feeling incapable from time to time, and experiencing a general loss of personal value. These experiences can seriously affect one's confidence and the maintenance of femininity or masculinity. Negative or hesitant reactions from life partners or family members who have become caregivers for the aging individual, health care professionals who do not understand geriatrics, and society in general can increase the vulnerability of one's self-esteem.

The transition from being a healthy adult to one who experiences traumatic or chronic illness or disability can be difficult for many (Trieschmann, 1987). Elderly individuals become keenly aware of their frailties. Inaccurately and inappropriately, society may increase the potential for guilt and shame, which it associates with aspects of aging. This can be directly experienced, for example, by a woman who is incontinent and vulnerable to conspicuous embarrassment in social situations, or by the man who experiences erectile difficulties due to aging or the presence of disease.

It is time that new horizons be recognized and that we cease to add further societal burdens on individuals experiencing natural aging difficulties. Medical and societal recognition of sexual health, sexual development, gender socialization, and fertility issues pertaining to persons with disabilities will serve to pave the way for all individuals to age with sexual dignity.

There has been progressive recognition of the need to liberate people with disabilities who are oppressed. The Rehabilitation Act of 1973 that has been updated and amended is an example of the recognition of the rights of individuals with disabilities. The community of people with disabilities is working together to better state what needs to be addressed by federal legislation. The Americans with Disabilities Act of 1990 (ADA) (PL 101-336) is a civil rights act and an advance for people with disabilities. The ADA does not deal specifically with sexuality, but it does empower the individual.

Sexuality and fertility concerns are natural experiences for persons with disabilities. We cannot artificially separate sexuality from the spectrum of life for anyone.

Civil rights, which are the rallying points of those who are oppressed, include the *right to reproductive information* that is comprehensive and accurate.

REFERENCES

Allgeier, E.R., & Allgeier, A.R. (1991). *Sexual interactions.* Lexington, MA: D.C. Heath.

Biklen, D. (1988). The myth of clinical judgment. *Journal of Social Issues, 44*(1), 127–140.

Blackwell-Stratton, M., Breslin, M.L., Mayerson, A.B., & Bailey, S. (1988). Smashing icons: Disabled women and the disability and women's movements. In M. Fine & A. Asch (Eds.). *Women with disabilities: Essays in psychology, culture, and politics* (pp. 306–333). Philadelphia: Temple University Press.

Bogdan, R., Biklen, D., Shapiro, A., & Spelkoman, D. (1990). The disabled: Media's monster. In M. Nagler (Ed.). *Perspectives in disability* (pp. 138–143). Palo Alto, CA: Health Markets Research.

Brolley, D.Y., & Anderson, S.C. (1990). Advertising and attitudes. In M. Nagler (Ed.). *Perspectives on disability* (pp. 147–151). Palo Alto, CA: Health Markets Research.

Cole, S.S. (1986). Facing the challenges of sexual abuse in persons with disabilities. *Sexuality and Disability 7*(3/4), 71–89.

Cole, T.M., & Cole, S.S. (1990). Rehabilitation of problems of sexuality in physical disability. In F.J. Kottke, G.K. Stillwell, & J.F. Lehmann (Eds.). *Krusen's handbook of physical medicine and rehabilitation* (pp. 988–1008). Philadelphia: W.B. Saunders.

Darling, R.B. (1988). Parental entrepreneurship: A consumerist response to professional dominance. *Journal of Social Issues, 44*(1), 141–158.

Deloach, C., & Greer, B.G. (1981). The third disabling myth: The asexuality of the disabled. In *Adjustment to severe physical disability: A metamorphosis* (pp. 65–99). New York: McGraw-Hill.

Ferreyra, S., & Hughes, K. (1982). *Table manners: A guide to the pelvic examination for disabled women and a health care providers.* Oakland, CA: Sex Education for Disabled People.

Fine, M., & Asch, A. (1985). Disabled women: Sexism without the pedestal. In M.J. Deegan & N.A. Brooks (Eds.). *Women and disability: The double handicap* (pp. 6–23). New Brunswick, NJ: Transaction Books.

Finklehor, D. (1979). *Sexually victimized children.* New York: Free Press.

Frank, G. (1988). Beyond stigma: Visibility and self-empowerment of persons with congenital limb deficiencies. *Journal of Social Issues, 44*(1), 95–117.

Goffman, E. (1963). *Stigma: Notes on the management of spoiled identity.* Englewood Cliffs, NJ: Prentice-Hall.

Gordon, S. (1975). *Living fully: A guide for young people with a handicap, their parents, their teachers, and professionals.* New York: John Day.

Gordon, S., & Gordon, J. (1983). *Raising a child conservatively in a sexually permissive world.* New York: Simon and Schuster.

Griffith, E.R., Cole, S.S., & Cole, T.M. (1990). Sexuality and sexual dysfunction. In M. Rosenthal, E.R. Griffith, M.R. Bond, & J.D. Miller (Eds.). *Rehabilitation of the adult and child with traumatic brain injury* (pp. 206–225). Philadelphia: F.A. Davis.

Hahn, H. (1981). The social component of sexuality and disability: Some problems and proposals. *Sexuality and Disability, 4*(4), 220–234.

Hanks, M., & Poplin, D. (1981). The sociology of physical disability: A review of literature and some conceptual perspectives. *Deviant Behavior: An Interdisciplinary Journal, 2,* 309–328.

Kinsey, A.C., Pomeroy, W.B., & Martin, C.E. (1948). *Sexual behavior in the human male.* Philadelphia: W.B. Saunders.

Miller, S., & Morgan, M. (1980). Marriage matters: For people with disabilities too. *Sexuality and Disability, 3*(3), 203–212.

Money, J. (1986). *Lovemaps: Clinical concepts of sexual/erotic health and pathology, paraphilia, and gender transposition in childhood, adolescence, and maturity.* New York: Irvington Publishers.

Mooney, T.O., Cole, T.M., & Chilgren, R.A. (1975). *Sexual options for paraplegics and quadriplegics.* Boston: Little, Brown.

Moses, A.E., & Hawkins, R.O., Jr. (1982). *Counseling lesbian women and gay men: A life-issues approach.* St. Louis: C.V. Mosby.

Mullan, P.B., & Cole, S.S. (1991). Health care providers' perceptions of the vulnerability of persons with disabilities: Sociological frameworks and empirical analyses. *Sexuality and Disability, 9*(3), 221–243.

Neistadt, M.E., & Freda, M. (1987). *Choices: A guide to sex counseling with physically disabled adults.* Malabar, FL: Robert E. Krieger Publishing Co.

Rabin, B.J. (1980). *The sensuous wheeler: Sexual adjustment for the spinal cord injured.* San Francisco: Multi Media Resource Center.

Reinisch, J.M. (1990). *The Kinsey Institute new report on sex: What you must know to be sexually literate.* New York: St. Martin's Report.

Robinault, I.P. (1978). *Sex, society, and the disabled.* New York: Harper & Row.

Romeis, J.C. (1990). Alienation as a consequence of disability: Contradictory evidence and its interpretations. In M. Nagler (Ed.). *Perspectives on disability* (pp. 47–57). Palo Alto, CA: Health Markets Research.

Rousso, H. (1988). Daughters with disabilities: Defective women or minority women? In M. Fine & A. Asch (Eds.). *Women with disabilities: Essays in psychology, culture, and politics* (pp. 139–172). Philadelphia: Temple University Press.

Ruffner, R.H. (1984). The invisible issue: Disability in the media. *Rehabilitation Digest, 15*(4).

Sandowski, C.L. (1989). *Sexual concerns when illness or disability strikes.* Springfield: Charles C. Thomas.

Sha'ked, A. (Ed.). (1981). *Human sexuality and rehabilitation medicine: Sexual functioning following spinal cord injury.* Baltimore: Williams & Wilkins.

Shapiro, J. (1983). Family reactions and coping strategies in response to the physically ill or handicapped child: A review. *Social Science Medicine, 17*(14), 913–931.

Sobsey, D., & Varnhagen, C. (1988). *Sexual abuse, assault, and exploitation of people with disabilities.* Ottawa, Ontario: Health and Welfare Canada.

Trieschmann, R.B. (1987). *Aging with a disability.* New York: Demos Publications.

18

Addressing the Needs of Lesbian and Gay Clients with Disabilities

Leslie C. McAllan and Deb Ditillo

As society in general, and the profession of rehabilitation counseling in particular, near the turn of the century, it is time to take stock of our history and our future. Counselors must ask the question, "Are we evolving into a profession which truly embraces diversity in the broadest sense and responds with sincere compassion and understanding to all who request services?" As a profession which is centered on working with persons with disabilities to achieve personal empowerment, and full and equal participation in society, rehabilitation counselors often have led the way in developing and implementing new teaching strategies, counselor roles, and innovative legislation and social programs. Rehabilitation professionals have a body of knowledge and experience which has helped to reduce stigma, advocate for individuals and groups, encourage service providers in the community to work together as effective teams, and help people who often have been rejected by society regain their status as participating members.

Historically, rehabilitation counselors have philosophically advocated for viewing the client from a holistic perspective, focusing on the assets of individuals, helping to promote coping behaviors, working together in teams, and actively promoting the participation of clients in the rehabilitation process (Jaques, 1970). Although the profession of rehabilitation counseling has come a long way, we continue to face circumstances which challenge the self-imposed boundaries of our profession. The purpose of this article is to discuss one such challenge facing the rehabilitation counseling profession, addressing the needs of clients with disabilities who also are gay or lesbian.

The authors wish to thank all of the consumers and/or practitioners who reviewed and edited this paper for their insightful and encouraging support. Special thanks to Dr. Gary Hollander of Sinai Samaritan Medical Center in Milwaukee, WI.

From *Journal of Applied Rehabilitation Counseling, 25*(1) (Spring 1994), 26–35. Reprinted with permission.

Why might this topic be particularly important at this time? Counselors have always had gay and lesbian clients in their caseloads, whether they knew they did or not; however, it is unlikely that rehabilitation counselors have been trained to deal with the needs of gay and lesbian clients effectively when sexual orientation is revealed. More persons are identifying themselves as gay or lesbian either because of social and political trends which have encouraged persons to "come out," or because AIDS and other health concerns have forced others to "come out" and ask for rehabilitation services. Kinsey, Pomeroy, and Martin (1948; 1953) concluded that one in ten persons interviewed in their study could be described as "homosexual" and that this figure did not include persons who admitted to having homosexual experiences at some point in their lives. More recently, Janus and Janus (1993) completed a national study, the results of which suggested that 9% of men and 5% of women surveyed could be considered to be homosexual, although they also admitted that the term "homosexual" is difficult to define. Others (*AIDS Conference Bulletin,* Friday, June 22, 1990) agreed that the term "homosexual" is confusing and that one must be careful to distinguish between a person who identifies him or herself as homosexual and one who admits to having participated in homosexual activities. Using the Kinsey et al. (1948; 1953) one in ten statistic for homosexuality in our society, as well as the same one in ten statistic for persons with disabilities, Wohlander and Petal (1985) estimated that there are approximately three million people who are both lesbian or gay and disabled. Recent media attention surrounding the presence of gays and lesbians in the military also has caused tensions to mount and the mental health professions to attempt responses. Finally, rehabilitation counselors might also be working next to colleagues who are gay or lesbian, or be helping employers deal with their fears about hiring someone with AIDS or someone they perceive to be lesbian or gay.

It has always been necessary for counselors to address same sex behavior on personal, professional, social and political levels, but there is an urgent need to take action now since many people who are lesbian or gay will not live until the year 2,000, in part because of the consequences of AIDS, anti-gay violence, and suicide resulting from the intense social stigma associated with being gay or lesbian.

Before proceeding, a brief discussion about vocabulary and the scope of this article is important to include here. Although the term "gay" can be used to refer to both males and females of homosexual orientation, we have chosen to use "gay and lesbian" throughout this article in order to emphasize the fact that we are referring to issues which both genders may have in common. The reader should be aware that there are issues relevant specifically to gay men or lesbians which will not be covered at this time. In addition, Kinsey et al. (1948; 1953) suggested that heterosexuality/homosexuality is not an either/or trait. A continuum was proposed which placed pure homosexuality at one end and pure heterosexuality at the other with a broad range of possibilities in between, including bisexuality. We have chosen to limit the scope of this article to persons who are primarily identified as homosexual in order to simplify the material presented.

Counselors should recognize the range of possibilities with regard to sexual behavior. Finally, we have chosen not to discuss issues related to persons who are transvestites or transsexuals since these manifestations of personality and behavior are not dependent on sexual orientation.

With these parameters in mind, we would like to emphasize that we are primarily advocating for a way of thinking and behaving as professional counselors which is applicable to persons with a variety of concerns beyond being gay or lesbian. In this period of change, values as private citizens and ethics as professionals are being challenged on a variety of issues. How can we, regardless of our own sexual orientation, respond to the challenges related to working with persons with disabilities who are gay or lesbian? 1) We can understand and counter the myths which seem to have been perpetuated from generation to generation regarding gays and lesbians in our society; 2) We can come to understand the reality of what it means to be gay or lesbian in modern American culture; 3) We can learn about ourselves and our own biases with regard to sexuality; 4) We can learn the skills and resources available to us which can help us more effectively work with diverse clientele; and 5) We can return to the roots of comprehensive rehabilitation practice.

MYTHS ABOUT GAYS AND LESBIANS IN SOCIETY

Myths have surfaced in a number of ways in society (see Table 18.1), and rehabilitation counselors should be aware of the power of myths. For many years counselors have helped dispel the myths that people with disabilities are dependent, childlike, asexual, sexually undesirable, sexually inadequate, and in need of protection (Wohlander & Petal, 1985). These myths may even be internalized by persons with disabilities and result in discounting and suppressing their own sexuality. All of the socialpsychological terminology used by Wright (1983) to help rehabilitation professionals understand social response to disability in our society can be applied to the experience of being gay or lesbian. For example, "shame" often results from people with disabilities and people who are gay or lesbian accepting the standards of the "normal" group as being ideal. Persons in either or both of these stigmatized groups may feel they have to act, or be forced to act, "as if" they are heterosexual in order to not be devalued by others. Persons who are gay or lesbian may try to compensate for what they are told is the "socially undesirable trait" of homosexuality by exaggerating heterosexuality, attempting to prove themselves through excessive achievement, and emphasizing other desirable traits in order to deemphasize sexual orientation. Wright added that "spread" may result when a socially undesirable trait erroneously results in other negative associations about a person or group. Spread occurs when persons assume simply on the basis of a label that all gay and lesbian people are immoral, sick, and AIDS infected; that all gay males are promiscuous, effeminate, flamboyant men who want to be women; and that all lesbians are masculine, sexually addicted women who want to be men.

TABLE 18.1 Myths About Gays and Lesbians in American Culture

"Gay men want to be women and lesbians want to be men."

"All pedophiles are gay."

"Gays recruit straights through intimidation."

"All gay people are males."

"Gay people are not people, not normal, not moral."

"Gay relationships are defined solely by sex."

"Gay people are only interested in sex and are promiscuous." "Lesbians are driven by sexual desires."

"Gayness is contagious."

"If you talk about gayness to young people, they will become gay." "Gay men are sissies, and lesbians are Tom boys."

"Gays become gay because of domineering mothers and nonexistent or weak fathers."

Another socialpsychological concept which Wright (1983) applied to persons with disability is "requirement of mourning." According to Wright, people often try to protect their own values and sense of well-being by devaluing another and insisting that a person they consider to be unfortunate should be suffering. An example of devaluing occurs when persons who represent the "majority" expect that minority persons should be kept in their "place." Persons who are gay or lesbian may be expected to mourn the loss of a heterosexual lifestyle, because if they do not mourn the loss it appears to devalue the heterosexual person's own lifestyle and values. However, if a person who is gay or lesbian excels in certain acceptable attributes, the "majority" may consider that person to be an exception to the rule and suppress the acknowledgement of that person's sexual identity. Another way that persons may try to protect their own values is by blaming a person with a disability, or the person who is gay or lesbian, for who or what they perceive them to be, rather than more appropriately examining the responsibility of environmental factors when trying to explain behavior which is not understood. For example, many of the problems faced by people who are gay or lesbian are due to the negative attitudes of employers, hostile attitudes about homosexuality in the media, and the lack of available public role models for younger people who are lesbian or gay.

Wright (1983) also wrote that persons may focus on the possible threatening aspects of a situation when they face the insecurity of new situations, especially when they feel their personal values are threatened. For instance, when people are unfamiliar with homosexuality they may react with a high degree of fear and hostility. Some individuals may associate homosexuality with sin and respond with negative behavior, and even punishment of gay and lesbian people.

People who are gay or lesbian may respond to their sexual orientation in healthy or unhealthy ways. Suicide has been a major response for many persons experiencing intense fears, especially gay and lesbian teenagers (O'Connor, 1992). Others may turn to addictive behaviors, become depressed, act out behaviorally, or get sick. On the other hand, many people have found healthy ways to respond through confronting societal norms, taking political action, challenging attitudes and behaviors, facing honest self-assessment, learning to use skills and resources, dealing with loss directly, finding support from others, and seeking therapy from skilled and sensitive counselors.

Societal norms make accepting one's own homosexuality a challenge for gay and lesbian clients. Norms exist which create double binds that can result in confusion. For example, a person who uses a wheelchair can get the double message that "you're welcome in this society, but we're not going to make it accessible." People who are gay or lesbian may similarly receive the message that, "your relationship would be legitimate if you were married, but we won't allow you to marry," or as the recent decision about gays in the military states, "you're welcome to be a part of the military, but don't talk about it or act on it." Recent newspaper editorial sections have been brimming with alarming comments which reflect the true extent of institutionalized homophobia in our society. Some of these mixed messages convey an overt message of hospitality and acceptance, but a covert message that who or what you are is bad.

The societal norm of fear toward homosexuals is expressed through fears of recruitment and guilt by association that seem to surface on a regular basis. In an editorial entitled "Dangerous Exposure" (Rucker, 1993, p. F2), the author expressed his overt homophobia by stating that, "our 'straight' children may be intimidated into becoming homosexuals" if our schools are allowed to condone homosexuality. Some parents of young children often are worried about homosexuals converting their young children to an immoral lifestyle. Little thought is given to the reality that most gay and lesbian adults were brought up by heterosexual parents in a heterosexual environment.

Because of the societal sanctions against homosexuality, many persons who are gay or lesbian learn to hide their sexual orientation very early in life and may expend a lot of emotional and physical energy in doing so. Hiding is an unhealthy psychological response and most gay and lesbian persons are experts at it, so the counselor must focus on teaching skills and exploring options related to expressing one's sexual orientation in ways that are healthy and empowering for that person. Counselors always have the opportunity to create what can be the fist safe environment in which a client may be able to express his/her sexual identity, whether they have chosen to do so or not.

Counselors need to recognize the role the environment plays in determining response to sexual orientation and be careful about scapegoating. In other words, gay and lesbian people are not a problem to be solved. Societal sanctions against homosexuality have resulted in reactions by some people which have fueled stereotypes and led to demands that homosexuals should seek a cure for their condition. However, persons who are being told that they are bad and must change, told that their healthy responses to sexuality are immoral, and who are physically threatened on a regular basis may learn behaviors which are self-destructive and socially unacceptable. These situations are realistic consequences of stigma, so counselors should not blame the person for her/his response to a very real and unhealthy social situation.

BEING GAY OR LESBIAN IN AMERICA

The political climate throughout the past two decades has been creating more awareness and controversy about gay and lesbian people. Progress was being made toward the possibility of full inclusion of gay and lesbian people in society. However, recent reactions to this progress have impacted on society in a number of ways. Attempts by gay and lesbian activists to advocate for "equal rights" were challenged by individuals and groups who believed that these activist were really seeking "special rights" and the legitimization of behavior they consider to be immoral. For example, during 1992, an organization calling itself the Oregon Citizens Alliance (OCA) attempted, among other things, to have books which presented a positive image of homosexuality banned from public libraries in the state. Although the OCA failed in its initial attempts to pass legislation on a state-wide measure, it continues to expand its anti-gay efforts through local city and county initiatives.

How do these political forces impact on rehabilitation? Probably the single most important factor that almost prevented the Americans with Disabilities Act from becoming law related to HIV Disease and irrational and illogical fears about indirectly legalizing homosexual behavior through this piece of legislation (McAllan & Hollander, 1992). Senator Harkin (1990) had to assure people that the ADA was not a "gay rights" bill and pointed out the fact that it specially excluded homosexuality and bisexuality from qualification as handicaps, disabilities, or behavior disorders. Also, it is important to note that there is no direct relationship between homosexuality and AIDS. In other words, not all people who are gay or lesbian have the disease and heterosexual incidence continues to increase rapidly. Much of the same language from the ADA was used when writing the 1992 Reauthorization of the Rehabilitation Act. Although the intent of the legal language was to prevent either piece of legislation from being used to legalize homosexual behavior, the result is legal documentation that homosexuality is not a disability, handicap, or behavior disorder.

Although political issues have been a focal point in recent years, Garnets and Kimmel (1991) identified the following more subtle social characteristics that they believe have influenced the development of lesbians and gay people in our society:

> 1) Gay men and lesbians discover their sexual orientation at a relatively late point in the process of identity development, often at the time sexual desire begins to be recognized; 2) Lesbians and gay men learn negative attitudes about homosexuality . . . ;

3) Because families of lesbians and gay men typically are heterosexual, they do not provide useful role models for normal transitions and developmental periods of gay and lesbian lives; 4) Family disruption often results when a gay or lesbian sexual orientation is revealed; 5) Because lesbians and gay men are diverse and the majority are not easily identifiable, most move in and out of gay and straight identities, and many hide their sexual orientation from public view; 6) Even when gay men and lesbians are open about their sexual orientation, they do not automatically invalidate stereotypes about other gays and lesbians in general because each individual can be discounted as an exception to the general pattern; 7) The lesbian and gay male community encompasses diversity in terms of gender, race, ethnicity, age, socioeconomic status, relationship status, parenthood, health, disabilities, politics, and sexual behavior; 8) Gay and lesbian people have had little awareness of any community history until relatively recently. Although the gay and lesbian community has a history, it is not passed on through family traditions; 9) Gay men and lesbians are often encouraged or permitted by their deviance from accepted norms to explore androgynous gender role behavior, independence, self-reliance, and educational and occupational options; 10) Lesbians and gay men raise issues that some members of the public may find potentially threatening, such as (a) anyone can be gay (stereotypes are inaccurate predictors), (b) same-sex sexual fantasies can be explored (everyone is not 100% heterosexual all of the time), and (c) relationships and sexual relations need not be based on gender role constraints (pp. 148–149).

How can rehabilitation counselors help to change attitudes and behaviors which need changing? To begin with, representatives of professional organizations should speak out. It has been suggested that professional organizations should remain neutral and not be politically involved in "controversial" issues. However, counselors can teach clients to advocate for themselves by letting them know that they have the right to have social institutions respond to their needs. Rehabilitation counselors also have the responsibility to learn advocacy skills themselves and find out about the advocacy organizations which exist in their communities. Finally, counselors can support legislation which actively protects the equality of all individuals by writing legislators and expressing concern when they see or hear of actions which are unjust.

In addition to counselors impacting on the social environment, here are some suggestions about how to approach dealing with clients directly in the counseling session: 1) Get to know your clients as individuals, not stereotypes; 2) Do not assume heterosexuality or homosexuality about your client; 3) Do not assume that marriage and children exempt a person from being gay or lesbian; 4) Do not assume disability causes gayness or that poor parenting or overprotection result in dependency and gayness; 5) Do not try to convince your client that she/he is not lesbian or gay and suggest that her/his sexual orientation is caused by limited social contact; and 6) Do not assume that sexual orientation is the basis of all of the psychological and social problems a client identifies.

Rehabilitation counselors can help to educate and dispel stereotypes about many gay, lesbian, and heterosexual clients. In addition, they can be careful about their own use of demeaning humor and jokes which often are done at the expense of clients. They can actively discourage intraoffice jokes, demeaning remarks, stereotypical gesturing, and other behaviors which make fun of clients. In other words, they can learn more appropriate ways to vent and express work frustrations and educate and dispel stereotypes among co-workers. To more clearly advocate for clients, provide effective counseling, and take a proactive position with colleagues and society in general, it is necessary that counselors start by assessing their own values and attitudes.

UNDERSTANDING OURSELVES

Self-assessment is the place to start when planning to assess one's ability to provide services to any client. Goodman (1985) suggested that counselors assess their own knowledge about the gay and lesbian culture; review their knowledge and understanding of racism, sexism, and homophobia in society; and ask themselves how and in what way they participate in the lesbian and gay community. Lack of self-awareness can lead to blatant heterosexism—the belief that everyone is heterosexual and that heterosexual relationships are necessary for the preservation of the family, particularly the nuclear family (Pharr, 1988). All too often counselors exhibit this heterosexism by assuming that their clients are heterosexual through the questions that they ask. They may also assume that a person they are counseling has the same values and attitudes that the counselor believes are important. Through these assumptions counselors may strip their clients of their identity on all levels. A disturbing discovery of attempting to understand our own biases may be that we are homophobic—an irrational fear response which can result in hatred of those who love and sexually desire persons of the same gender (Pharr, 1988). Pharr reported that homophobia is powerful enough to keep the sexual identity of 10-20 percent of the population hidden and living in fear of danger. Pharr concluded that homophobia works effectively when joined with heterosexism by dictating the mandatory heterosexuality of all.

The potential impact of heterosexism and homophobia on the quality of care of a person seeking medical attention in a hospital setting is evident in the following example. A younger female client was admitted for a few days of tests and observation due to a back injury from playing a game of volleyball. During a pelvic exam which was completed in the emergency room, this young woman stated that she was lesbian. From that point on, every entry into her hospital chart started off with the following label, "a 22 year old lesbian." Not only was that entry made by each resident, intern and her attending physician, but by nursing staff as well. Although it may have been potentially important for the patient to tell the physician that she was lesbian, it did not have to become a primary identifying label for that client. In this case, hospital staff would not routinely state that a person is "a 22 year old heterosexual, female." As a consequence of this labeling, there were some nurses who did not want to care for the client, even though she required and requested very little. It is possible that the nurses thought that her "homosexuality" was contagious and avoided her. Is it any wonder that gays and lesbians often will not reveal their sexual orientation under these circumstances?

Fear may be the driving force behind "routine" labels. The behaviors of the hospital staff are heterosexist because the process of consistently labeling this person as homosexual implies that she deviates from the "norm" of heterosexuality. The staff behaviors are homophobic because the motivation behind these actions and comments were based in irrational fear and ignorance about homosexuality.

When used by society in general, the labels gay, lesbian, homosexual or bisexual tend to reduce a person's identity to only sexual behavior. Counselors must be careful to recognize that sexual activity is only a small part of one's identity. Counselors must understand the nature of sexuality in general, and their own bias and limitations with regard to sexuality specifically when interacting with a client. Perhaps a counselor expects the person to be just like he/or she is in all ways, or maybe feels uncomfortable with his/her own sexuality. If this is the case, clients might not be willing to be open and honest. If counselors cannot address their own needs in a holistic fashion, clients may have difficulty identifying who is important to them, who they love, or who their support system is in their rehabilitation process.

Rehabilitation professionals must learn to openly address sex and sexuality with clients. Counselors can learn to speak frankly using appropriate sexual terminology (see Table 18.2). They can recognize that there is no difference between heterosexual sex acts and homosexual sex acts except for the sex of the partner; in other words, homosexual sex is not bizarre or even all that different. In order to talk about sex comfortably, counselors must fist acknowledge that discussions about sex and sexuality are within the realm of counselor activity, and then take responsibility for becoming comfortable talking about sex. This may require learning more about a variety of sexual practices, including "safer sex practices." Counselors can assess their own attitudes about disability and sexuality by attending workshops on sexuality, accepting personal counseling and supervision as options for themselves, practicing talking about sex with friends and relatives, and utilizing the many resources available to counselors and the general public (see Resource List). Since sexuality is a natural part of life, it should become a natural part of conversation and counseling.

In addition, counselors can acknowledge that heterosexism is a problem in our society and take responsibility for their part in it. Counselors should always respect client boundaries with regard to discussion of personal issues, but they should note that sex is a private issue, not a secret one. Respecting a person's privacy involves acknowledging a person's "freedom to choose for themselves the time and the circumstances under which and the extent to which their beliefs, behavior, and opinions are to be shared or withheld from others" (Siegel, cited in Corey, Corey, & Callanan, 1988, p. 179).

Rehabilitation counselors must be careful not to project their own discomfort with discussing sex onto clients. Sometimes the client is more comfortable

TABLE 18.2 Common Terminology Regarding Gays and Lesbians

Heterosexism: Heterosexism is the belief that everyone is heterosexual and that heterosexual relationships are necessary for the preservation of the family, particularly the nuclear family. Heterosexism is institutionalized through religion, education and the media and leads to homophobia (Pharr, 1988).

Homophobia: Homophobia is the irrational fear of anyone gay or lesbian, or of anyone perceived to be gay or lesbian. Homophobia is a weapon of sexism because it works to keep men and women in rigidly defined gender roles (Pharr, 1988).

Internalized homophobia: Internalized homophobia is produced by the negative messages about homosexuality that gays and lesbians hear from early childhood on. Because gays and lesbians are stereotyped, kept isolated and uninformed, or fed inaccurate distorted information about homosexuality, the messages are internalized and result in low self-esteem. Internalized homophobia leads to self-hatred and often to psychological problems (Dworkin & Gutierrez, 1992).

Coming out: Coming out is the process whereby a gay man or lesbian comes to accept a gay or lesbian identity as his or her own identity (Dworkin & Gutierrez, 1992).

Sexual orientation: This term refers to the partner with whom one has or would have sexual relations. It encompasses heterosexual, homosexual, and bisexual orientation. Heterosexual is the cultural and statistical norm and is not considered as a sexual minority category (Klein, 1991).

Bisexual: This term refers to sexual orientation to both genders. Bisexual persons are considered to be outside of the cultural norm, although it is sometimes suggested that we all would be bisexual if it were not for societal constraints, socialization, or channeling into either homosexuality or heterosexuality (Klein, 1991).

Homosexual/lesbian/gay: These terms refer to individuals who have sexual relationships with individuals of the same sex. The terms "homosexual" or "gay" are usually applied to males and "lesbian" to females. However, the term "gay " is often used to refer to both female and male homosexuals. The term "lesbian" refers only to female homosexuals (Klein, 1991).

Non-sexual, asexual: "Non-sexual" means no sexual activity. "Asexual" is defined biologically. In its application to people, asexual can be said to include absence of sex identity or orientation as well as activity (Klein, 1991).

Gender identity: This term refers to that social and anatomical gender which a person conceives him/herself to be; being recognized as this self definition with the pronoun "he" or "she." There are also persons who see themselves as both male and female simultaneously or at different times. Then again, there can be people who see themselves as neither. The term gender identity includes males, females, and transgenderals (Klein, 1991).

Transgenderal/transsexual: These terms refer to biologically described males and females whose psychological orientation lies with the other gender. These individuals are persons who, at times, may surgically have their external biological sex changed to fit with their psychological identification (Klein, 1991). Note: Transsexuals may be heterosexual, bisexual, or homosexual after reassignment—gender identity issues are different from issues of sexual orientation.

Transvestite: This term refers to persons who assume the dress of the opposite sex, a man who wears women's clothing for example, as a significant aspect of that person's sexuality. This includes male, female, heterosexual and homosexual persons but in the vast number of instances, occurs in male heterosexuals (Klein, 1991).

addressing sex in the proper context than is the counselor. The counselor must learn how and when to take the initiative when discussing sexuality. People who are gay or lesbian often look and listen for cues from the counselor that it is safe to reveal sexual orientation concerns. It is especially important that counselors be assertive regarding discussions about sexuality, AIDS and sexuality transmitted diseases since sexual behavior can result in life-threatening consequences. The counselor can help let the client know that his/her surroundings are safe by discussing where records are going to be kept, what is going to be said about him/her and to who, and who will have access to files. Finally, it may be important for a counselor to know that a person is lesbian or gay, but it may not be necessary to record that information in the client's file if it is not relevant to the vocational rehabilitation planning—and it rarely is.

Following are examples of ways to approach the topic of sexual orientation in the counseling session:

Don't ask, "Are you married?" "Do you have a wife (or husband)" (even if the person has stated that she/he has children)

Do ask "Do you have a primary partner/relationship?" "Tell me about this relationship" or "Tell me about the people who are important in your life." "Are you currently involved in a sexual relationship with someone?"

Rehabilitation professionals may be the first authority figure to whom a gay or lesbian client may decide to reveal their sexual orientation. How the counselor reacts, through acceptance or nonacceptance, may influence how comfortable the person will be in discussing their orientation with others. Being deprived of someone who "knows" their sexual orientation can mean that the client may remain in a world of isolation, missed experiences and lost relationships. The world of isolation is one in which a great amount of mental energy is devoted to self-defeating behaviors, and the feeling of self-wholeness has been shattered. In order for a counselor to assist a gay or lesbian client in dealing with the internal and external conditions described in this article, the counselor must have competent skills and know the resources available.

SKILLS AND RESOURCES

The first problem faced by mental health professionals is case finding and assessment. Many times counselors work under the mistaken perception that they have no lesbian or gay clients because no client has ever confided that information to the counselor. Kus (1990) suggested that the majority of gay and lesbian people will not seek out helping professionals to aid them in their coming out process because they have little faith in the competence of the helping professional in this area. Clients will often come into contact with professionals because of alcoholism, depression, and inability to relax, which makes assessment a critical part of the rehabilitation process. Counselors can also encourage clients to meet other gays and lesbians, suggest that they read positive gay or lesbian literature, learn what resources might be available in the community for their clients, be willing to refer their clients to other professionals, and give positive reinforcement and encouragement to the client who is actively working on self-acceptance (see Resource and Reading Lists). Finally, Kus recommended that counselors create a safe environment by gently letting homophobic clients and staff know that anti-gay rhetoric will not be tolerated in the professional work environment.

Ryan (1985) suggested that counselors avoid assuming that everyone is heterosexual (heterosexism); avoid using language that is biased, sexist or judgmental; contact the lesbian and gay caucuses within the professional orga-nizations to which they belong (see Resource List); and attend workshops on les-bian and gay issues. With regard to the rehabilitation setting, Ryan recommended that counselors review applications, informational pamphlets and forms to make sure that they are not heterosexist. Examples which are easy to implement include, "*marriage* can be changed to read *primary relationship; husband* or *wife* can be phrased as *significant other, partner, lover;* and so on" (p. 67). Goodman (1985) added that the following questions should be asked with regard to agency practices: "1) Does the waiting room have lesbian/gay magazines and literature? 2) Does written material describing agency services include lesbian/gay people and their needs? 3) How many staff meetings are devoted to lesbian/gay issues? 4) How many open lesbian/gay professionals/workers are on the staff of the agency? 5) Does the agency encourage clients to feel free to ask for a coun-selor/therapist who is knowledgeable about lesbian/gay culture and who has been retrained to recognize homophobic attitudes, values and practices? (p. 143)" Counselors and agency administrators must watch for homophobic, heterosexist, disabling attitudes in forms, agency policies, agency literature, agency practices, and staff meetings.

An important skill that needs to be addressed when dealing with persons with disabilities and persons who are gay or lesbian is the ability to talk about death and loss. Surprisingly, these issues often are overlooked in some rehabili-tation training programs and workshops. It is very difficult to encourage people to focus on death because the subject can be anxiety provoking. In a study of 81 beginning counselors, Kirchberg and Neimeyer (1991) asked participants to cre-ate their degree of comfort with fifteen counseling scenarios, five of which con-cerned death or loss and ten of which concerned other focal issues. The new counselors rated situations involving death and dying as substantially more uncomfortable than other presenting probes. Clients presenting with HIV/AIDS, other forms of terminal illness, threats of self-destruction, and bereavement were consistently placed at or near the top of the hierarchy of distressing client diffi-culties. The subject of death may confront the counselor's fear and finiteness. When conjuring up thoughts of death, many individuals tend to think about why they exist, what they mean in relationship to the world, and sometimes more importantly, what comes after death? These questions and concerns can chal-lenge the counselor's beliefs, judgments, and assumptions. Some counselors may tend to think of death as fearful, inescapable situation; yet, counselors and clients who have experienced the death of another often come to see that death can be a peaceful and moving experience.

Rehabilitation counselors must recognize and deal with other types of loss as well, since loss may always be involved in the counseling and adjustment process. Typical losses for persons who are lesbian or gay can include the physical consequence of AIDS, the loss of sexual freedom, multiple personal losses due to AIDS, loss of family of origin, and loss of a perceived "normal" life. For example, a person may be unable to participate in socially sanctioned activities such as marriage, hospital visitation, certain friendships, certain jobs, "couples" oriented activities, housing, or having children (for some). It also is important to remember that loss of a significant other is just as emotionally painful as loss of a heterosexual husband or wife.

An equally emotional issue in rehabilitation counseling is spirituality and religion. For gays and lesbians with disabilities, problems related to sin and punishment may be exacerbated. When a person is told that he or she is immoral often enough, that person can easily come to believe that punishment and mistreatment by others is deserved. Rehabilitation counselors can help lesbian and gay clients find positive and accepting clergy, and congregations where lesbian and gay clients can participate fully, as well as use counseling skills to facilitate the client's sense of wholeness.

Rehabilitation counselors can create a place for all clients to feel safe, free of discrimination, and free of fear. A primary difficulty a person who is lesbian or gay faces is the person whose intolerance excludes other human beings. Pharr (1988) suggested an exercise that can be used by heterosexual counselors to develop an awareness of the pain and difficulty involved in the process of "coming out." A counselor writes a letter to someone he or she loves so much that losing that person would be devastating. In this letter, the counselor is instructed to tell the other person that he or she is gay or lesbian and then explore the fears that writing this letter may bring up and the power disclosing sexual orientation can have over one's life. However, it must be remembered that persons who are lesbian or gay often face a wide range of responses to their disclosure which can include laughter, shock, disgust, nervousness, and rejection, acceptance, joy, relief, and love.

Since disclosure can be a difficult and critical experience for a client it is important that the counselor be aware of what not to say or do when a client discloses sexual orientation. Although the counselor may view "no response" as acceptance, the client may view "no response" as not caring or apathy. The counselor should be careful about the "standard" responses:

"Why are you telling me this?"
"Oh, I knew that. I could tell by the way you act."
"Oh, that's OK. I have lots of friends who are gay."
"I can accept that in you, but that's not a choice I would make for myself."
"That's OK for you but I just want you to know that I'm not interested in that kind of stuff."

"Oh, can you wait a minute please. I'll be right back."

"If you turn this over to God, He will fix it." (At least not without assessing the person's religious inclinations).

"How can you be sure that you are gay, have you ever tried heterosexuality?"

More appropriate ways for a counselor to respond when a client discloses sexual orientation could include:

"Tell me what being gay has been like for you" or "Tell me what you've experienced as a gay person"

"How do you feel about calling yourself gay or lesbian?"

"Who are the important support people in your life at this time?"

"How did you feel telling me that you are gay or lesbian" (say the words)

"Have you ever talked about being gay with someone else? If so, what were their reactions?" "What have you experienced when disclosing to others?"

"I understand that this might have been difficult to say to me and I really appreciate your trust in me and our relationship—I appreciate getting to know you as a whole person."

In addition to verbal statements, counselors often are reluctant about the use of nonverbal contact when discussing sexuality because it tends to be more ambiguous. Touching can still be an important part of an appropriate response, since counselors can set limits and boundaries as part of the therapeutic process. Touching is not always a form of "coming on" to a client, although this may be a fear of many counselors. People who are gay and lesbian do not "come on" to other people any more than persons who identify as heterosexual, and perhaps even less because of deeply conditioned fears of discovery.

With regard to client empowerment, counselors can learn to provide assertiveness training for clients. Persons who are gay or lesbian may have internalized anger to address. The counselor can help people explore the underlying feelings and resultant behaviors by role playing situations in which a person asserts needs and desires, "comes out" to a significant person in his/her life, or responds to both negative and positive comments about his/her sexuality with self-enhancing rather than demeaning language. The more a person rehearses using uncomfortable or unfamiliar words and expressing difficult or important feelings in the counseling setting, the more that person will become comfortable talking about these same concerns outside of the counseling setting because it becomes a natural part of who he/she is. Gay or lesbian clients must also learn to discern to whom and when to discuss their sexual orientation. Knowing the right time is based primarily on visceral reactions like comfort and safety needs. Assertiveness training helps persons learn that they have the right to be who they are, while also encouraging persons to accept personal responsibility for how and when to act upon this right. Becoming more comfortable with sexual orientation, becoming knowledgeable about resources, and increasing self esteem also help make clients become better consumers of resources.

Client empowerment also means the ability to locate and develop healthy social support systems. Social support is a critical element in the development of self-esteem, and the reduction of isolation through a sense of belongingness. Social support has been defined as, "Support accessible to an individual through social ties to other individuals, groups, and the larger community" (Lin, Ensel, Simeone, & Kuo, 1979, p. 109). After a thorough review of the literature related to social support, Billings and Moos (1981) concluded that low levels of social support are ascoiated with psychological distress. To reduce this type of distress, the counselor can encourage clients to become involved with therapy, peer support, political action, and social groups. To do so, the counselor must know about the community support services available including the population served, functions, and the quality of personnel and programming. The counselor must be sure to follow-up with the client after having referred him/her to these services. In addition it can be very difficult for a person to take her/his first step into these groups, so it may be necessary for the counselor to take an active role in the referral process. The counselor could first contact, or set up a buddy system to support clients in taking the initial step. Counselors should not automatically assume that involvement in gay and lesbian oriented bars be considered a social support system in and of itself (see Resource List).

Perhaps the most crucial form of social support is family involvement, including significant others. Family ties have been found to reduce the likelihood of stress, but more recent research suggests that effective support may be provided through extrafamilial ties and groups as well (Lin et al., 1979). The term "family" could broadly be defined as the nuclear family, extended family, friendship systems, and non-married couples. Ideally, it is the nature of these relationships, and not the actual biological connection, which is important. The family potentially aids in the healing and acceptance of the self, including acceptance of disability and sexual orientation. The counselor must acknowledge the importance of all types of family and support groups, and not discount the reactions clients describe from nuclear families by simply stating, "I can't believe a mother would reject her son or daughter." Clients should be encouraged to invite the supportive people in their lives to participate in the rehabilitation plan. However, the counselor must not assume that it will be the person's parents or nuclear family who will be involved. Often the client's immediate support system will know her/him best and will be active participants in the rehabilitation process. Most rehabilitation counselors have been trained to work with persons who have not always been accepted by society as a whole, and it is these basic skills which can be transferred to issues related to sexual orientation.

RETURN TO THE BASIC PHILOSOPHY
OF REHABILITATION

To answer the question, "Are we evolving into a profession which truly embraces diversity in the broadest sense and responds with sincere compassion and understanding to all who request services?" The answer is probably "no" for most rehabilitation counselors, especially with regard to lesbian and gay clients with disabilities, but counselors can learn how to respond more appropriately and with compassion. Rehabilitation counselors should not forget the basic philosophical roots of what we learned as counselors. We do not look for limitations, we look for assets within each individual. We acknowledge the importance of both environmental and personal factors with regard to the development of self-esteem and eventual inclusion in society. We have been taught to recognize our own strengths and limits and to work with a team of qualified professionals using multiple resources to accomplish total rehabilitation. We have been taught not to judge, preach, moralize, or discount what a person is telling us. Finally, rehabilitation counselors have been taught to acknowledge cultural differences among people and how different cultures may view disability differently. We can maintain the tradition of the profession by affording all clients dignity and respect.

Even though we have been taught these principles, we have not always been able or willing to find practical ways of applying them in working with persons with disabilities or persons who are gay or lesbian. Professional rehabilitation counselors need to look back at the past and begin applying the wealth of knowledge and experiences gained throughout the history of rehabilitation of persons with disability towards the empowerment of gay and lesbian clients, and full and equal participation in society.

REFERENCES

AIDS Conference Bulletin (Friday, June 22, 1990). Sixth International Conference on AIDS, June 20–24, 1990; Bunn Communications International, Inc.

Billings, A. G., & Moos, R. (1981). The role of coping responses and social resources in attenuating the stress of life events. *Journal of Behavioral Medicine, 4,* 139–157.

Corey, G., Corey, M. S., and Callanan, P. (1988). *Issues and ethics in the helping professions* (Third Edition). Pacific Grove, CA: Brooks/Cole.

Dworkin, S. H. & Gutierrez, F. J. (Eds.). (1992). *Counseling gay men & lesbians: Journey to the end of the rainbow.* Alexandria, VA: American Association for Counseling and Development.

Garnets, L. & Kimmel, D. (1991). Lesbian and gay male dimensions in the psychological study of human diversity. In Goodchilds, J. (Ed.). *Psychological perspective on human diversity in America.* Washington, D.C.: American Psychological Association.

Goodman, B. (1985). Out of the therapeutic closet. In Hidalgo, H., Peterson, T. L., & Woodman, N. J. (Eds.). *Lesbian and gay issues: A resource manual for social workers.* Silver Spring, MD: National Association of Social Workers.

Harkin, T. (1990, July 26). *Responses to issues raised about the Americans with Disabilities Act of 1990.* Chair, Senate Subcommittee on Disability Policy: Washington, DC (202) 224-6265.

Janus, S. S. & Janus, C. L. (1993). *The Janus report on sexual behavior.* New York: John Wiley & Sons, Inc.

Jaques, M. E. (1970). *Rehabilitation counseling: Scope and services.* Boston: Houghton Mifflin Company.

Kinsey, A. C., Pomeroy, W. B., & Martin, C. E. (1948). *Sexual behavior in the human male.* Philadelphia, PA: W. B. Saunders.

Kinsey, A. C., Pomeroy, W. B., & Martin, C. E. (1953). *Sexual behavior in the human female.* Philadelphia, PA: W. B. Saunders.

Kirchberg, T. M. & Neimeyer, R. A. (1991). Reactions of beginning counselors to situations involving death and dying. *Death Studies, 15*(6), 603–610.

Klein, C. (1991). *Counseling our own: The lesbian/gay subculture meets the mental health system* (2nd Ed). Seattle, WA: Consultant Services Northwest.

Kus, R. J. (1990). *Keys to caring: Assisting your gay and lesbian clients.* Boston: Alyson Publications.

Lin, N., Ensel, W. M., Simeone, R. S., & Kuo, W. (1979). Social support, stressful life events, and illness: A model and an empirical test. *Journal of Health and Social Behavior, 20,* 108–119.

McAllan, L. C. & Hollander, G. (1992). AIDS/HIV disease and employment. In Hablutzel, N. and McMahon, B. T. (Eds.). *The Americans with Disabilities Act: Access and accommodations (implications for human resources, rehabilitation, and legal professionals).* Orlando, FL: Paul M. Deutsch Press.

O'Connor, M. F. (1992). Psychotherapy with gay and lesbian adolescents. In Dworkin, S. H. & Gutierrez, F. J. (Eds.). *Counseling gay men & lesbians: Journey to the end of the rainbow.* (pp. 3–21). Alexandria, VA: American Association for Counseling and Development.

Pharr, S. (1988). *Homophobia: A weapon of sexism.* Little Rock, AR: The Women's Project.

Rucker, R. D. (1993, Sunday, Feb. 14, F2). Dangerous exposure. *Arizona Daily Star.*

Ryan, C. C. (1985). Gay health issues: Oppression is a health hazard. In Hidalgo, H., Peterson, T. L., & Woodman, N. J. (Eds.). *Lesbian and gay issues: A resource manual for social workers.* Silver Spring, MD: National Association of Social Workers.

Wohlander, K. & Petal, M. A. (1985). People who are gay or lesbian and disabled. In Hidalgo, H., Peterson, T. L., & Woodman, N. J. (Eds.). *Lesbian and gay issues: A resource manual for social workers.* Silver Spring, MD: National Association of Social Workers.

Wright, B. A. (1983). *Physical disability—A psychosocial approach.* 2nd Edition. New York: Harper and Row.

ADDITIONAL READING RESOURCES

Dworkin, S. H. & Gutierrez, F. J. (Eds.). (1989). Gay, lesbian, and bisexual issues in counseling [Special issue]. *Journal of Counseling and Development, 68*(1).

Evans, N. J. & Wall, V. A. (1991). *Beyond tolerance: Gays, lesbians and bisexuals on campus.* Alexandria, VA: American College Personnel Association

Hidalgo, H., Peterson, T. L. & Woodman, N. J. (Eds.). (1985). *Lesbian and gay issues: A resource manual for social workers.* Silver Spring, MD: National Association of Social Workers.

Stone, G. L. (Ed.). (1991). Counseling the HIV-infected client [Special issue]. *The Counseling Psychologist, 19*(4).

RESOURCE LIST

American Association of Physicians for Human Rights, P.O. Box 14366, San Francisco, CA 94144.

American Psychological Association, Division 44, Lesbian and Gay Issues, 1200 Seventeenth St., NW, Washington, D.C. 20036-3090.

Association for Gay, Lesbian, and Bisexual Issues in Counseling (AGLBIC), P.O. Box 216, Jenkintown, PA 19046.

Campaign to End Homophobia, P.O. Box 819, Cambridge, MA 02139, 617-868-8280.

Directory of Gay and Lesbian Professional Groups. GTLF Library Information Clearinghouse, 491 Seminole Ave., #14, Atlanta, GA 404-577-4600.

Education in a Disabled Gay Environment (EDGE), P.O. Box 305, Village Station, New York, NY 10014. 212-246-3811 x 292.

Handicapped Gay Correspondence Club, Para-Amps, P.O. Box 515, South Beloit, IL 61080.

Human Rights Campaign Fund, 1012 14th St., NW, Suite 600, Washington, DC 20005. 202-628-4160.

Parents and Friends of Lesbian and Gays (P-FLAG), P.O. Box 27605, Washington, DC 20038, (202) 638-4200.

Sex Information and Education Council of the United States (SIECUS), 130 West 42nd St., New York, NY 10036. 212-819-9770.

19

Sexual Abuse and Persons with Disabilities: A Call for Awareness

Lee Ann Watson-Armstrong,

Barbara O'Rourke, and John Schatzlein

While issues of sexuality and disability have been recognized for many years within the rehabilitation literature (Wright, B., 1983; Vash, 1981; Wright, G., 1980), these issues are still addressed inadequately within the counseling relationship (Fowler, O'Rourke, Wadsworth & Harper, 1992; Marinelli & Dell Orto, 1991). Indeed, regarding the topic of sexuality, a conflict seems to exist between the attitudes and behavior of rehabilitation professionals. For instance, in a survey of rehabilitation professionals at a Boston area hospital (Gill, 1988 [cited in Ducharme & Gill, 1991]; Ducharme & Gill, 1991), 79 percent of the rehabilitation professionals stated that sexual adjustment is as important to clients as any other area of the rehabilitation, yet only 9 percent indicated that they regularly included sexuality in their rehabilitation plans. Furthermore, 51 percent of the rehabilitation professionals in the study reported that sexuality is discussed in the counseling relationship only if the client first initiates the conversation (Gill, 1988). The lack of focus on sexuality creates a situation that may have many serious implications for the client. Perhaps the most dangerous of these implications being that rehabilitation professionals may overlook or ignore the issue of sexual abuse completely.

Since the definition of sexual abuse can be difficult to fully conceptualize, it may be helpful to define it by using a continuum of behavior with actual use of physical force lying on one end. All behavior associated with sexual abuse however, involves abuse of power within the areas of physical, emotional, economic, or employment status (Goodman, Koss, Fitzgerald, Felipe Russo, & Puryear Keita, 1993). Sexual abuse, which is defined here as ". . . any form of unwanted

From *Journal of Applied Rehabilitation Counseling,* 25(1) (1994), 36–42. Reprinted with permission.

sexual touching, nonconsensual sexual intercourse, other ongoing sexual exploitation, or perhaps [an] isolated incidence of physical harassment which is experienced as sexual intent" (Cole, 1986; p. 71), is a serious issue that regrettably has received little attention from both researchers and practitioners. While a paucity of accurate data still exists, a small but significant amount of research on the topic of sexual abuse among persons with disabilities is beginning to emerge. The results of these studies show the presence of a startling trend; persons with disabilities are at an increased risk for both sexual assault and sexual abuse (Sobsey & Varnhagen, 1991; Sobsey, Gray, Wells, Pyper & Reimer-Heck, 1991; Seattle Rape Relief Development Disabilities Project, 1987).

Even though recent studies clearly suggest that sexual abuse is occurring among persons with disabilities, health care professionals in general still tend to lack awareness of the increased risk this population faces. This overall lack of awareness is perhaps based in a lack of education among health care providers with regard to the issues of sexual abuse which then leads to inadequate treatment being available for people with all types of disabilities.

Since awareness and understanding are the first steps to intervention as well as prevention of the problem, this article will present an overview of sexual abuse issues and the impact of that abuse on persons with disabilities. The following topics will be addressed: the prevalence of sexual abuse, issues of vulnerability, sexual abuse reporting issues, and barriers to services and treatment. Case studies describing various types of sexual abuse, as well as recommendations for rehabilitation professionals will also be presented.

PREVALENCE OF SEXUAL ABUSE
AMONG INDIVIDUALS WITH DISABILITIES

Because of the lack of reported cases (Sobsey & Doe, 1991), it is difficult to determine accurately the incidence of sexual abuse among persons with disabilities. While national statistics regarding abuse among persons with disabilities are lacking, other studies provoke awareness of devastating possibilities. Prevalence studies in the field of psychology have suggested that between 21% and 34% of women in this country will be physically assaulted by an intimate partner (Browne, 1993). Further, Sobsey and Varnhagen (1991) estimated that the likelihood of sexual abuse among persons with disabilities is about one and a half times higher than that for people without disabilities of the same age and sex. Analysis from data collected over a 10 year period by Seattle Rape Relief indicates that reported sexual abuse of people with cognitive disabilities is four times the national rate for people without disabilities (Seattle Rape Relief Disabilities Project, 1987). Furthermore, sexual abuse appears to be related to gender since it is especially prevalent among women with disabilities (Brown, 1989; Asch & Fine, 1987; Doucette, 1986; Hard, 1986). Indeed, findings from the Sexual Abuse and Disability Project (Sobsey & Doe, 1991) conducted at The University of Alberta analyzed from 162 reports of persons with disabilities show that a large majority of those who reported being sexually abused in the study were women (81.7 percent) with most of the offenders being men (90.8 percent). A smaller but still important number of those who reported sexual abuse in the study were male (18.3 percent) and offenders were female (9.2 percent). In addition, of those individuals who reported abuse, a high percentage (79.6 percent) stated that they had been victimized on more than one occasion (Sobsey & Doe, 1991).

According to the results of the Sobsey and Doe (1991) study, sexual abuse consisted of vaginal or anal penetration in 53.1 percent of the reports, fondling or masturbation in 41.4 percent, and oral-genital contact in 24.7 percent (7.4 percent to the victim's genitalia and 17.3 percent to the offender's) of the cases. While these statistics provide some idea of the nature and type of sexual abuse, a presentation of several case examples of abuse will further illustrate the types of sexual abuse as well as the serious effects sexual assault and abuse have on persons with disabilities.

CASE ONE

Woman with Post Polio Syndrome
Living in an Abusive Environment

Feeling the need to constantly have a man in her life, this woman, who used a wheelchair, initially lived with several different men. The need for male companionship was believed to have developed from her functional limitations as well as a personal sense of not feeling capable of making life choices or controlling her own economic stability. She stated that she initially felt wanted and needed within these different relationships and received some mutual pleasure, both emotionally and sexually. However, she quickly became victimized within these relationships, experiencing both physical and sexual abuse. At the time the abuse was occurring, no accessible safe houses or counseling groups were available. Only through her own determination and strength was she able to get the help she desperately needed.

CASE TWO

Male with Cerebral Palsy Raped
by a Male Attendant

This mid twenty's individual, who used a wheelchair, was dependent on others for assistance in dressing, bathing and other activities of daily living. After several months of appropriate contact, this individual was forcibly raped by his personal care attendant. This individual had tremendous difficulty trying to get health care professionals to accept his experience as serious. The case lasted more than two years, but did not result in a conviction of the personal care attendant. This individual is still working through the devastating effects of his experience. He reports that his ability to be touched tenderly and to trust others has been seriously effected by the sexual abuse. While he has had counseling, counselors experienced and educated in dealing with rape cases among males with disabilities are not readily available to all individuals who may need the service.

CASE THREE

Nineteen Year Old Female with Cerebral Palsy Taken Advantage of by Residence Staff

This young woman moved to a large urbanely located transitional residence center from a small rural community. Coming from a small town where she had dated no one, she was vulnerable to males showing any interest in her. Within months of her arrival at the residence, she was invited to various parties both at the residence and at staff members' homes. Even though she was under aged, she was given drinks at these parties and was eventually sexually assaulted at one of the parties. A male fondled her breasts and externally touched her labia. He further manipulated her into rubbing his groin. She originally expressed guilt and feelings of confusion and believed that she was to blame for the incidence.

VULNERABILITY OF PERSONS WITH DISABILITIES

Brown (1989), in her discussion of interpersonal victimization states that "members of any culturally disenfranchised group, men as well as women of color, the poor, people with physical or intellectual [as well as emotional] disabilities, elders, sexual minorities, are all more likely than members of the culturally dominant group to have experienced victimization" (p. 2). Why do persons with disabilities experience an increased risk of sexual abuse? Although little empirical research has been conducted to determine if there is a causal link between certain characteristics of persons with disabilities and sexual abuse, intuition has lead many to contemplate several common elements, all of which have to do with diminishing the humanness of persons with disabilities (Crossmaker, 1991; Waxman, 1991). These common elements are both directly and indirectly associated with the disability and include: financial and physical dependence, isolation and lack of sex education, as well as societal attitudes toward sexuality and disability. Even though these common elements appear to increase the risk of sexual abuse among persons with disabilities, it must be understood that important differences exist between persons with disabilities based on the type and nature of the disability present (i.e.: congenital or acquired, stable or progressive, early or late onset) as well as race, age, class, gender and sexual preference that may further increase the risk of abuse for some individuals. An example of this interaction is evident in the high incidence of sexual abuse among women with disabilities (Sobsey & Doe, 1991; Doucette, 1986).

Dependency on others for assistance with activities of daily living, and therefore the inability to be spontaneous in protecting oneself, appears to increase the risk of sexual abuse. Indeed, research shows that persons with disabilities are likely to be abused by the very people they entrust with their care (Crossmaker, 1991; Sobsey & Doe, 1991). According to Mansell, Sobsey and Calder (1992), offenders were likely to be paid care givers or personal care attendants in 26.3 percent of the sexual abuse cases reported in their study. Being dependent on others for survival, coupled with communication, cognitive or mobility difficulties may result in an inability to escape abuse,

Social isolation may also increase the vulnerability of persons with disabilities. Isolation due to mobility or communication difficulties, parental inability or reluctance to provide social opportunities outside the home, or an individual's inability to take social risks due to one's own fear of their disability, are all factors which reduce an individual's opportunity to grow and test one's self socially and sexually in a safe and reasonably guided manner. This lack of social interaction may lead an individual to accept professed 'affection' from another who is in fact exploiting the vulnerability of that individual. In addition, individuals may continue to be victimized believing that sex is an expression of love or that an abusive relationship is better than no relationship at all (Crossmaker, 1991).

The identification or understanding of what actions are abusive or assaulting is not always readily apparent to those who are being abused or assaulted. This is particularly of concern for persons with developmental disabilities (Shaman, 1986). If rehabilitation professionals view persons with disabilities as asexual, then they are not likely to discuss sexuality with them. Such a lack of discussion in turn prevents the client's acknowledgment of what constitutes appropriate affectionate or sexual behavior and increases vulnerability to sexual abuse. In fact, while rehabilitation professionals may recognize sexuality as a component of rehabilitation planning, sexuality information and educational materials are seriously lacking. Most of the focus on sexuality for persons with disabilities concentrates on how to contain one's sexuality or cope with limitations on sexuality rather than exploring it as part of being an adult in a real world. For example, often what is available for women with disabilities is limited to material on birth control or child delivery, not issues of sexual desire (O'Toole & Bregante, 1992).

The above factors, while certainly contributing to the vulnerability of persons with disabilities, may not be sufficient to fully explain why sexual abuse occurs more often among this population. In fact, relying solely on the factors discussed above as the cause of abuse may result in the conclusion that victims of abuse, due to their behaviors and attributes, provoke and invite abuse (see for example: Waxman, 1991; Brown, 1989), thereby sharing responsibility for their maltreatment. The fact that offenders do not generally abuse those who are respected or seen as equal (Bart & O'Brien, 1985; Groth, 1979) suggest a more plausible explanation for the relationship between sexual abuse and disability may lie in society's negative attitudes and discrimination towards persons with disabilities. Indeed, Sobsey and Varnhagen (1991) point out that "in many cases it may not be the actual disability that contributes to the increased risk, but rather (it is) a function of society's expectations and treatment of disabled (sic) people." (p. 202).

While still lacking creditability as such, persons with disabilities constitute a minority group (Hahn, 1989). Similar to other minority groups, persons with disabilities face patterns of oppressive treatment, with personal difficulties stemming not from within themselves but rather from a disabling and discriminatory social and physical environment (Waxman, 1991). When an individual is subjected to hatred, discrimination or demeaning attitudes, vulnerability to sexual abuse is increased. Indeed, offenders choose potential victims who are both unlikely to resist attack based on their lack of social and physical power and unlikely to report since they will often not be believed. As Crossmaker (1991) suggests, anytime an imbalance of power exists, there is a potential for abuse. Indeed, "all unequal power relationships must, in the end, rely on the threat or reality of violence to maintain themselves" (cited in Crossmaker, 1991; p. 208). Therefore, sexual abuse can be seen as a highly effective social control mechanism. Sexual abuse may be the means society uses to assert and reinforce the power of the majority group and remind the minority group that they are indeed the inferior group. It may then be that negative attitudes and stereotypes towards persons with disabilities increase the risk of sexual abuse, with physical vulnerability only providing an opportunity for offenders to express their negative feelings.

Negative attitudes and discrimination may also contribute to a lack of awareness and recognition of its occurrence and therefore an under reporting of cases. Despite major social reform, negative attitudes toward persons with disabilities still persist in our society. These negative attitudes often take the form of myths which portray persons with disabilities as helpless and dependent, dangerous, damaged, asexual, inhuman or insensitive to pain (Sobsey & Mansell, 1990). Indeed, because persons with disabilities are often considered by society to be undesirable and asexual, many individuals may not believe or want to believe that abuse is occurring. Unfortunately, rehabilitation professionals may not be immune to these negative attitudes. Indeed, research has shown that rehabilitation institutional staff members often hold the same negative attitudes and beliefs as the general public (Taylor, 1987; Mirabi, Weinman, Magnetti, Keppler, 1985).

ISSUES AFFECTING REPORTING OF ABUSE

As mentioned earlier, due to a lack of reporting, the extent of sexual abuse among persons with disabilities is difficult to determine (Sobsey & Doe, 1991). Indeed, reporting the incidence of sexual abuse appears difficult for people in general and persons with disabilities in particular, for many reasons. Koss, Dinero, Seibel, and Cox (1988) suggest that, in part, due to reporting difficulties public authorities have underestimated rape rates in the general population by as much as 10-15 times the actual rate. Difficulties include such factors as vague and ambiguous screening for issues of sexual abuse, interview features that may impede rapport, lack of confidentiality; for an extended discussion see Koss (1992; 1993). A combination of the following issues results in many cases of sexual abuse going unreported, allowing for the continuation of the abuse.

Obviously, sexual abuse can not be reported if an individual does not identify it as such. But, even when one is able to identify abuse, issues of reporting are still problematic. For instance, individuals who may attempt to report sexual abuse may be seen as attention seeking or manipulative and are therefore not believed by a system that lacks awareness. This in turn results in further victimization (Aiello, Capkin & Catania, 1983).

Furthermore, if a person with a physical disability, relies on the abusive person for activities of daily living assistance (i.e. survival) there is significant pressure on the abused individual to ignore what is really occurring. Indeed, reporting may be viewed as a highly undesirable alternative. The individual who reports the abuse may risk losing essential services and potentially end up in an institution with a corresponding lack of independence and risk for further abuse (Crossmaker, 1991).

Treatment accessibility and availability is also a factor that effects reporting. While clearly identified channels for reporting and processing claims of abuse may not be available, functional limitations and isolation of persons with disabilities often makes reporting sexual abuse extremely difficult, even when these channels are available. For instance, the communication abilities of many persons with disabilities may prohibit them from explaining what has occurred. Furthermore, lack of accessible transport to services, physical inaccessibility of the rape or crisis center, lack of TTY's and interpreters at rape and crisis centers, as well as a lack of funding during the emergency for attendant care or equipment are all problems experienced by persons with disabilities.

While safe houses, residential facilities for battered individuals, and clinic services may be required to comply to the recently passed Americans with Disabilities Act (U.S. Congress, 1990), structural accessibility alone is not adequate to assure that treatment or services are appropriate for persons with disabilities. Indeed, the unavailability of appropriate treatment for this population will most likely still be an issue. While finances are certainly a contributing factor, lack of available treatment persists because of many professional's inadequate education and experience in the area of sexuality and sexual abuse. Indeed, rehabilitation professionals, while being educated in the general area of sex education for persons with disabilities, receive little to no education in sexual abuse, victim behavior or abuse protection. Furthermore, sexual abuse specialists are most likely to have no education or even a basic understanding of the impact a disability can have on an individual's life. It is indeed difficult to treat an individual with a disability who has been sexually bused without a clear understanding of the relationships between stigma, vulnerability, adjustment issues, as well as communication difficulties and mobility limitations. In addition, Cole (1991) has pointed out that there is no mutual language by which detection of sexual abuse, reporting and treatment issues can consistently be discussed among these different health care specialties. This results in a lack of interaction to share expertise, information and resources thereby resulting in the problem of sexual abuse going unnoticed and untreated.

THE ROLE OF REHABILITATION PROFESSIONALS

It is clear that persons with disabilities are at increased risk for sexual abuse and that this situation needs immediate attention. It is incumbent upon rehabilitation professionals to join other disciplines in a systematic, research-based approach to sexual abuse that examines the varying levels of professional involvement (i.e., individual treatment intervention, as well as, policy making).

In order to adequately identify and understand sexual abuse among persons with disabilities, studies which address issues of sexual abuse among adults with all types of disabilities are needed in addition to the more recent emphasis on children with developmental disabilities. Further, studies must be undertaken to explore the relationship between sexual abuse and disability and what can be done to improve mechanisms for reporting abuse. Perhaps most important, appropriate treatment models need to be identified and made available for persons with disabilities. However, this treatment can not occur without professionals realizing the importance of screening clients for sexual abuse and feeling comfortable enough to address issues of sexuality and sexual abuse within their counseling relationships.

Awareness among professionals can be raised through preprofessional educational programs within rehabilitation counselor education and continuing educational seminars. While not all rehabilitation professionals need be, or even should be, experts in the area of sexuality and sexual abuse, all rehabilitation practitioners should possess enough knowledge to be able to identify potential abuse or past abuse, discuss sexuality, and refer individuals to appropriate treatment centers. In addition, public awareness of sexual abuse among persons with disabilities can be encouraged and addressed in a number of ways. Brown (1989) has suggested that public awareness efforts need to incorporate education aimed at eliminating both the stigma and blame attached to persons experiencing sexual abuse and relocating the blame on the perpetrators of this type of violence and those cultural institutions that encourage or enable the abuse among persons with disabilities.

To assist clients who have been sexually abused, rehabilitation practitioners must first become aware of the potential for sexual abuse among persons with disabilities, as well as the unique situations which create this increased vulnerability. As part of the awareness of sexual abuse, professionals need to be able to recognize the signs of sexual abuse. Cole (1986, p. 81) has provided some guidelines which may be helpful in determining the presence of sexual abuse (Table 19.1).

TABLE 19.1 Indications of Possible Sexual Abuse

- bloody or stained clothing
- reports of neglect or injury by the parents, care takers or other health care providers
- a diagnosis of venereal diseases of the mouth, eyes, anus or genitalia
- reports of pain or itching, bruises or bleeding in the genital area
- presence of overadaptive behaviors that meet other individual's needs not those of the client
- presence of extreme fearfulness, withdrawal or fantasy
- inappropriate dress
- seductive behavior
- a past history of abuse by parents or care givers
- an unwanted pregnancy
- mood swings, feelings of humiliation, anger, nightmares, eating pattern disturbances, fear of sex, development of phobias about the attack
- sleep disturbances
- severe emotional conflict at home or place of residence
- fear of intervention   (Cole, 1986, p. 81)

The following can also be indications:
- depression
- substance abuse
- increased interest in discussing sexual issues
- the presence of bruises or lacerations
- appearance of a dramatic change in the individual's behavior
- low or lowered self esteem

While these indicators of sexual abuse were originally developed to identify sexual abuse among children, they are applicable for identification of past or currently occurring abuse among all individuals.

Feelings of shame and guilt as well as fear of rejection may make it difficult to reveal sexual abuse to anyone, including a professional. In fact, many individuals do not volunteer this information unless specifically asked (Rosewater, 1985). Therefore, without careful inquiry, abuse may go unnoticed and unreported. Further, being aware of the signs of abuse may not be enough, especially since many persons with disabilities who have been institutionalized often share outward characteristics which indicate a history of abuse (Assault Prevention Training Project, 1983). As Cole (1986) has pointed out, the emotional reactions and adjustment of individuals who have been denied their personal integrity through sexual abuse are similar to those of an individual who has been denied personal integrity by being institutionalized. Indeed, both share characteristics of dependency based on the lack of personal freedom. Because of the difficulty associated with disclosing abuse as well as the similarity between the behavior of persons with disabilities who have been institutionalized and those who have been abused, rehabilitation practitioners need to also provide a supportive environment for the discussion of sexual issues.

As Ducharme and Gill (1991) have pointed out, rehabilitation practitioners can function as both educators and counselors when it comes to issues of sexuality. In order to prevent sexual abuse, practitioners must provide persons with disabilities with adequate and appropriate information regarding sexuality. Included in the topic of sexuality should be education aimed at preventing sexual abuse before it occurs. Persons with disabilities must be informed of their right to trust their own feelings; to say "no"; to tell someone if they are currently being or have been sexually abused; to live in a safe environment; and to not permit any touch or behavior that frightens, confuses or hurts them in any manner (Cole, 1986). Further, rehabilitation practitioners can prepare their clients to identify issues of vulnerability and sexuality. Sobsey and Doe (1991) have suggested that persons with disabilities should be taught to distinguish between appropriate occasions for compliance and for assertiveness; not generalized compliance for all situations. In this manner, persons with disabilities will be empowered through knowledge. Rehabilitation practitioners must let their clients know that they are in fact sexual beings, with sexual needs and feelings, and that it is ultimately their responsibility to learn their limitations and abilities.

Further, if sexual abuse is disclosed, it is extremely important that the rehabilitation practitioner take the statements seriously, since this may be the only time the individual will chance revealing the abuse (Cole, 1986). After disclosure, the rehabilitation practitioner must be sensitive to the needs of the client. Is the individual in crisis? Is abuse ongoing? Is medical attention necessary? Does the individual need to be transported to an accessible safe house with an available care attendant? The rehabilitation practitioner must also assess the emotional stability of the individual. Is the individual in need of crisis counseling intervention? Is the individual blaming themselves? This is an opportunity for the practitioner to assure individuals that they are not at fault, and validate any feelings of fear and anxiety (Cole, 1986).

To assure that professionals are prepared for disclosure of sexual abuse by one of their clients, they will need to be familiar with the sexual abuse reporting guidelines and requirements in their state and take responsibility for handling the situation appropriately. Further, the practitioner needs to identify community resources available for sexual abuse counseling and treatment. However, it is important to remember that in order to empower the client, the professional must fully discuss all the actions that are necessary or are being considered in reporting the sexual abuse and treating the effects of such abuse (Aiello, 1985).

Because skillful intervention is necessary for ethical and effective treatment of sexual abuse, the rehabilitation practitioner who suspects abuse is advised to provide a referral for specialized psychological treatment to a sexual abuse program or a specific clinician who is trained in rape trauma specific to disability if possible (Baladerian, 1991). It is indeed the rehabilitation practitioner's responsibility to assure that clients who reveal sexual abuse receive appropriate referrals to treatment what is both physically accessible and appropriate for the client's individual needs. However, because appropriate referrals may not exist the rehabilitation practitioner may need to work in unison with a rape crisis center or related agency. Because of expertise with disability issues, a rehabilitation practitioner can guide such programs in a fundamental understanding of the implications of a disability, thereby maximizing treatment effectiveness.

Treatment is extremely important for individuals who have been sexually abused since it is generally believed that the aftermath of sexual abuse is more severe than the actual abuse itself (Brown, 1989; Cole, 1986; Koss, 1993). However, in order to be attuned into the psychological and behavioral effects of sexual abuse and therefore aware of treatment needs, rehabilitation practitioners need to understand the impact of sexual abuse on an individual (Sarnacki, Canfield, & Sgroi, 1982). Fitzgerald (1993) and Koss (1993) concur that the empirical date on the impact of various interventions remains limited and are often insensitive to the ethnic diversity of the individual regarding abuse. Koss (1993) does offer a succinct summary of intervention issues that are salient to the treatment of survivors of rape.

Sexual abuse does have a serious impact that is both immediate and long term. Browne and Finkelhor (1986) identified several effects of sexual abuse which occurred in childhood. Brown (1989) identified similar effects among women who are victimized. According to Browne and Finkelhor (1986), initial effects of sexual abuse include anger, anxiety, depression, fear and inappropriate sexual behavior. Long term effects include feelings of isolation and stigma, depression, poor self-esteem, self destructive behavior, tendencies toward re-victimization, substance abuse, difficulty trusting others and sexual maladjustment. These symptoms are often treated without identifying or addressing the underlying cause as sexual abuse. This is indeed likely since many individuals who are sexually abused do not seek treatment for their sexual abuse per say, but instead the symptoms of that abuse, such as depression and substance abuse (Craine, Hensen, Colliver & MacLean, 1988).

Therefore, to assure that appropriate treatment is provided, rehabilitation practitioners must be able to identify and confront the issue of sexual abuse among their clientele, but they must also know the limits of their competency. If the psychological needs of a client are beyond the limits of the practitioner's competency, a referral is in order. An adaptation of the PLISST model (Annon, 1976) may provide rehabilitation professionals with a useful framework to follow in addressing sexual issues as well as sexual abuse. This model provides the practitioner with four levels of involvement in working with client's sexual issues or problems and further allows rehabilitation practitioners to rate their own competence and to determine the level of intervention with which they feel most comfortable (Ducharme & Gill, 1991).

As rehabilitation professionals begin to construct a systematic approach to sexual abuse among persons with disabilities, their focus on the individual must not obscure problems within the social and cultural dimensions. One such dimension is public policy. Koss (1993) offers a succinct outline of public policy implications regarding rape. Another is sexual harassment in the workplace which has been characterized by Fitzgerald (1993) as so pervasive to be a "fixture" (p. 1070) of our workplaces. Also, as Goodman, Koss, Fitzgerald, Felipe Russo, and Puryear Keita (1993) point out, fundamental work is needed to change attitudes that perpetuate violent acts. These authors highlight the legislative efforts of Senator Joseph Biden (The Violence Against Women Act) as one example of broad based work in abuse which attempts to shape attitudes by "sending a powerful message that violence based on gender—like violence based on race or religion, [or disability]—assaults an ideal of equality shared by the entire nation" (Biden, 1993, p. 1060).

CONCLUSION

Persons with disabilities appear to be at an increased risk for both sexual assault and sexual abuse (Sobsey & Varnhagen, 1991). Despite this fact, many health care professionals lack awareness of the potential for this problem, which further results in a lack of accessible, available and appropriate sexual abuse treatment for persons with disabilities. In order to begin to improve this situation, acknowledgment and awareness of the issue is needed through available sexual abuse education for all health care professionals, particularly including rehabilitation professionals. According to Sobsey and Mansell (1990) sexual abuse education may improve a professional's detection skills, encourage sexual abuse reporting, and promote the implementation of sexual abuse prevention strategies. Rehabilitation professionals must realize that negative attitudes and lack of knowledge concerning sexuality and sexual abuse only serves to impede the rehabilitation process. Only when rehabilitation professionals play an active role in the discussion of sexuality, will identification and therefore reporting of sexual abuse occur, which in turn will increase the availability of accessible treatment for persons with disabilities. Because of their knowledge of disabilities, rehabilitation professionals are in a unique position to begin much of the needed awareness and treatment of sexual abuse among persons with disabilities.

REFERENCES

Aiello, D. (1985). Issues and concerns confronting disabled assault victims: Strategies for treatment and prevention. *Sexuality and Disability, 7*(3–4), 96–101.

Aiello, D., Capkin, L., & Catania, H. (1983). Strategies and techniques for serving the disabled assault victim: A pilot training program for providers and consumers. *Sexuality and Disability, 6*(3–4), 14–16.

Annon, J. S. (1976). The PLISST model: A proposed conceptual scheme for the behavioral treatment for sexual problems. *Journal for Sex Education Therapy, 2*(1), 1–15.

Asch, A., & Fine, M. (1987). Beyond pedestals. In M. Fine & A. Asch (Eds.) *Women with disabilities: Essays in psychology, culture and politics.* Philadelphia: Temple University Press.

Assault Prevention Training Project: Women Against Rape (1983). P.O. Box 82024, Columbus, Ohio 43202.

Baladerian, N. J. (1991). Sexual abuse of people with developmental disabilities. *Sexuality and Disability, 9*(4), 323–335.

Bart, P. B., & O'Brien, P. H. (1985). *Stopping rape: Successful survival strategies.* New York: Pergamon Press.

Biden, Jr. J. (1993). Violence against women: The congressional response. *American Psychologist, 48*(10), 1059–1061.

Brown, L. S. (1989). *The contribution of victimization as a risk factor for the development of depressive symptomatology in women.* Paper presented at the 97th Annual Convention of the American Psychological Association, New Orleans, LA, August, 1989.

Browne, A. (1993). Violence against women by male partners: Prevalence, outcomes, and policy implications. *American Psychologist, 48*(10) 1077–1087.

Browne, A., & Finkelhor, D. (1986). Impact of child sexual abuse: A review of the research. *Psychological Bulletin, 99,* 66–77.

Craine, L. S., Henson, C. E., Colliver, J. A., & MacLean, D. G. (1988). Prevalence of a history of sexual abuse among female psychiatric patients in a state hospital system. *Hospital and Community Psychiatry, 39*(3), 300–304.

Cole, S. S. (1986). Facing the challenges of sexual abuse in persons with disabilities. *Sexuality and Disability, 7*(3–4), 71–88.

Cole, S. S. (1991). Preface to the special issue on sexual exploitation of persons with disabilities. *Sexuality and Disability, 9*(3), 179–183.

Crossmaker, M. (1991). Behind locked doors—institutional sexual abuse. *Sexuality and Disability, 2*(3), 201–219.

Doucette, J. (1986). *Violent acts against disabled women.* Toronto, Canada: DAWN (DisAbled Women's Network).

Ducharme, S., & Gill, K. M. (1991). Sexual values, training, and professional roles. In R. P. Marinelli & A. E. Dell Orto (Eds.) *The psychological and social impact of disability* (3rd Ed.) (pp. 201–209). New York: Springer Publishing.

Fitzgerald, L. F. (1993). Violence against women in the workplace. *American Psychologist, 48*(10), 1070–1076.

Fowler, C., O'Rourke, B., Wadsworth, J., & Harper, D. (1992). Disability and feminism: Models for counselor exploration of personal values and beliefs. *Journal of Applied Rehabilitation Counseling, 23*(4), 14–19.

Goodman, L. A., Koss, M. P., Fitzgerald, L. F., Felipe Russo, N., & Puryear Keita, G. (1993). Male violence against women: Current research and future directions. *American Psychologist 48*(10), 1054–1058.

Groth, A. N. (1979). *Men who rape: The psychology of the offender.* New York Plenum Press.

Hahn, H. (189). Theories and values: Ethics and contrasting perspectives on disability. In B. Duncan & D. E. Woods (Eds.), *Ethical issues in disability and rehabilitation: Report of a 1989 international conference.* New York: World Rehabilitation Fund/Rehabilitation International.

Hard, S. (1986). *Sexual abuse of the developmentally disabled: A case study.* Paper presented at the National Conference of Executives of Associations of Retarded Citizens, Omaha, Nebraska.

Koss, M. P. (1992). The under detection of rape. *Journal of Social Issues, 48,* 63–75.

Koss, M. P. (1993). Rape. *American Psychologist, 48*(10), 1062–1069.

Koss, M. P., Dinero, T. E., Siebel, C., & Cox, S. (1988). Stranger, acquaintance, and date rape: Is there a difference in the victim's experience? *Psychology of Women's Quarterly, 12,* 1–24.

Mansell, S., Sobsey, D., & Calder, P. (1992). Sexual abuse treatment for persons with developmental disabilities. *Professional Psychology: Research and Practice, 23*(5), 404–409.

Marinelli, R. P., & Del Orto, A. E. (Eds.) (1991). *The psychological and social impact of disability* (3rd ed.). New York: Springer Publishing Company.

Mirabi, M., Weinman, M. L., Magnetti, S. M. & Keppler, K. N. (1985). Professional attitudes toward the chronic mentally ill. *Hospital Community Psychiatry, 36*(4), 40–405.

O'Toole, C. J., & Bregante, J. L. (1992). Lesbians with disabilities. *Sexuality and Disability, 10*(3), 163–172.

Rosewater, L. B. (1985). Schizophrenia, borderline, or battered? In L. B. Rosewater & L. E. A. Walker (Eds.) *Handbook of feminist therapy: Women's issues in psychotherapy,* (pp. 215–225). New York: Springer.

Sarnacki, P. F., Canfield, B. L., & Sgroi, S. M. (1982). Treatment for the sexually abused child. In S. M. Sgroi (Ed.), *Handbook of clinical intervention in child sexual abuse* (pp. 109–145). Lexington, MA: Lexington Books.

Seattle Rape Relief Developmental Disabilities Project. (1987). *Information concerning sexual exploitation of mentally and physically handicapped individuals.* Seattle, Washington: Seattle Rape Relief Project.

Shaman, E. J. (1986). Prevention for children with disabilities. In M. Nelson & K. Clark (Eds.), *The educator's guide to preventing child sexual abuse* (pp. 122–125). Santa Cruz, CA: Network Publications.

Sobsey, D., & Doe, T. (1991). Patterns of sexual abuse and assault. *Sexuality and Disability 9*(3), 243–259.

Sobsey, D., Gray, S., Wells, D., Pyper, D., & Reimer-Heck, B. (1991). *Disability, sexuality, and abuse: An annotated bibliography.* Baltimore, MD: Brookes.

Sobsey, D., & Varnhagen, C. K. (1991). Sexual abuse, assault, and exploitation of individuals with disabilities. In C. Bagley & R. J. Thomlinson (Eds.) *Child sexual abuse: Critical Perspectives on prevention, intervention and treatment* (pp. 203–216). Toronto, Canada: Wall and Emerson.

Taylor, S. J. (1987). "They're not like you and me": Institutional attendants' perspectives on residents. *Qualitative Research and Evaluation in Group Care,* New York: Haworth Press, pp. 109–125.

U.S. Congress. (1990). *Public Law 101-336: The Americans with Disabilities Act.* Washington, DC: 101st Congress.

Vash, C. L. (1981). *The psychology of disability.* New York: Springer Publishing Company.

Waxman, B. F. (1991). Hatred: The unacknowledged dimension in violence against disabled people. *Sexuality and Disability, 9*(3), 185–199.

Wright, B. A. (1983). *Physical disability: A psychosocial approach* (2nd ed.). New York: Harper Collins Row.

Wright G. (1980). *Total rehabilitation.* Boston: Little, Brown.

RESOURCES

American Association of Sex Educators, Counselors and Therapist, 435 N. Michigan Ave., Suite 1717, Chicago, IL 60611, (312) 644-0828.

CHOICES: Self Protection Workbooks for Persons with Physical, Visual and Hearing Impairments. (1985). Seattle Rape Relief.

O'Day, B. (1983). Minnesota Program for Victims of Sexual Assault: Preventing Sexual Abuse of Persons with Disabilities: A Curriculum for Hearing Impaired, Physically Disabled, Blind and Mentally Retarded Students Network Publications, Santa Cruz, CA.

Sexuality and Disability Training Center, Boston University Medical Center, 88 E. Newton St. Boston, MA 02118, (617) 638-7358.

Sexuality and Disability Training Center, University of Michigan Medical Center Department of Physical Medicine and Rehabilitation, 1500 E. Medical Center Dr., Ann Arbor, MI 48109, (313) 936-7067.

20

Sexuality Ascending

Carolyn L. Vash

"A bad thing happened to me when I was sixteen. After several days of feeling more peculiar than ill, I noticed the first signs of weakness. Within hours I was totally paralyzed. After a year I asked for hard facts and got them. Three days later an important matter hit me. I called my two best friends over for a conference: 'What if I can't *do* It?' I wailed. We were all virgins but were pretty sure girls have to hold their knees up during intercourse, and I *couldn't*! For hours we giggled—I, very nervously—inventing Rube Goldberg contraptions to solve the problem.

"The next day they solemnly reported that they had made a decision. I had their permission to do it before I was married, since I needed to find out if I could, but I had to promise to tell them absolutely everything. That was in 1951, and I couldn't bring myself to take advantage of their offer. Instead, I ran away with my boyfriend and got secretly married exactly two weeks after learning that I would be permanently paralyzed. I soon found out I could do it; but it would be many years before I'd learn what my *feelings,* ignoring them and plunging ahead as if nothing had happened, could do to my happiness.

"The marriage ended five years later, after I was accepted for doctoral studies at a school away from home. My husband refused to let me go so I left him, and was soon remarried to someone who respected my goals. But again, I'd married for practical reasons and an unfulfilled part of me was insisting on experiencing love. I had affairs with other men, felt inconsolably lonely, and made a good man miserable for ten years before this marriage dissolved, too.

"I was terrified at first. How could I bear being alone for the rest of my life? now that I was not only disabled—and therefore 'damaged merchandise' on the marriage market—but was also approaching 35 years of age and whatever youthful beauty had helped me snag two husbands was rapidly fading. Plenty of men wanted to play, but no one would want me on a lifetime basis. I foresaw my future, when I was too old to attract lovers any more, alone. I contemplated suicide. That scared me. The next day I went to see a psychologist.

"The most important thing he did was help me see that my fears of being alone, severe self criticism, and tendency to ignore my emotions until they overpowered me were not related to disability. Like everyone else, I had other reasons for hangups,

From *Sexuality and Disability, 11*(2) (1993), 149–156. Reprinted with permission.

too. Once I sorted the disability issues from the problems that came from other sources, the fog began to clear. I began to like my life. The prospect of living alone stopped causing panic. I had me.

"As so often happens, when you stop trying so hard to get something, it comes to you. After about a year of living single and liking it, I finally met a man I loved. He fell in love, too, but was not overjoyed about the problems I posed. I hoped he'd want to marry me, but knew I could still be happy if he opted out. After several months of weighing whether *he* wanted to accept my disability, he opted in.

"There's no fairy tale ending. After fifteen years of marriage, the angry arguments, stony silence, and sheepish apologies all go on. But they're the usual marital frictions. It's my personality that makes him crazy sometimes, not my disability."

Since I wrote the foregoing, the fifteen years of marriage have grown to twenty-three and counting. The passage is the closest I've come to writing a sexual autobiography until now—a snapshot taken at a crucial moment in time. I'll flash back, then forward, to tell a fuller story. My intent is to reflect on personal experience in order to better understand the functions and effects of sexual energy in my own life and in the lives of people generally—with or without disabilities.

FLASHBACK

Since the sexual revolution began, few people confess to having only average sex drive. Most will admit to subnormal intelligence before acknowledging modest libido. However, as far as I can tell, the degree to which my behavior is driven by my hormones is in the middle of the average range. My head and heart have usually wanted sex more than my genitals.

This should not imply an absence of impassioned eras and episodes. At sixteen the battle between suppressive programming and physiological urges to *experience* were fierce. My virginity may have been saved until I was seventeen, not by repressive social forces, but by catastrophically disabling polio. (In a forthcoming book I examine the coincidence of coming down with polio exactly the duration of the incubation period after the only family fight ever to occur over my sexual behavior.)

As a teenager, my sex drive may have been average, but my desire to procreate was not. While my peers looked for the best college in which to find a good man so they could marry and raise children, I tried to choose between psychology and choreography careers. I had no interest in child rearing and—to my present chagrin—recall saying, "I'll get married when I'm fifty . . . too old to do anything else." An acting-out style of reacting to my prognosis changed that. I was the first in the crowd to be married, but I stuck to my word on kids.

MOVING FORWARD

I'd been attracted to my first husband at age 14 but by age 17, when we married, the magnetism was gone. I married him for three reasons. I wanted to find out if

I could do intercourse. He worked hard to convince me that he was the only one who'd want me now, and in my vulnerable condition I believed him and felt grateful. Choreography was out as a career and, in 1951, believing no one would trust an old-maid psychologist, I decided to put a "Mrs." before my name—which I would keep, after a preplanned divorce, to gain credibility. (The use of "Dr." to obfuscate the matter didn't occur to me.)

Over my husband's protestations, I attended community college. Within two weeks I knew he had lied to me. I was asked for dates by guys who hadn't noticed my wedding ring, and told of more who'd said they would "trade places with him any old day." "That rat!" said I, "He tricked me into marrying him!" I cancelled my vow of fidelity and started shopping for my 'real' husband. I believed I could do it more effectively married than single since my disability put men on guard against falling for me. Married, I could sneak up on them, make them fall in love before they mobilized their defenses. And that's what happened, time after neurotically repetitive time. I was about as mature as you'd expect for someone whose psychosexual development was fixated at the 1951-high-school level. I had about a dozen love affairs between my 1952 marriage and 1957 divorce and never put out.

In those days a divorce required a year of waiting, during which I narrowed the husband shopping from six to three and finally one contender. Actually, my mother made the final choice and it occurred to me a decade later that *she* should have married him. He supported my career, but our chemistry was lacking. For two years I was faithful, then the urge to experience true love, or at least true passion, overtook me again. I had matured sexually if not socially, and my affairs for the remainder of this marriage were worthy of the name. I was in search of rapture and found it. The affair that ended two marriages was pure rhapsody for three years. When we became single, the enchantment disappeared.

This was when I got into therapy and started growing up. A man I was dating was worried about me and tired of my craziness so he took me to *his* therapist and said, "Fix her, she's broke." I got a lot of help from my friends. One man's tough love stands out in memory. He'd been my supervisor years earlier and we'd never acted on the attraction between us until I was single. After making love he asked languidly, "Why do so many men want to make love to you?" I wisecracked, "It must be I'm a great lay." He shot back fast "Can the crap. Don't make fun of yourself. Sex-wise you're lousy and you know it . . . you're almost totally paralyzed for Chrissake. There's only one reason men want you. A lot of us love you."

Chastised, embarrassed, and overwhelmed by the loving friendship expressed, I recognized a blessing I'd never noticed. Among all the men I'd been involved with over so many years, there had not been one bad apple. They were all good men, good people, many of whom remained friends after dalliance was spent. I wasn't fixed yet, but I was on my way. A few months later I ended therapy and went about enjoying my single life.

I was still dating the man who took me to his therapist when I met my "real" husband twenty-four years ago. I had one date and fell madly in love. We did not go to bed. Then I had a date with the other man. We did go to bed, like always—well, not quite like always. If explicit sexual descriptions offend you, skip to the next heading because the rest of this paragraph will make you grind your teeth. My genitals had made a unilateral decision without informing my head; they were going to be faithful to my newly-found true love. They expressed this decision by evincing what is called "vaginismus." That means the guy can't get in. I mean *can't*. After a bit of a struggle my friend and erstwhile lover lay back and said, "Girl, I think you've found someone else! I'm going to miss you, but I wish you happiness." I admitted he was right, and was amazed and grateful at the immediacy of his intuition.

THROUGH THE MAGNIFYING GLASS

An analysis of the foregoing will be more useful if focused through the lens of theory. Because my theoretical grounding is atypical for rehabilitation psychologists, I will describe it and my reasons for adopting it. Most modern psychological theories derive from science based on the materialist assumption—"what you see is what you've got". Consequently, they usually arise from observations of other people's behavior, even when they postulate an invisible personality that develops, unfolds, matures over time. Introspection is being readmitted to scientific respectability via new enthusiasm for "qualitative research" and the development of a "post-modern" paradigm by eminent scientists and philosophers of science. (2) Still, making room in personality theory for a psychospiritual dimension is widely considered beyond the pale.

Carl Jung's solution was to turn to theories of consciousness embodied in the sacred and esoteric belief systems of ancient religions, philosophies, and psychologies to help us understand our own nature and its lawful relationships within a larger context of existence. These traditions assume that the developing personality is intended to serve as an increasingly adequate instrument of expression for a higher Self which extends beyond the limits of the personal ego and participates in the divine. Another pioneer in the synthesis of modern scientific and ancient sacred psychologies is Abraham Maslow, whose best-known conceptualization came to be known as "Maslow's need ladder". Based on the "Chakras" of yoga psychophysiology, the rungs comprise a hierarchy of centers of personality or energy wherein each is construed as the seat of a higher state of consciousness than the one just below it. This forms a kind of Jacob's ladder of developing consciousness with rungs we may or may not choose to climb.

Theories accommodating both personality and a higher Self seem to be needed on the subject of sexuality. We are confused about sex and mainstream (*exo*teric) religious doctrines—which focus more on controlling outer behavior and conditions than clarifying inner realities—are implicated. I need a theoretical matrix that accommodates *eso*teric philosophical and religious ideas as well as scientific psychological findings. To comprehend sexual energy as it relates to life energy generally, I need a paradigm open to more possibilities than materialist science admits. Although I respect and use the modern science model when it can respond to the data, I'm not willing to ignore issues it cannot address. I have broadened my worldview beyond the boundaries of modern science because I can no longer endure the unnecessary handicap of limiting my thinking to a model that excludes the one thing of which I am certain—consciousness.

SEXUALITY UP THE LADDER

Maslow's need ladder focused on the first five of seven centers described. Moving upward you progress from (1) consciousness focused on brute level survival of the physical organism, to (2) replicating your DNA and taking sensual pleasure where you may, to (3) gaining ascendancy over your fellow creatures and the environment in order to fancy you're having it your way, to (4) feeling love for the fellow creatures and environment you once just wanted to control, to (5) feeling reverence, awe, joy, and gratitude for all that life is, to (6) seeing the whole drama of life played out and accepting your own pain as a necessary part of it, to (7) a state of cosmic consciousness said to have been experienced by a sprinkling of prophets, saints, and sages throughout the ages. The experience is so rare that no cultures have developed language by which to talk about it. People who have not devoted their lives to attaining the upper reaches of evolving consciousness can probably not expect to identify, much less differentiate, them. Maslow's solution is to lump levels five and six together and to pretty much ignore level seven.

Level One

This is the mere awareness of being alive and the drive to stay that way which we share with all animals. Whatever we're here for won't get done unless we survive, so this comes first. Maslow stressed the needs for safety, protection, and security. In many mythologies it is symbolized as a coiled serpent—the Kundalini—libidinal energy, wound tight like a clockwork mechanism. It is voltage—potential—ready to do work, whenever it is released, as it unwinds. At this first level, libido—arguably sexual energy but the only life energy there is—represents raw, instinctive craving to survive. A great deal of sexual activity takes place in the service of survival—not procreation, not love, not any function commonly associated with sex. The record suggests that for at least three millennia female humans have found reason to believe that biological survival might depend on putting out when what was really needed was groceries and shelter.

This writer's disability experience highlighted another way in which sexual behavior can reflect survival strategy, not lust. Had the latter been the prime motivator of all those affairs, one lover at a time would have been sufficient. But my fears of being abandoned were all-consuming—I think because my father wrote me off when my mother divorced him plus disability-related insecurities. I worried my way into feeling I'd better have a back-up to my lover in case my husband and lover defected at once. Talk about self-fulfilling prophecies; my second husband grew tired of being cuckolded and left me.

Level Two

The second rung of the ladder is the center of consciousness with which sexuality is most commonly associated. It involves the urge to get your genes into the gene pool and enjoy the pleasure of doing so. Sensual pleasures involve all five sense channels and extend from the crassest gluttony to the loftiest art appreciation. To Maslow, this rung added a need to experience life consciously and emotionally to the first step's need to keep the biological organism alive.

I've already labeled myself 'average' on sensual drive and 'far below average' on desire to procreate. However, once I almost got carried away with the romantic notion of 'having *his* baby'. The first year of my present marriage saw heroic efforts to produce a symbol of our love. By the time I realized that if I wanted to get pregnant I'd better see a fertility specialist, it also hit me that this flesh-and-blood souvenir was going to need parenting that no one was volunteering to deduct from their career time. I regained my reason and sense of responsibility, and never pursued finding out what the problem was. I just redefined it as a solution—free contraception. Later, my husband directed his paternal instinct into the Big Brothers program and he says this met his needs.

Level Three

Whereas Freudian psychology has been associated with second rung functioning, the third is said to be the natural home of Adler's theory. Freud saw libido, life energy, as virtually identical with sexual energy and his theories related much of human behavior to sexual motivation. Adler saw superiority over others as the primary motivator, thus moving his personality theory up a rung to the center relating to power and the intellect, humanity's most advanced tool. Maslow translates that into the drive for self esteem. At this third level of consciousness we feel okay about ourselves by comparing: what we have with what others have, how we're doing with how others fare.

I feel shame over a phase of third-rung power-tripping when I indulged hostile egotism in a cruel game of 'Lady, if you act like you consider me asexual, you'll see how fast I can get your man into bed.' To an infuriated, wounded ego, this didn't seem like over-reacting. Today, it seems like using a steamroller to swat a fly. I can no longer remember the fears that made patronizing attitudes hurt and enrage me that much. It was a shabby way to treat a sister and a shabbier way to treat a brother. The husband or boy friend was only a pawn in a transaction between her and me. Again, I got a little help from a true friend, the kind who tells you what you don't want to know. In response to self-justifying blah-blah about proving I was still desirable even though disabled, she said, "Why don't you worry about being a grown-up woman instead?" "Thanks," said I, after a few days of stunned silence. "I needed that."

Level Four

Just as Adler raised personality theory from the second to the third rung, Jung raised it to the level four. We have now crossed the great divide between the 'lower' centers of the consciousness associated with the basic functioning of the smart animal, and the 'higher' centers associated with love, self actualization, and transcendence. When your consciousness operates at level four, you no longer need to prove you are somebody by besting others, you just love them. This is the center associated with the merciful consciousness of the Chasidim, Christ-consciousness, and Buddha-consciousness, by a sampling of religious traditions.

Sexual relationship expressed at or influenced by this level of consciousness ceases to fall into any problem category. Once is all it takes to know that 'having sex' and 'making love' are not synonyms. Sexual intercourse may or may not be involved. In *The Psychology of Disability* I mentioned a couple who were both so severely disabled that they could only lie side by side touching hands. Their descriptions of love-making reminded me of accounts of 'yab yum' by tantric yoga practitioners. At this level, I prefer not to share personal experiences. At the levels cited next, I simply have nothing authentic to say.

Levels Five, Six, and Seven

The fifth center is described by Maslow as the step of self realization and by transpersonal psychologists as the seat of transformative consciousness. This can be interpreted as realizing the promise of one's mundane talents and aptitudes, or in terms of the potentialities of a higher Self that partakes of the divine. At this level, sensual and egotistical cravings have been largely transformed into longings to 'follow one's bliss', as Joseph Campbell puts it, toward some higher purpose, the exact nature of which may still be unclear.

At the highest levels of consciousness, one can identify with the higher Self instead of the personality. One can be in the dramas of life but not of them, grasping and accepting how life has to be in an evolving galaxy of firestorms without judging 'good' or 'evil' aspects of it. I've met a few people who claim to have spent moments at these rarified levels of consciousness and have read about many more. There is a great deal of sexual symbolism in reports of elevated consciousness and contacts with the divine. I'll close with a speculation as to why this might be.

SEXUALITY AND SPIRITUAL SYMBOLISM

Life energy, libido, is available for us to express in many ways: to maintain the species, enhance the influence of our gene pools, produce sensual pleasure, bring forth children to nurture, gain ascendance over others, express love, and, I believe, to experience intimations of contact with the divine. I've long suspected that one of Life's purposes for the little urge to merge, sexual union with a human partner, is to give us a hint of what the big urge to merge, cosmic Union with the Source, is all about. Sexual ecstasy may be a faint fore-shadowing of this. It may be the nearest approximation to sublime ecstasy that most of us will experience while we're here on planet Earth in bodies.

This idea distresses people with attitudes that sex is unmentionable in context with the divine. But if ever we are godlike, it must surely be when we participate as co-creators in bringing forth new life. Derogating what may be our loftiest function—a snickering as if it were naughty or denouncing it as evil—is a potential blasphemy I intend to avoid. Our cultural obsession with sex may reflect intuitive recognition of it as a physical symbol of the ecstasy of re-uniting with our Source.

Our abilities to understand and use symbols are impaired by the over-developed reasoning and under-developed intuition that characterize us today. Weak intuition cannot interpret the significance of our observations. When distorted by benighted cultural doctrines about sexuality, the intuition is put at still greater disadvantage. This is the situation we may be in when we are amused or confused by accounts of mystics who describe their experiences of God in sexual terms. When the Beloved is God, in cultures that call God 'he,' confusions can be expected. When we think the poet's language is funny, the hangups may be ours.

Part V: *Study Questions and Disability Awareness Exercise*

1. How is sexuality impacted by the existence of a disability?
2. What are the unique sexual issues people with the following disabilities must address?

   - Facial disfigurement
   - Traumatic brain injury
   - Alzheimer's disease
   - Down syndrome
   - AIDS
   - Spinal cord injury
   - Chemical dependency
   - Severe obesity
   - Chronic mental illness

3. Should birth control and abortion information be part of a rehabilitation program for persons with a disability?
4. Discuss the issues generated by a rehabilitation center's policy that has rules against intimate sexual contact.
5. The directors of the rehabilitation agency/facility for whom you work is completely opposed to sex education for any of the unmarried clients. They believe that sex is inappropriate outside of marriage and providing sex education promotes sexual activity. How would you respond to their concerns?
6. Your legally competent adult client, with borderline intelligence, informs you that she is pregnant and, regardless of anyone else's opinion, she plans to abort her child and have a hysterectomy? What is your response? Does her disability make a difference?
7. Why is touch an important issue for children with disabilities?
8. Are sexual issues related to disability more or less important to people with disabilities in their 50s, 60s, & 70s, as compared to their 20s, 30s, and 40s?
9. What do you believe results in more discrimination for a person with a disability who is gay or lesbian—their disability or their sexual orientation? What are the reasons for this?
10. Why is information about sexual abuse of people with disabilities of limited awareness to rehabilitation practitioners?
11. Why are individuals with disabilities more prone to sexual abuse?

12. What disabilities would tend to have more increased vulnerability to sexual abuse.
13. What does Vash mean by sexuality ascending?
14. Is it possible for you to expand your world view of issues beyond the boundaries of modern science as Vash has done? Why or why not?
15. At what level of Maslow's model do you believe most people function sexually? Why?

I AM JUST LIKE EVERYONE ELSE

Sexuality is a complex reality for all people. When developmental issues, values, and parenting concerns are considered as they relate to the disability experience, many issues emerge. The following exercise explores some of these issues from a parental perspective.

Goals

1. To explore different perspectives related to the sexuality of persons with disabilities.
2. To consider gender-related issues.
3. To discuss the differential impact of different disabilities.

Procedure

Imagine you are the parent of a 16-year-old adolescent who has both a physical and emotional disability. When she asked you for birth control information:

1. What would be your response?
2. What would be the response of your spouse or significant other ?
3. Would there be a difference if the child was a male?
4. Would your response vary if the adolescent had a chronic mental illness, brain injury, multiple sclerosis, AIDS, or was terminally ill?
5. What would you say if your child was dating a person with one of these disabilities and was sexually active?

Part VI

Interventions in the Rehabilitation Process

The primary goal of rehabilitation is to help persons with disabilities to overcome, as much as possible, their deficits; to capitalize on their assets; and to achieve their optimal functioning. Although this assistance may be provided by peers, professionals, or family members, a common denominator in the helping process is the ability to assist others to achieve and maintain personal and rehabilitation goals. Therefore, an understanding of therapeutic strategies is important in the fulfillment of team roles and in the implementation of relevant interventions.

Livneh, in 1986, provided a model of adaptation to disability that consisted of five stages: initial impact, defense mobilization, initialization, realization, and integration. Stewart, in chapter 21, combines Livneh's model with Beck's cognitive therapy (CT), an approach that focuses upon changing dysfunctional beliefs and, through this change, dysfunctional behavior. Recommended CT interventions for each phase of adaptation within Livneh's model are provided in addition to a case example for each phase.

Depression and denial in psychotherapy of persons with disabilities is the focus of chapter 22. Psychological, social, and physical losses secondary to disability are major contributing factors to depression within the population of people with disabilities. Denial and countertransference processes and their role in assisting clients to integrate loss and preserve a sense of meaning in life are emphasized.

Encouragement in helping people with disabilities to gain empowerment is the focus of chapter 23. The concept of courage is discussed in relation to its role in encouragement. Using an existential perspective, processes that may enable courage to emerge are discussed.

Family involvement in the rehabilitation of persons with disabilities will become more important in the 21st century. The family's role in assisting a family member to recover from mental illness is the focus of chapter 24. Contemporary perspectives incorporating family resilience and family burden are presented as a bridge to discussing family interventions. A range of family interventions including support and advocacy groups, consultation, education, psychoeducation, and psychotherapy are discussed as are ethical concerns, particularly confidentiality.

In chapter 25, Albert Ellis, noted psychotherapist, theorist, and founder of Rational Emotive Behavior Therapy (REBT), and a person who has coped with a variety of significant physical disabilities during most of his 82 years, presents a personal perspective on how he has used REBT to accept his limitations, overcome frustration, and avoid self-degradation. His article provides us with the unique perspective of how Ellis's serious physical problems from the age of 5 years onward have contributed to his development of the theory and practice of REBT.

21

Applying Beck's Cognitive Therapy to Livneh's Model of Adaptation to Disability

Jay R. Stewart

INTRODUCTION

Individuals with disabilities experience a range of mental and emotional reactions in adapting to traumatic physically disabling conditions (Livneh, 1986a). Rehabilitation counselors have responded to these reactions through identifying affective counseling as a "significant activity in all settings" (Rubin et al., 1984, p. 215). Rehabilitation counselors also focus on counseling clients to help them realistically assess problems and accept limitations resulting from their disabilities (Rubin et al., 1984). Both private and state rehabilitation counselors see a substantial part of their job as affective counseling (Beardsley & Rubin, 1988; Rubin & Puckett, 1984); confirming that working with persons with disabilities requires a reduction of negative emotional states. It would be helpful for counselors to possess a unified and convenient approach that addresses emotional and cognitive issues in the counseling process.

Curiously, cognitive therapy (CT), the most requested addition to Corsini's and Wedding's (1989) recent compilation of counseling theories, is rarely theoretically addressed in rehabilitation counseling literature (Bowers, 1988; Livneh & Sherwood, 1991). Promising experimental results of applying CT to rehabilitation settings (Larcombe & Wilson, 1984) have not been followed by many investigations to lend credibility to using CT in rehabilitation counseling. A possible explanation for this may be that most rehabilitation counselors and researchers are not fully aware of the latest innovations in CT and the relative

From *Journal of Applied Rehabilitation Counseling, 27*(2), 40–45. Reprinted with permission.

ease of its application in a rehabilitation setting. Also, because CT was originated to manage depression (Beck, 1967), rehabilitation researchers limit their investigation of CT to reducing depression (Livneh, 1986a; Thomas, Thoreson, Butler, & Parker, 1992). Recently, CT has been made more diverse in its ability to both help with emotional difficulties and help clients manage their lives over the entire rehabilitation process (Kuehlwein, 1993). This paper will discuss the applicability of CT to clients with disabling conditions and their problems in each of the phases of adaptation, theorized by Livneh (1986a).

CT and Livneh's theory of adaptation to disability seem to be moving toward focusing on similar populations. CT, first developed as an intervention for clinical depression in psychiatric settings (Beck, 1967), has been recently extended to work with other emotional states, many disabling conditions, and in a variety of settings (Kuehlwein & Rosen, 1993). Bowers (1988) appeared to be the first to discuss CT as an effective and comprehensive counseling model for rehabilitation counselors. He made a strong case for rehabilitation counselors to use CT for individuals with disabilities; however, he did not refer to a model of adaptation to disabilities. Through an extensive review of theories of adaptation to disability, Livneh (1991) synthesized a five-phase model of adjustment to physical disability. In each phase, Livneh and Sherwood (1991) described defense mechanisms and affective, cognitive, and behavioral correlates. Livneh (1991) also identified phase specific interventions, including CT, for rehabilitation counselors.

There appears, however, to be a need for going beyond Livneh's discussions of CT. Livneh (1991), in his reviews of counseling theory's application to phase interventions grouped together Rational Emotional Therapy (RET) (Ellis, 1973) and CT, as if they were nearly the same approach. Unlike RET, CT states that each type of emotional state is caused by a unique cognitive pattern (Thomas, Thoreson, Butler, & Parker, 1992), leading to a wide range of interventions. There are also unique cognitive patterns in addiction (Beck, Wright, Newman, & Liese, 1993) and personality disorders (Beck, Freeman, & Associates, 1990).

Descriptions of CT theory, assessments, and interventions are presented below. A strategy for differentially applying CT in each phase of adaptation to disability will also be presented.

THE THEORY OF COGNITIVE THERAPY

Beck (1967) developed the concept of schemas: fundamental beliefs and assumptions about self, others, and how the environment works (Beck & Weisharr, 1989). Schemas can be latent until activated by certain situations, such as stress (Beck, Rush, Shaw, & Emery, 1979), or, in the case of personality disorders, can operate continually (Beck, Freeman, & Associates, 1990). The schemas are responsible for filtering and interpreting experiences. To Beck (1976), changing schemas from dysfunctional to functional was key to permanent improvement in clients. Schemas could not be seen, only inferred by clients' automatic thoughts, interpretations of experiences, and reactions to situations.

Resulting from dysfunctional schemas, systematic errors in thinking, called cognitive distortions, can cause emotional and behavioral problems (Beck, Freeman, & Associates, 1990). Beck (1967) identified three cognitive patterns associated with depression: interpreting experiences as negative, viewing oneself negatively, and anticipating endless suffering. In depression, the (a) negative schemata lead to (b) negative automatic thoughts that result in (c) depressed mood that prompts (d) negatively biased recall and perception that produce (e) more negative automatic thoughts (Freeman, Pretzer, Fleming, & Simon, 1990). This creates a downward spiral toward severe depression. Counselors can modify all five components that lead to depression, through cognitive and behavioral interventions. The process can be applied to other problems found in rehabilitation. It would be helpful to use a model of adaptation to disability to understand phase-specific client behavior and focus interventions on cognitions that are likely to be present. Livneh's model of adaptation to disability seems to be a useful framework for the application of CT.

LIVNEH'S MODEL OF ADAPTATION TO DISABILITY

Livneh's (1986a) model consists of five phases. In two phases, initial impact and defense mobilization, the individual resists awareness of the disability. In the other three phases, initial realization, retaliation, and reintegration, the individual moves from realizing to fully accepting the disability. The cognitive defenses, and emotional components are seen as markedly different in each of the phases.

In the **initial impact** phase, the individual experiences shock and uses depersonalization to defend against anxiety and dissolution (Livneh, 1991). The thought processes are marked by confusion and alienation from self. As the shock dissipates, anxiety sets in with cognitive flooding and disorganization often present. In the **defense mobilization** phase, bargaining and denial keep from awareness the consequences of the disabling condition, resulting in euphoric or carefree emotions. The cognitive correlates are rigidity and selective attention. **Initial realization** phase contains mourning with a period of internalized anger, self blame, and obsessive thought processes. The **retaliation** phase involves projecting anger and bitterness outward. The last phase, **reintegration,** contains three subphases: **acknowledgment**—cognitive, but not emotional admitting of the disability, laying the groundwork for **acceptance** and **final adjustment.**

Treatment needs in each phase can be understood as being in three main areas. The first is psychological defenses, protection from trauma; the second, emotions, includes anxiety, euphoria, depression, and anger; the third, the cognitive processes, ranges from disorientation, to rigidity and selective attention, then self-blame.

LIMITATIONS OF LIVNEH'S MODEL OF PHASES
OF ADJUSTMENT TO PHYSICAL DISABILITY

Although there has been partial confirmation of Livneh's phase model (Livneh & Antonak, 1991; Antonak & Livneh, 1991), his model should be viewed as a tentative set of characterizations about how one is **likely** to react to disability over time and to consider Livneh's phases as place markers, not absolute and complete descriptions of what a counselor should see and do in each treatment session. Moreover, there is evidence that the type of disability affects the pattern of reactions and final adjustment if any (Antonak & Livneh, 1995). More research is needed to decide if Livneh's model, or any model, is the definitive, accurate, and useful description of how individuals adjust to their disabilities. The value of using his model is having a systematic approach for researchers and counselors to investigate reactions to traumatic disabilities. Finally, while there is still debate over the order of reactions to traumatic disabilities and achievement of adjustment to disabilities, there is much more consensus about the high incidence of cognition, behaviors and emotions described in each of Livneh's phases. Thus, it appears fruitful to investigate phase specific reactions and apply CT to those reactions.

Combining Livneh's and Beck's insights to create innovative rehabilitation counseling interventions appears possible; however, there are issues between the two that need attention. Although Livneh (1991) does not state a causal link among cognitive processes and emotional states, CT does. In CT, the cognitive processes affect the emotional state, which maintains the cognitive processes (Freeman, et al. 1990). Livneh also does not state **how** or **if** specific therapeutic interventions facilitate progress through each phase to a **final** resolution, or that each person must experience each phase in a specific order. Thus, counselors applying CT to his model must confirm the model's applicability and CT's effectiveness for each client.

REHABILITATION COUNSELOR'S APPLICATION
OF CT TO LIVNEH'S PHASES OF ADAPTATION

As Livneh (1986a) presents his phases, several implications are made. The first is that there is a **tendency** to progress through the phases (individuals can also skip or regress to phases), but no description of what could be motivating the quality, speed, and direction of that progression. The second is that previous or ongoing cognitive and emotional conditions are not important as the power of the disability to overwhelm the psychological state of the individual. If rehabilitation counselors embrace this phase approach and not work with cognitive problems pre-dating the injury, they are likely to neglect significant problem areas. Thus, individuals are helped to manage their disabilities, but not their lives. A third key issue is that each phase could be viewed as self protection, avoiding a complete breakdown of functioning, gradually confronting the disability and creating a new set of coping mechanisms, including a new view of the world and the self. Those who do not resolve a phase adequately may not achieve total adaptation. CT appears to offer empathy and support to aid in adequately resolving each phase.

CT is also action oriented with an approach similar to rehabilitation counseling. Client activity is promoted when client and counselor engage in hypothesis testing. Hypothesis testing begins with counselors creating tasks for clients to complete (Thase & Beck, 1990). The tasks intended to refute dysfunctional thought and promote realistic cognitive self-appraisals, can increase self-confidence.

In working with individuals who have experienced recent physical trauma, CT could be useful in the area of maladaptive schemas. Livneh's model implies that the most significant emotional issues are caused by the physical trauma; counseling is primarily for the trauma's overpowering consequences. However, the CT model also works with schemas (Bricker, Young, & Flanagan, 1993) formed before the trauma. Maladaptive schemas related to dependency, abandonment, unlovability, and social undesirability can exacerbate negative emotions that follow the trauma.

Livneh's Phases of Adaptation to Disability with Case Examples

The five phases of adaptation to disability are presented below with their application to case examples by Barbara, a rehabilitation counselor trained in CT. Counselors are encouraged to view and work with each client as he/she presents unique problems and situations. The case examples are intended to show a common scenario, not the only manner of adapting to disabilities.

Initial impact phase. If the rehabilitation counselor begins working with the client at this phase, the approach must be initially slow and limited to relationship building and information gathering. During the early phases of CT, Beck encourages counselors to provide reassurance, delivered at the level clients are able to accept (Beck, 1967). The clients are helped to explore positive aspects of past or present life. Ventilation and catharsis may either not be possible or performed in a disjointed and detached manner. The counselor would serve the client best by just being there, listening, and not pushing the client to initiate or process emotional material. The listening is more than just supportive: the counselor identifies recurrent statements about self and others that reflect automatic thoughts and how information is processed. The counselor works at relationship and trust building, essential in treatment.

Because this first phase is physiologically determined and self limiting, the counselor lets this phase run its course and provides a safe psychological environment. This includes educating significant others about reactions to disabilities. Family members may be interviewed to get a complete picture of clients' prior cognitive processes, behaviors, and difficulties.

As the shock reaction leaves the body, anxiety sets in, bringing cognitive flooding (Livneh, 1991). CT counselors must now shift gears. Before, there was little client thought or action; now clients are overwhelmed with fear and anxiety. The counselors rely on the established relationship and trust to help clients recognize that anxiety is the result of cognitive processes creating catastrophic interpretations (Freeman et al., 1990) about the disabilities. The counselors also warn clients about the potential for their defenses mobilizing as a method for managing anxiety. The forewarning is not intended to prevent the defense mobilization (a critical self-protection element), but to educate the clients on how their cognitive processes operate. Counselors should talk in generalizations, avoiding specific predictions for their clients' progress.

Case Example 1

Cal, a 38 year-old, self-employed carpenter was shot in a robbery and sustained a spinal cord injury. In the emergency room he was contacted by Barbara. She was present when the surgeon informed Cal that his injury resulted in loss of limb mobility. Cal appeared dazed and talked haltingly. Barbara spent time listening to Cal describe his carpentry business and the robbery. Over the next two sessions she introduced the concept of adaptation to disability and how there would be changes in the way that Cal thought and felt about his injury.

In their fourth session, Barbara found Cal to be anxious and talking rapidly. He feared losing his company. She told him that his cognition determined his feelings, and helped Cal to view his situation more realistically.

Defense Mobilization

Bargaining and denial are the prominent defenses used in this phase (Livneh, 1986a). Awareness of disability is lost to escape anxiety. Clients appear carefree, even euphoric, making it unlikely that they will ask for help in stopping the feelings. The therapist can best intervene by concentrating on cognitive processes, including how the filtering of information distorts reality (Beck & Weirsharr, 1989). Short-term goals can be formed with the patient to develop a collaborative working relationship, promote client activity, and teach the client how to create and follow through on therapeutic goals.

The two most common defenses in this phase, denial and bargaining (Livneh, 1986a), should also be confronted. The value in the confrontations lay in training clients to realize when they are screening out negative material by denial and engaging in illogical thought processes (Beck, 1989). Counselors instruct clients on the negative consequences of keeping the defenses for too long. As counselors become successful in eliminating the defenses, a potential for crises occurs. Clients, realizing that they have been deprived of protection and feel anxious, may blame counselors for their newly acquired discomfort. Counselors should inform clients that the removal of errant cognitive processes leads to negative feelings, but will benefit clients in adapting to their disability.

The concept of selective attention should be taught to clients, exploring how they exclude negative information.

Case Example 2

Barbara was called in for an emergency consultation by nursing staff for her client Rosario. Although both legs were recently paralyzed from an industrial accident, he demanded to be discharged, because he could walk and the nurse would not let him. Rosario appeared elated, laughing and singing. He described his plans for returning to masonry work. He stated that he would walk again, because he had made a deal with God. Barbara confronted Rosario with his medical condition and connected his thoughts to his denial process. She described the tendency for clients to make deals to get better. Rosario stated that God knew more about his condition than she did. He told her to leave if she had nothing positive to say. Understanding that Rosario was protecting himself form his condition, Barbara stopped confronting his defenses and provided supportive counseling, preparing for when he could accept her help. She urged him to cooperate with the medical staff, even though he did not agree with their diagnosis. She encouraged him to stay in the hospital to rest up. She presented herself as being on his side, but seeing it necessary that he not hurt himself.

Initial Realization

As individuals become aware of their disabilities and their consequences, they view their counseling relationship in a different context, seeing the counselor as a resource in dealing with their disabilities. The most prominent emotional issues in this phase are mourning and depression (Livneh, 1986a). Clients also become more introspective, even obsessive with their thoughts. The counselor now can bring the full force of CT into action. Clients in this phase are more vulnerable to major depression and may require anti-depressants. According to Murphy, Simons, Wetzel, and Lustman (1984), CT works well in conjunction with anti-depressants.

Thus, the first task of the counselor is to assess the presence and type of depression (Beck, 1973). If clients have been seen by a psychiatrist or psychologist, a diagnosis of depression may be available. However, in many cases a diagnosis has not been made. This leaves the counselor with the task of assessing the client's emotional state in the context of CT, including patterns of depressive episodes and events that initiate or deepen depression. Training in the DSM-IV (American Psychiatric Association, 1994) can provide a foundation for adequate diagnosis. The Beck Depression Inventory (BDI) is another tool for identifying and understanding client depression (Beck, Riskind, Brown, & Steer, 1988).

The BDI (Beck, 1978), a 21 item multiple choice questionnaire is a helpful CT assessment. It is constructed to measure the cognitive and somatic components of depression that are dealt with in CT (Beck & Beamesderfer, 1974). It can be self administered in written form or orally administered. Counselors with the appropriate education, license, and supervision can administer and interpret this test. Some CT counselors have clients take the BDI before each session, then discuss responses to salient items (Freeman et al., 1990). Not intended to be used as the sole measure of depression, it can be helpful when used with a diagnostic clinical interview (Kendall, Hollon, Beck, Hammen, & Ingram, 1987).

Treatment of depression begins with reviewing the life history to determine maladaptive patterns (Beck, 1973). A reconstruction of depression throughout their lives helps clients to identify early childhood experiences that have created attitudes and sensitization to stress. The objective is to create a complete picture of how the depression is manifested. As clients view their depression in a broader context, they can detect depression-generating automatic thoughts and understand how their disabling conditions prompt automatic thoughts that cause depression.

After clients are more aware of their cognitive processes, counselors can use other CT techniques, including checking clients' observations, responding to depressive cognition, and modifying mood through image modification (Freeman, et al., 1990). Counselors assist clients in reflecting on their observations to determine if they are correct and complete. Clients can recast memories in a more positive light. As clients identify cognitions that lead to depression, they can develop statements to neutralize the cognitions (Beck, 1967).

Because of the self-blame in this phase (Livneh, 1986a), counseling should center on schemas and identifying the more pervasive cognitive processes that initiate and deepen depression through distorting perceptions (Beck, 1973). Since clients are already obsessed with their thought processes, they are more open to discussing negative aspects of their inner world. Gentle confrontation and cooperative attempts at neutralizing these schema can be initiated.

Case Example 3

Ben asked to see Barbara because he was feeling depressed. He told her how angry that he was at himself. Ben confessed that he was made blind by using cocaine. He feared that his wife would discover the truth and leave him. Barbara requested a diagnosis from a psychiatrist and administered the BDI to Ben. Barbara worked with Ben to see how his cognitive processes led to his pre-injury depression and drug use. Before each session, Ben would complete the BDI and Barbara would cover items that he rated as high, including the need for punishment and suicidal thoughts.

Retaliation

This phase can be frustrating for counselors who are subject to projected anger (Livneh, 1986a). Despite this, the client, pulling out of malaise, now has energy to engage the outside world. In the techniques developed by Beck and his colleagues (Beck, Freeman, and Associates, 1990) and refined by Muran and Safran (1993), anger is contained or resolved through assuming a moderate view of the world and confronting the automatic thoughts prompting the emotion. When clients see others more realistically (less hostile and more supportive), they are less threatened by their limitations, lowering projection of anger towards others.

When clients view the counselor as less threatening, a more cooperative and positive relationship ensues (Young, 1992). Clients should work to insulate themselves against reoccurrence of anger and the projecting of that anger. The CT approach can also neutralize anger that was present before the disability. Individuals with borderline, narcissistic, or passive aggressive personality disorders, have schemas centered on justifying anger at others and exhibit frequent and unconfined anger (Young, 1992). Clients need to comprehensively explore and change negative schemas. Freeman (1993) offers three approaches to changing schemas as follows:

1. Schematic modification: maintaining the structure, but making changes to better handle specific situations. Clients are taught to limit displaced anger.
2. Schematic reinterpretations: understanding schemas in ways that are more functional. Anger could be seen as a source of energy for rehabilitation purposes.
3. Schematic camouflage: behavior changes so the client will appear changed, but not think differently. Mistrust of treatment is concealed to get services.

Case Example 4

Sifu started the session yelling about the doctors who could have fixed him, but did not. Sifu, 70 years old, had been a Tai Chi instructor and the loss of movement due to arthritis was difficult for him. He missed his students and his status as Master Instructor. Though a wheelchair user, he refused physical therapy. When he immigrated from China, he promised that he would always care for his family. He was angry at Barbara because she could not help him care for his wife. He wanted to strike out, but could not even make a fist. His physical and mental training had not prepared him for this loss of status and ability to care for others. Barbara helped Sifu to view the negative schema that were causing his anger as a source of motivation that would enable him to teach again (schematic reinterpretation). They devised ways for him to contain his anger by working with his hands, using splints, in recreational therapy (schematic camouflage), a form of work hardening for Sifu, who returned to his academy as a "technical instructor." She helped him to see how he still could give to others (schematic modification).

Reintegration

There are three subphases: cognitively admitting the disability, fully accepting the disability, and the final adjustment (Livneh, 1986b). This is where the action orientation of CT is most beneficial. As clients' depression and anger diminish, they have the energy and motivation for new behaviors. Homework assignments test the accuracy of automatic thoughts and develop social skills. They can be vocationally oriented to improve the work personality.

When clients are in the acknowledgment subphase, they verbalize their disabilities. This provides CT counselors with opportunities to investigate more deeply cognitive reactions to losses from the disability. The clients can connect their immediately available thought processes to less available schemas and emotions. Negative higher order schemas can hinder making the profound changes in philosophy, attitude, and behaviors for their new lifestyle.

In the acceptance and final adjustment subphases, clients have emotionally accepted their disabilities. CT can move from disability issues to daily living issues (Beck et al., 1993). Clients are free to face emotional problems that had been kept in the background, develop new and healthy relationships, identify new goals, and then resume self-actualizing behaviors. A positive, supportive, and insightful counseling relationship provides needed follow-up work.

Case Example 5

James, a firefighter, had severe facial burns and loss of his left hand from a drug related accident at work. After seven months of treatment and CT, he was discharged from the hospital. He maintained monthly contacts with Barbara. While in the hospital he realized the depression that he experienced after the accident was there before the fire; he had simply covered it with drug use. A schema was related to how he felt about his own unattractiveness as a child and rejection by his mother, an alcoholic. He had worked hard to escape those feelings only to have them return with a vengeance after his accident. Barbara continued to help change his depressive and substance use schema to limit thoughts leading to depression and substance abuse. He returned to work as an instructor for new firemen. As he progressed, he accepted his physical disability with its limitations. When he was able to verbalize his physical condition to himself, Barbara helped him connect his feelings and his cognitive reaction to his disability. He also understood the need to work to prevent depression and substance abuse.

SUMMARY

Rehabilitation counselors need to look at both theories that describe the adaptation to disabilities and counseling approaches that are most likely to attend to the problems encountered while adapting to the disabilities. Livneh's phase model and Beck's CT approach seem an excellent combination to consider. The advantages include a comprehensive understanding of adaptation processes, how individuals react to and manage problems in each phase, and intervention techniques that fit the context of rehabilitation counseling. It is hoped that research on coordinated applications of these two systems will ensue as rehabilitation counselors and researchers are made more aware of the benefits of this approach.

REFERENCES

American Psychiatric Association (1994). *Diagnostic and statistical manual of mental disorders* (4th Ed.). Washington DC: Author.

Antonak, R.F., & Livneh H. (1991). A hierarchy of reactions to disability. *International Journal of Rehabilitation Research, 14,* 13–24.

Antonak, R., & Livneh, H. (1995). Psychosocial adaptation to disability and its investigation among persons with multiple sclerosis. *Social Science & Medicine, 40,* 1099–1108.

Beardsley, M.M., & Rubin, S.E. (1988). Rehabilitation service providers: An investigation of generic job tasks and knowledge. *Rehabilitation Counseling Bulletin, 32,* 122–231.

Beck, A.T. (1967). *Depression: Clinical, experimental and theoretical aspects.* New York: Harper & Row.

Beck, A.T. (1973). *The diagnosis and management of depression.* Philadelphia: University of Pennsylvania Press.

Beck, A.T. (1976). *Cognitive therapy and emotional disorders.* New York: Meridian.

Beck, A.T. (1978). *Depression inventory.* Philadelphia: Center for Cognitive Therapy.

Beck, A.T. (1987). Cognitive model of depression. *Journal of Cognitive Psychotherapy, 1,* 2–27.

Beck, A.T. (1989). Foreword. In J. Scott, J.M. Williams, & A.T. Beck (Eds.) *Cognitive therapy in clinical practice: An illustrative casebook* (pp. vii–xv). New York: Routledge.

Beck, A.T., & Beamesderfer, A. (1974). Assessment of depression: The depression inventory. In P. Pichot (Ed.), *Modern problems in pharmacopsychiatry* (pp. 151–169). Basel, Switzerland: Karger.

Beck, A.T., & Weishaar, M.E. (1989). Cognitive therapy. In R.J. Corsini & Wedding, D. (Eds.), *Current psychotherapies* (4th Ed.) (pp. 285–320). Itasca, IL: F.E. Peacock.

Beck, A.T., Freeman, A., & Associates (1990). *Cognitive therapy of personality disorders.* New York: The Guilford Press.

Beck, A.T., Riskind, J.H., Brown, G., & Steer, R.A. (1988). Levels of hopelessness in DSM-III disorders: A test of the cognitive model of depression. *Cognitive Therapy and Research, 12,* 459–469.

Beck, A.T., Rush, A.J., Shaw, B.F., & Emery, G. (1979). *Cognitive therapy of depression.* New York: Guilford Press.

Beck, A.T., Wright, F.D., Newman, C.F., & Liese, C.F. (1993). *Cognitive therapy of substance abuse.* New York: The Guilford Press.

Bowers, W.A. (1988). Beck's cognitive therapy: An overview for rehabilitation counselors. *Journal of Applied Rehabilitation Counseling, 19,* 43–46.

Bricker, D., Young, J.E., & Flanagan, C.M. (1993). Schema-focused therapy: A comprehensive framework for characterological problems. In K.T. Kuehlwein & H. Rosen (Eds.), *Cognitive therapies in action: Evolving innovative practice* (pp. 88–125). San Francisco: Jossey-Bass Publishers.

Corsini, R., & Wedding, D. (Eds.) (1989). *Current psychotherapies* (4th ed.). Itasca, IL: F.E. Peacock.

Ellis, A. (1973). *Humanistic psychotherapy: The rational-emotive approach.* New York: McGraw-Hill.

Freeman, A. (1993). A psychosocial approach for conceptualizing schematic development for cognitive therapy. In K.T. Kuehlwein & H. Rosen (Eds), *Cognitive therapies in action: Evolving innovative practice* (pp. 54–87). San Francisco: Jossey-Bass Publishers.

Freeman, A., Pretzer, J., Fleming, B., & Simon, K.M. (1990). *Clinical applications of cognitive therapy.* New York: Plenum Press.

Kendall, P.C., Hollon, S.D., Beck, A.T., Hammen, C.L., & Ingram, R.E. (1987). Issues and Recommendations Regarding use of the Beck Depression Inventory. *Cognitive Therapy and Research, 11,* 289–299.

Kuehlwein, K.T. (1993). A survey and update of cognitive therapy systems. In K.T. Kuehlwein & H. Rosen (Eds.), *Cognitive therapies in action: Evolving innovative practice* (pp. 1–32). San Francisco: Jossey-Bass Publishers.

Kuehlwein, K.T., & Rosen, H. (Eds.) (1993). *Cognitive therapies in action: Evolving innovative practice* (pp. 1–32). San Francisco: Jossey-Bass Publishers.

Larcombe, N.A., & Wilson, P.H. (1984). An evaluation of cognitive-behaviour therapy for depression in patients with multiple sclerosis. *British Journal of Psychiatry, 145,* 366–371.

Livneh, H. (1986a). A unified approach to existing models of adaptation to disability: Part I: A model adaptation. *Journal for Applied Rehabilitation Counseling, 17*(1), 5–16.

Livneh, H. (1986b). A unified approach to existing models of adaptation to disability: Part II: Intervention strategies. *Journal of Applied Rehabilitation Counseling, 17*(2), 6–10.

Livneh, H. (1991). A unified approach to existing models of adaptation to disabilities: A model of adaptation In R.P. Marinelli, & A.E. Dell Orto (Eds.), *The psychological and social impact of disability* (3rd ed.). New York: Springer Publishing Company.

Livneh, H., & Antonak, R.F. (1991). Temporal structure to disability. *Rehabilitation Counseling Bulletin, 34,* 298–319.

Livneh, H., & Sherwood, A. (1991). Application of personality theories and counseling strategies to clients with physical disabilities. *Journal of Counseling and Development, 69,* 525–538.

Muran, J.C., & Safran, J.D. (1993). Emotional and interpersonal considerations in cognitive therapy. In K.T. Kuehlwein & H. Rosen (Eds.), *Cognitive therapies in action: Evolving innovative practice* (pp. 185–212). San Francisco: Jossey-Bass Publishers.

Murphy, G.E., Simons, A.D., Wetzel, R.D., & Lustman, P.J. (1984). Cognitive therapy versus tricyclic antidepressants in major depression. *Archives of General Psychiatry, 41,* 959–967.

Rubin, S.E., & Puckett, F.D. (1984). Roles and functions of the rehabilitation counselor. *Rehabilitation Counseling Bulletin, 27,* 225–231.

Rubin, S.E., Matkin, R.E, Ashley, J., Beardsley, M.M., May, V.R., Onstott, K., & Puckett, F.D. (1984). Roles and functions of certified rehabilitation counselors. *Rehabilitation Counseling Bulletin, 27,* 199–224.

Thase, M.E., & Beck, A.T. (1990). Overview of cognitive therapy. In J.H. Wright, M.E. Thase, A.T. Beck, & J.W. Ludgate (Eds.), *Cognitive therapy with inpatients: Developing a cognitive milieu* (pp. 3–35). New York: The Guilford Press.

Thomas, K., Thoreson, R., Butler, A., & Parker, R.M. (1992). Theoretical foundations of rehabilitation counseling. In R.M. Parker & E.M. Szymanski (Eds.), *Rehabilitation Counseling* (2nd ed.) (pp. 207–247). Austin, TX: PRO-ED.

Young, J. (1992). An integrative schema-focused model for personality disorders. *Journal of Cognitive Psychotherapy, 6,* 11–23.

22

Depression and Denial in Psychotherapy of Persons with Disabilities

Karen G. Langer

INTRODUCTION

Psychotherapy may play a vital role in easing the suffering of a patient with disability. Physical losses are not the only ones sustained by a patient who becomes acutely or progressively disabled; the losses involving definitions of self and personhood are often critical to adjustment.

On a fundamental level, the losses incurred in disability are losses of aspects of oneself; certainly body parts and functioning are altered, but psychological entities that accompany (or subsume) them may be wounded as well. Indeed, as Nemiah states:

> Hopes and aspirations must be modified, income and security for his family and himself are threatened; his position in the social structure is altered; feelings of helplessness and weakness replace his former sense of strength and competence. All that . . . forms a person's concept of himself is jeopardized . . . loss may involve physical objects . . . and psychological entities—self-concepts, ideals, social status, etc.[1] (p. 151).

In this paper, we shall first examine, rather broadly, the nature of the psychologic impact of disability and some of the more subtle but implicit losses that may ensue. Those losses are not so obvious or concrete as the physical or functional losses, but equally as broad-reaching with regard to effect on the patient's

The author gratefully acknowledges the continued support of Dr. Leonard Diller and Dr. Frank Padrone, the technical assistance of Dr. Gregg Salem, and the inspiration of all those who have taught and from whom I have learned.

From *American Journal of Psychotherapy,* 48(2) (Spring 1994), 181–194. Reprinted with permission.

experience. Next, we shall consider one primary reaction to disability and loss, namely, depression. Although certainly depression is only one of the many possible emotional responses to disability, the fundamental connection between loss and depression leads to a natural conceptual bridge that warrants attention. Denial is, too, only one of defensive strategies that may commonly be used after the onset of disability. We consider it here because of its relatively common appearance in many patients after onset of disabling loss and because it may be one of the most challenging and countertransference-provoking reactions to encounter in practice. The special psychotherapeutic treatment considerations posed by disability (broadly speaking) will be outlined. Lastly, the uniqueness of the countertransference reactions to the patient with a disability consists in part in the enormity of the losses and their power to evoke the therapist's own sense of vulnerability and humanity.

With regard to the experience of suffering by the patient with disability, phenomenological accounts of disability[2] provide a clear distinction between illness or disability as viewed by the practitioner as opposed to the patient's experience. Cassell[3,4] has likewise underscored the distinction between distress (viewed clinically) and suffering (as a personal human phenomenon); patients who, in medical terms, are in "no acute distress" may yet be suffering. Suffering may result from internal psychic conflicts involving sense of self, self-esteem, altered ability to fulfill expectations, negative perceptions of self or others regarding disability,[1] etc., along with other losses, some unique to disability (cf. below). Suffering results from violation or impending threat to the integrity of the person, not simply the body and its functions, nor is suffering limited to physical pain. The psychotherapist may play a unique part in the healing process itself. Many aspects of the experience of illness, loss of function, and treatment can be profoundly dehumanizing; in early phases, the onset of disability may be fundamentally disintegrating to the sense of unity of self. The patient's experience of disorder may result from "changing relations between body, self, and world"[2] (p. 82). Cassell[4] notes that a therapeutic goal includes maintaining or restoring the integrity of the person. Exploration of individual values,[2] which is so much a part of the exploration of personal valence and meaning in psychotherapy, can also help preserve the sense of self in the face of the threat of minor or catastrophic disruptions posed by disability.

Disability may challenge some fundamental assumptions that are often implicit about living. Disruptions posed by disability may result in an altered sense of significance of time or space;[1] future goals and projections may be shattered, as may certainties about the present that become replaced by anxieties for the imagined future. Even space itself may become a harsh reminder of loss and restrictions to a person with a disability. The invitation to experience life is fraught with the considerations of accessibility; effort and limitations may be continual reminders of loss, resulting in suffering. The body itself may be viewed as an opponent to intention, where disability renders volition, physical effort, and will incapable of carrying out intended actions.

Among the losses that ensue with adult-onset disability is the myth of invulnerability and assumptions regarding the world. In some sense, even as adults, on a primitive level we may retain a childlike fantasy about justness in the world: "If I'm good—good things will happen" which leads to its corollary—"If I'm bad—bad things happen", and (erroneous) deductive reasoning leads to the assumption, "If bad things happen—I must be bad" or "If bad things happen—it's not fair (or just)." We believe that our very assumptions about the world are valid, which helps provide an anchoring sense of consistency of meaning and constancy of experience, but which may be as subjective as perception. However, to the person who has lost the meaning provided by assumptions about the world living itself can become a frightening ordeal of the unknown. Depression can quickly ensue when assumptions about "fairness" are interpreted as if shattered. The dashed sense of expectant entitlement can lead to a frustration that produces anger and rage or hopeless futility and despair, rather than growth or maturely renegotiated assumptions.

With regard to the context in which disability is experienced, let us note that it has been rare to encounter a patient who had been comforted by the notion that others at the same age or stage in life were equally as disabled. There have been, perhaps, a few. But certainly it seems true that when disability is catastrophic or is worse than the norm for others at the same stage in life, there is potential for greater grief and mournfulness. In other words, one can derive a sense of perspective from knowing that many others are in the same boat, so to speak, although the individual's personal sense of loss is not diminished. But if one incurs a (catastrophic) disability when others of the same age/stage do not, one may feel more alienated or different from others, which can itself increase the psychic pain.

Depression: Conceptual and Diagnostic Issues

There are certain predictable human responses to loss, including potential shock, sadness, anger/bitterness, and pining for the lost object that are well described in the literature on trauma and loss. Freud's[5] own early conceptualizations describe the process of mourning as involving gradual (but sometimes stormy) relinquishment of emotional attachment to the lost object over time. Depression (clinical) as a postbereavement response was thought to be the result of reactions to the lost object. Karasu[6] summarizes the diverse perspectives of such classic writers as Freud, Klein, Jacobson, Kohut, Bowlby, Sullivan, and Arieti and proposes a "developmentalist metatheory" for the treatment of depressive disorder that integrates the many prior conceptual and theoretical approaches to the phenomenon and etiology of depression.

In the *DSM,*[7] bereavement is characterized by feelings of depression and may include vegetative signs, but prolonged functional impairment with a morbid sense of worthlessness and marked psychomotor retardation may point to a clinical (major) depression. In bereavement, the feelings of guilt and thoughts of death tend to be circumscribed. However, much cultural variability exists in bereavement patterns and duration.

Bowlby[8] and Parkes[9] have provided rich clinical insight into the process of mourning and adaptation to loss in states of grief and bereavement. Bowlby has outlined four basic phases of mourning: numbness, yearning/pining, depression, and recovery, each characterized by different attachment behaviors and emotional responses. Kübler-Ross'[10] clinical descriptions of terminally ill persons has sparked much work in the area of anticipatory loss and dying. In distinguishing depression from grief and bereavement, in working with persons with catastrophic loss and disability, the question of what is "normal" emerges. Horowitz[11] has constructed a model that depicts the phases of response to serious or catastrophic life events that may characterize the early stages of response to sudden catastrophic or progressive disability. These stages are: outcry, denial, intrusiveness, working through, and completion. The specific pathologic signs and symptoms of each phase are identified, along with the nature of cognitive and emotional processing in "normal" bereavement and successful versus unsuccessful use of controls or defenses in coping; the interested reader is referred for an excellent exposition of the proposed modes of human cognitive and emotional responses to serious life events.

Depression as a clinical phenomenon may be a bit of a challenge, however, in patients with a disability since the features of depression may be difficult to distinguish from somatic features of disease in those who are concomitantly medically ill.[12,13] Depression, too, may present with symptoms that mimic medical illness,[14,15] further complicating differential diagnosis.

From another perspective, the misdiagnosis of depression as grief in acute settings[16] and overdiagnosis of depression in chronic settings has been discussed. The challenge of differential diagnostic assessment is important for the treatment of clinical depression and for therapeutic management of grief in an institutional (rehabilitation) setting.[17]

Impact of Disability upon Coping Mechanisms

The adaptive functions of the defense of sublimation are well-known even at a common-sense level; the ability to "work the tension off," to channel the energy into an alternate interest or activity may spur creativity as well as alter the manifestations of the personality. When restrictions posed by a disability interfere with work or leisure activities, they may interrupt the directions into which energy and interest had been sublimated before.

Traditional means of coping with sadness and loss may be disrupted by the disability itself, (e.g., long walks on the beach, leisure activities that distract, etc.). Activities that used to provide a sense of needed relief or escape may be compromised or inaccessible because of the disability. It is not simply the enjoyed activity itself that may be sadly interrupted, but the psychic function that it represents as well (i.e., adaptive coping or sublimation).

One man who had acquired quadriplegia due to a cervical spinal tumor aptly described his dilemma. On the rehabilitation unit, he had frequent outbursts of explosive and often physically violent rage, which alternated with despair. Before the onset of his physical condition, he said he would run miles a day, or go boating to discharge tension and numb dysphoric feelings. (We also knew that he had abused alcohol.) Not only could he not enjoy his favorite pastimes, but he had significant and major losses that intensified prior developmental and interpersonal conflicts and he had good reason to feel depressed. As he said, the very ways he would have chosen to deal with his situation were not available because of the losses causing depression; he felt, understandably, as if he were trapped.

DEPRESSION AND DISABILITY

The complex and multifactorial relationship of disability to depression in some persons with similar physical disabilities[18] leads to the suggestion that depression is not a univariate corollary of disability and that personal psychodynamic, intercurrent situational, social, and historical factors should be considered for individual patients before psychotherapy commences.

Factors to consider in treating depression in the case of patients with disabilities, include:

a. the future course of the condition, (i.e., progressive vs. stable, chronic vs. acute, dynamic/episodic vs. static, and issues of prognosis); each new loss or decline can symbolize dreaded disintegration and each new blow can revivify the initial horror all over again;

b. the amount of time since onset;

c. the issue of accompanying physical pain or discomfort;

d. personal (premorbid) affective and cognitive style;[19]

e. the social resources available to the person, versus the depletion of social resources (due to factors of aging, personal style, the ability of significant others to cope themselves with disability, or other factors);

f. the meaning of the disability to the patient in considering both narcissistic colorations and the actual or perceived impact on functioning;

g. the meaning to others in society—social strangers in cultural/subcultural or social networks;

h. the personal ability to sustain hope regarding opportunities for the future as well as about any aspect of experience in life (present and future) and find some sense of purpose or meaning in it;

i. the "domino" effect of disability on other factors (see Vignette below) including financial status, environmental accessibility, quality of living, stress on existing social networks, and stressors to future social contacts, etc.;

j. the prior experience with, and meaning of, disability (and loss in general) that may render disability meaningful as a life challenge or simply add to the strain of preexisting multiple chronic stressors upon coping resources, or may act as the straw that broke the camel's back.

Vignette 1

M., a 52-year-old man, had sustained a spinal cord injury resulting in C_5 quadriplegia 10 years prior to psychotherapy treatment. He had been a successful businessman before the injury, but had not worked since because of the "financial disincentive"; he had depleted all personal resources, and depended on state funds in order to pay for his personal aides to assist in daily care routines. He felt that he could not earn enough by working to pay for the amount of yearly assistance he needed. As a result, he was cut off from social and vocational contact that he had enjoyed and became more isolated. Indeed, his wife had left him shortly after the accident. M. had been attempting to expand his business to a corporation, but his plans were interrupted by his injury. The national prominence of his major business competitor brought into sharp focus reminders of all that the patient had lost and/or the plans and dreams that were tragically not to be realized.

In psychotherapy, this articulate and generally insightful man stated that he often felt that his own body got in his way. At one point, he even suggested that he would be better off if his "head were cut off and put on a platter," a symbol of the degree to which he felt dissociated from and encumbered by his body. The sense of mutilation and fantasies about personal defeat are also reflected in his choice of words, as are features of significant depression.

Countertransference Issues with Depression and Disabling Loss

One risk in psychotherapy is for either patient or therapist to assume that things (i.e., mood states) must be the way they are. It may well be that without the disability, the person might not be depressed. However, the comprehensibility of the cause ought not to engender complacent validation of the existence of depression, whether to the patient (via depressive inertia or attempt to normalize the experience) or to the therapist. Sometimes, the novice therapist may feel overwhelmed by the disability or assume that "of course, the person is depressed" given his/her disability. The "of course" should be used to express empathy, but not to cloud the suffering of the patient or the need for clinically established psychotherapeutic means for treating the depression. The issue here again is one of preconceived expectancy or what is "normal," as well as the ability of the therapist to monitor countertransferential reactions of identification with, or emotional distancing from, the patient in response to the therapist's own sense of horror about the patient's losses, disfigurement or prognosis.

Denial and Loss

In clinical practice, we sometimes encounter patients with traumatic or catastrophic disabling losses who are not so distressed as might be realistically expected, even when considering individual differences. The question in these instances is whether the person simply has not yet realized the full emotional impact and/or implications of these losses, whether they are simply not so distressed by what they do realize or whether they are in some state of denial.

Since grief after major loss and some form of (time-limited) depression are treated as "normal" in classic psychoanalytic and psychodynamic literature[5,8] as well as in everyday culture, it is widely believed that distress and depression are to be expected and that their absence is the sign of pathology, if not denial. Wortman[20] has challenged these beliefs in reviewing research on loss and argues that there is probably more interindividual variability in emotional response to loss that is "normal" than traditional theorists believed; she suggests that attention to his individual variability will enhance nonjudgmental sensitivity and empathy.

In this section, the focus will be upon the phenomenon of denial of losses in physical disability, as a defensive process and on the question of its adaptiveness.

Defensive Nature of Denial

Denial, as we know, operates on different levels. The amusing anecdote of a five-year-old boy who adamantly asserts to his kindergarten teacher, when congratulated on the birth of his sister, "No, I have no sister, it's just me and my brother," reveals the boy to be neither unobservant nor crazy in denying the reality of his new baby sister. The denial serves to protect him from panic on a level of reality that he can modulate, a purely subjective reality that operates in his own mind. Anna Freud,[21] in her study of the ego and its defensive activities, describes how the processes of denial in act and in fantasy correspond to and deviate from the constraints of external reality, and how denial may threaten the ability to test reality. Conversely, the adaptive role of denial has fueled determination in creative or scientific endeavor[22] without which odds might have seemed insurmountable. Denial has provided hope to cope with illness and has fueled courage for heroic deed. But, blinded by a reality that is true only to its conceiver, the larger physical reality of nature may be ignored in ways that put the person at risk.

Breznitz[23] postulates seven kinds of denial that may operate, each one related to a different stage of processing threatening information; these are denial of: information, threat, personal relevance urgency, vulnerability/responsibility, affect, and affect relevance. The degree to which reality is distorted varies in each of these stages. We have found this schema clinically useful in specifying the locus of denial in our patients, particularly when conceptualizing the meaning of denial in teaching or in consultation roles.

Denial of Disability

Progressive illness as a condition, or perhaps terminal illness, concerns imped-ing or future projections of something that has not yet happened. In contrast, when patients deny disability, they deny that which may be sensorially perceived. The phenomenon of denial in chronic medical illness has been well reviewed and summarized elsewhere.[24] The striking aspect of denial as may be in evidence when noted in persons with disability is the contrast with sometimes marked lim-itations and visible inability. In extreme forms, patients with visual-perceptual losses or hemianopsia may state that they "see just fine"; the possible neurogenic origins of this "denial," or more correctly unawareness, versus psychologic fac-tors, has been discussed.[25-28] But patients with gross, even longstanding, physi-cal disabilities may deny aspects of the disability itself, if not the implications. [Full denial of all aspects of significant disability is usually a sign of either a post-traumatic state (i.e., acuteness) or a psychotic distortion of reality.]

Vignette 2

L., a 34-year-old man, had acquired paraplegia ("complete" spinal lesion) since age 19 due to a gunshot injury. L. had a history of nondescript trouble with the law and clinical history suggested psychopathic and narcissistic fea-tures. The details of the intake history itself were difficult to verify and some were contradictory. Five years after living with a disability that included full motor and sensory loss below the waist, L. still maintained that he had "full sensation." Compensatory bravado invoked to defend against a fragile and disrupted sense of self led to distortions at many levels, including his report of avocational success, physical functions, and level of independent func-tioning, etc. Although these distortions were not in keeping with the physi-cal reality, they were in keeping with the psychic narcissistic image. Understanding the narcissistic image helped us to predict where breakdown in reality testing might occur for this patient, so that realistic planning could take place concomitant with treatment of the narcissistic vulnerabilities and defective sense of self.

Horowitz[11] stresses the phasic nature of denial (and intrusion), and cautions that these processes or stages do not follow a prescribed pattern or sequence and oscillate idiographically for each person. Patients may also show fluctuating con-scious attention to disability. Family and staff may be exasperated (at least) in their attempts to make the patient "aware" of that which they believe is denied. As such, they may feel puzzled (or frustrated) at fluctuations in denial; the patient may ask with an explicit request for help with a function that cannot be performed, while the implication of living with the disability is avoided or dis-avowed.

Psychotherapeutic Considerations in Denial of Disability

In treating the patient who is "denying" the reality of disabling loss, some fundamental issues should be considered, including:

a. the risk/benefit ratio of denial versus "knowing," or alternately put, at which price is the subjective world of the patient maintained;
b. what needs are being served, and what would happen if denial were to be punctured?
c. analysis of whose needs would be met by having the patient faced with the external reality (e.g., those of the family, other treatment providers, or psychotherapists themselves); who is presuming the best interests of the patient, and how are these best interests determined?

Other dimensions of denial of disability include the dynamic nature of, and natural temporal fluctuations in, the defense over time, and the factors of content of denial (i.e., what), magnitude (severity) of defense, and the extent of disability (i.e., part/whole) denied.

A recent case was a patient who had sustained a right hemisphere CVA with left hemiplegia and hemianopsia, and severe left visual neglect. Judgment was generally adequate. The patient had been an experienced pilot. Needless to say, one might think twice now about having the patient anywhere near the airfield. Fluctuations were noted day-to-day between psychotherapy sessions: during one session, the patient stated that he knew he could not work as a pilot; during the next session he offered, "Well, I'm sure I can't continue to teach others," and during the next session stated, "Maybe I can go back to work, I'll have to see."

The fluctuations over time suggest that a patient must "know," but may at different moments in time have more or less ability to tolerate what is known and to integrate the knowledge into a meaningful reality. Often of importance in psychotherapeutic treatment involving denial of disability is the role of *a priori* knowledge. Cultural, educational and informational factors may play a role in awareness or understanding.

As in any clinical setting, a patient may show variability in aspects of denial of the relevance of disability and its personal meaning (hence, the part/whole nature of denial and distinctions between "intellectual" and "emotional" understanding). One young dancer was left with massive injuries and scars after a skiing accident that resulted in quadriplegia. Although she was both psychologically well-adjusted and medically sophisticated, it was only weeks later that she became struck by the horror of her scars and deformities as the numbness wore off and she began to struggle with the issues of appearance and feminine identity. As the issues were worked through, she was well able to make choices that reflected an integrated and healthy understanding of her own dynamic needs in the context of her disability.

Adaptiveness of the Defense

The adaptive or maladaptive quality of the defense is a primary consideration. In the initial response to the trauma, a fair amount of denial may serve to protect the patient from becoming psychologically overwhelmed and may be a psychic equivalent of shock. This denial may then facilitate posttraumatic functioning, so that an adaptive coping function is served. As time passes and the patient begins to integrate the emotional meaning of the losses, defensive denial may diminish. We tend to thing of denial and depression in an inverse relationship that may at times be true, but patients who show some signs of denial may still be depressed. A case example may illustrate.

Vignette 3

K., a 38-year-old divorced man, had a five-year history of a rare demyelinating disease that resulted in paraplegia. His prior history was significant for childhood asthma. K. had a very stormy and conflicted relationship with his widowed mother, whom he experienced as controlling and infantilizing. Despite his overt contempt for her, he moved into her home when his symptoms became rapidly progressive. His ongoing developmental conflict was represented in his continual defiance of her; he actively included "not telling my mother" as a step in all plans. There was a developmentally primitive quality inherent in the rigidity of the defiance. His plans became more wildly grandiose and unrealistic, suggesting that his need to defensively deny his progressive decline was multiply determined. First, he was becoming more desperate and despairing as his physical status worsened and second, the physical dependence triggered the conflict-laden representation of "mother." Mother began to symbolize all thwarting of independence. What he could not win in the battle against increasing disability (although he tried, insisting on using a cane and falling rather than using a walker), he could attempt to win by defying mother. He displayed his bruises after falling with the defiant pride of triumph in a symbolic victory (not a real one) over progressive disability. The real triumph, of course, was the battle he had (temporarily) won to protect the desperately vulnerable sense of self from further attack; our therapeutic question concerned the price he paid and we were reminded of the metaphor about "winning the battle but losing the war."

In treatment, the temptation to directly confront the obvious maladaptive effects of his denial was avoided (it would have resulted in rageful resistance to continue treatment). Instead, interpretations were gently titrated, with underlying narcissistic vulnerabilities concurrently addressed.

The above vignette also highlights the psychotherapeutic imperative of determining, in a sense, the risk/benefit ratio of denial. The price at which the subjective world of the patient is maintained must be weighed against the danger were denial to be punctured prematurely; particularly if the defense is serving to protect the person from psychic decompensation or disintegration.

Countertransference Issues

The psychotherapist who works with a patient who is denying aspects of disability may experience significant countertransference reactions, including anxiety, anger or frustration, especially if the therapist allows him/herself to be swayed by the needs of those other than the patient (i.e., family, other treatment providers or institutional and administrative staff, or therapist him/herself). This situation may be particularly prevalent in institutional settings where multiple agendas operate sometimes veiled from view. The key for the psychotherapist is to consider the underlying (nontherapeutic) sources of pressure to have the patient right away just accept "reality" as it is.

To conclude this section on issues of denial and disability in psychotherapy, as has been so well highlighted clinically in other contexts,[26] (p. 66) let us suggest that our patients first develop awareness based on their subjective reality and on the relevance to them of the information we want to impart. The ability to tolerate losses depends, in part, on what the losses mean. Second, they need time to adapt to and integrate any loss. Therapists need patience; patients need time. We cannot force a "reality" upon our patients; it must exist for them, and we must try to understand their reality so they can maximize its correspondence to that of the world-at-large. Lastly, we have often been reminded by patients themselves, at a moment of less-than-ideal clinical sensitivity, of the importance of hope and of maintaining hope, both in warding off despair and in preserving a sense of continuity and meaningfulness in life itself.

SUMMARY

Disability may challenge some basic assumptions about the world, and some psychological aspects of self may be profoundly violated, particularly when onset is sudden and functional changes seem catastrophic. The losses incurred in disability, broadly defined, whether minimal or major, physical, psychologic, symbolic, or all of the above, may lead to some predictable human emotional responses, although individual patients' responses do vary. Factors including prior life history, concurrent life stressors, social and financial resources, intrapsychic functions, psychodynamic issues, and personal/subcultural issues may influence the experience of disability.

Depression, as a natural concomitant to loss, may present in clinical form or in bereavement and grief patterns, and warrants full consideration (both diagnostically and therapeutically). In treating the patient with a disabling loss, the dynamic nature of denial must also be considered. The often visible inability or disability may stand in sharp contrast to that which is denied. The risk/benefit ratio of denial is a consideration when the psychotherapist weighs the need to maintain denial defensively versus the advisability of confronting the denial in an attempt to soften its brittleness. Countertransference reactions are also of prime importance and may differ from more typical reaction by virtue of the enormity of the patient's losses and their tendency to evoke the psychotherapist's own sense of vulnerability, morality, and humanity.

REFERENCES

American Psychiatric Association. (1980; rev. 1987). *Diagnostic and Statistical Manual of Mental Disorders, 3rd Edition.* Washington, D.C.: Author.

Bisiach, E., Valler, G., Perani, D., et al. (1986). Unawareness of disease following lesions of the right hemisphere: Anosagnosia for hemiplegia and anosagnosia for hemianopia. *Neuropsychology, 24,* 471–482.

Bowlby, J. (1980). *Attachment and loss* (Vol. 3). *Loss. Sadness and depression.* New York: Basic Books.

Breznitz, S. (1985). The seven kinds of denial. In S. Breznitz (Ed.), *The denial of stress* (pp. 257–280). New York: International Universities Press.

Cassell, E. J. (1991). *The nature of suffering.* New York: Oxford University Press.

Cassell, E. J. (1992). The nature of suffering and the goals of medicine. *New England Journal of Medicine, 306,* 639–645.

Freud, A. (1966). *The ego and the mechanisms of defense* (rev. ed.) In *The writings of Anna Freud.* (Vol. 2.) New York: International Universities Press. (Original work published 1936)

Freud, S. (1957). Mourning and melancholia. In J. Strachey (Ed. and Trans.), *The standard edition of the complete psychological works of Sigmund Freud* (Vol. 14, pp. 327–260). London: Hogarth Press (Original work published 1917).

Gans, J. S. (1981). Depression diagnosis in a rehabilitation hospital. *Archives of Physical Medicine and Rehabilitation, 62,* 386–389.

Hartmann, H. (1939). *Ego psychology and the problem of adaptation.* New York: International Universities Press.

Horowitz, M. J. (1983). Psychological response to serious life events. In S. Breznitz (Ed.), *The denial of stress* (pp. 129–159). New York: International Universities Press.

Karasu, T. B. (1992). Developmentalist metatheory of depression and psychotherapy. *American Journal of Psychotherapy* (Special Section: Minor Depression, T. B. Karasu, Ed.), *46,* 37–49.

Kübler-Ross, E. (1969). *On death and dying.* New York: Macmillan Co.

Langer, K. G., & Padrone, F. J. (1992). Psychotherapeutic treatment of awareness in acute rehabilitation of traumatic brain injury. *Neuropsychological Rehabilitation, 2,* 59–70.

Langer, K. G. (in press). Depression in disabling illness: Severity and patterns of self-reported symptoms in three groups. *Journal of Geriatric Psychiatry and Neurology.*

Lesse, S. (1983). The masked depression syndrome—Results of a seventeen year clinical study. *American Journal of Psychotherapy, 37,* 456–475.

Levine, D. N. (1990). Unawareness of visual and sensorimotor defects: A hypothesis. *Brain and Cognition, 13,* 233–281.

Lewis, L. (1991). Role of psychological factors in disordered awareness. In G. P. Prigatano & D. L. Schacter (Eds.), *Awareness of deficit after brain injury: clinical and theoretical issues.* (pp. 223–239). New York: Oxford University Press.

McGlynn, S. M. & Schacter, D. L. (1989). Unawareness of deficits in neuropsychological syndromes. *Journal of Clinical and Experimental Psychology, 11,* 143–205.

Nemiah, J. C. (1961). *Foundations of psychopathology.* New York: Oxford University Press.

Parkes, C. M. (1975). Psycho-social transitions: Comparison between reactions to loss of a limb and loss of a spouse. *British Journal of Psychiatry, 127,* 204–210.

Plumb, M. M., & Holland, J. (1977). Comparative studies of psychological functions in patients with advanced cancer. I. Self-reported depression symptoms. *Psychosomatic Medicine, 39,* 264–276.

Salzman, C., & Shader, R. I. (1978). Depression in the elderly. I. Relationship between depression, psychologic defense mechanism and physical illness. *Journal of The American Geriatrics Society, 26,* 253–260.

Schwab. J. J., Bialow, M., Brown, J. M., et al. (1967). Diagnosing depression in medical patients. *Annals of Internal Medicine, 67,* 695–707.

Shapiro, D. (1965). *Neurotic styles.* New York: Basic Books.

Stewart, T., & Shields, C. R. (1985). Grief in chronic illness: Assessment and management. *Archives of Physical Medicine and Rehabilitation, 66,* 447–450.

Toombs, S. K. (1992). *The meaning of illness: A phenomenological account of the different perspectives of physician and patient.* Dordrecht, The Netherlands: Kluwer Academic Publishers.

Wortman, C., & Silver, R. C. (1987). Coping with irrevocable loss. In G. R. VandenBos & B. K. Bryant (Eds.), *Cataclysms, crises, and catastrophes.* (Vol. 6, Master lecture series, pp. 185–235). Washington, D.C.: American Psychological Association.

23

Encouragement as a Vehicle to Empowerment in Counseling: An Existential Perspective

Richard J. Beck

INTRODUCTION

A major recent emphasis in disability rights and rehabilitation counseling is that of empowerment. The way that empowerment is generally viewed in this arena is that the experience of disability leads to the experience of viewing life differently, and to the creation of a new perspective that is less concerned with body image and ability, and focuses rather on living interdependently with the full use of one's assets (Hahn, 1989). The position of this paper is that the element of courage is involved in the creation of this new perspective, and that rehabilitation and independent living counselors can facilitate this process through the use of encouragement. For example, the word "encouragement" is used several times by both Emener (1991) and Vash (1991) in their articles on empowerment.

Rehabilitation counseling involves several components including evaluation (assessment), guidance (teaching new ways of living) and confrontation (removing blocks to and challenging the client to use resources). However, practitioners also frequently encourage clients particularly when they want them to try things which are new, or threatening, or for which the person has low confidence. Courage is a philosophical construct that belongs to the field of ontology and has been discussed in depth in the existential psychology literature (May, 1967, 1969, 1975). Thus, the author believes that the study of existence (existentialism) can elucidate courage as construct, and that conceptual bridges can be built to specific strategies in counseling that can "encourage" the creation of new life perspectives in persons with disabilities. Indeed, this paper will purport to

From *Journal of Rehabilitation,* 60(3) (1994), 6–11. Reprinted with permission.

demonstrate that courage is the stuff of everyday life and is a measure of how we live that life. As Rollo May (1967) puts it in *The Art of Counseling:*

> To live the life of self-expression requires courage. To love greatly, to admit one's hate without having it destroy one's equilibrium, to express anger, to rise to heights of joy and to know deep sorrow, to go on far adventures in spite of loneliness, to catch lofty ideas and carry them into action—in short, to live out the infinite number of instinctual urges that rise in glorious challenge within one—this requires courage (p. 193).

Courage has been defined in the philosophical and psychological literature (May, 1975; Walton, 1986) as generally occurring in the presence of the following conditions: (a) a careful presence of mind and deliberate action; (b) the presence of difficult, dangerous, and painful circumstances; and (c) a morally worthy intention. Tillich (1952) adds another dimension that underlies courage, which is that the person is engaged in an act that has existential meaning for him or her. Without that existential meaning, daily efforts become nothing but the drudgery of the slave.

Disability is sometimes accompanied by giving in, or, as Wright (1983) calls it, succumbing. Depression is the most frequent concomitant of this, but certainly other characteristics are also associated. External locus of control, failure identity, low self-esteem, and substance abuse often are the result of a person's succumbing to a disability experience (Beck & Lustig, 1990). In the area of substance abuse and alcoholism, several theories seem to imply that abuse and addiction result from a breakdown in courage as it is defined above. The degree of difficulty of a person's life (social strain), as exemplified by barriers to educational and employment opportunities, as well as escapism through addiction to give meaning to our existence, is reviewed by Simon (1986) in an article on alienation and alcohol abuse. And May (1975) states that courage is moving ahead with one's life in spite of despair. There is ample evidence that the emptiness that gives rise to addiction is seen in failures of courage, or, as May (1975) implies, victories of cowardice. When a client is confronted in counseling who has succumbed to addiction or who is in a state of deep self- or societal-estrangement because of the disability experience, it seems that sooner or later we, as counselors, must confront the courage issue. This is what is usually meant by encouragement, or, *giving* courage to our clients. We *give* the client the courage to take up their treatment as his/her own. Some counselors and therapists use the term "confrontation" for the same process, although "confront" is similar to "encounter," which implies a minor battle, whereas "encourage" implies inspiration with hope, courage, or spirit. The former is related to control, and may be appropriate in that stage of counseling whose object is destructive, to break down defenses, whereas the latter is constructive, and urges the person to own and attempt new ways of being and living.

Of course we as helpers have always encouraged our clients, but we often do so intuitively and pragmatically, and without a theoretical basis. The purpose of this paper is to attempt to give a description of courage and its conditions that hopefully will enable the reader to conceptualize efforts at encouragement, and therefore to "give" courage more effectively.

Courage as a Concept in the Counseling Professions

"Courage" is an ontological construct, which means it is generally about the nature of being, and specifically the metaphysical or spiritual being. This partially explains why the field of psychology has not addressed this construct, except for the existentialists (e.g., May, Frankl, and other isolated theorists such as Adler). Rehabilitation has begun to deal with the spiritual aspects of empowerment, and the importance of courage (Emener, 1991; Vash, 1991).

Another reason why courage may not have been employed as a construct in the writings on empowerment generally is that it goes against modern egalitarian ethics. According to Walton (1986):

> This theoretical bent toward an "economic" and "democratic" view of ethics as equal distribution of goods is mirrored by a popular suspicion and cynicism about anything that seems to derive value from heroic excellence As a result of the influence of the social sciences, altruistic acts are no longer likely to be taken at face value, and may be thought to be irrational in one way or another once deeper motives are explored . . . To many of us, then, courage as a virtue may seem but a tattered remnant of outdated ideals of chivalry—a macho-military quality that has outgrown its usefulness in civilized society (p. 18).

Courage, then, is on the same footing with another ontological concept, free-will, in the sense that in some branches of the helping professions we may act as though it doesn't exist or doesn't matter, then we go ahead and use it in counseling with clients in the sense that we try to encourage them to choose to make changes in their lives. We generally do this through refocusing a client's verbalizations in counseling towards a general responsibility-taking stance (for example, we use the phrase "client ownership" of feelings, goals, plans, behaviors, etc. that we all learn in counseling theories classes). We are on the side of their self-affirmation, or, choosing life rather than death, and as such, we actively engage ourselves in the battle for the client's *being.* In fact, paternalistic intervention and limit setting *against a person's will* has been justified by some (e.g., Bratter, 1985) with the argument that counselors are on the side of life-affirmation and are set against self-destruction. Indeed, if we as therapists are on the side of self-affirmation, then we cannot deny the role of courage lest we demean the struggles of clients and misunderstand their task.

Because those who have either an addiction or are convinced that they are failures because of a disability (Glasser, 1965) at least have *some-thing,* though that some-thing is destructive. The client has clung to that some-thing and has invested it with immense personal meaning (which is why many recovering alcoholics experience a profound question, "who am I?" when they abstain from alcohol). To let go of an addiction, a dependency, or a failure identity, though negative, means risking replacing it with nothing, except that which the client may identify as an alternate good, something worth risking and living for. If we do not admit the role of courage in this the client is indeed alone in their task.

Just before his death from cancer in 1991, Dr. Paul Lustig of the University of Wisconsin's Rehabilitation Counseling Psychology department discussed courage with the author in the context of the idea of putting together the present paper. His comments (Lustig, January 15, 1991) are reflected in the following several paragraphs that spell out his ideas regarding the conditions of courage, and its relationship to faith and support.

Lustig's Conceptualization of Courage

As was postulated in the introduction, one of the key elements of courage is that it involves doing something of positive value, despite full awareness of its possible negative consequences. The degree of courage is directly related to the degree and possibility of negative consequences of which one is fully aware. Thus, courage has a relationship to informed consent, in the knowing of the potential dire consequences and agreeing to proceed. Proceeding may entail risking the abyss of abandoning a known though uncomfortable life-style and replacing it with the new, which is the stuff of which ambivalence is made. With respect to ambivalence, it is a full recognition that not proceeding is less dangerous than proceeding.

Awareness of consequences can be based on factual knowledge or on belief. For example, if one believes that dangerous gremlins are inhabiting a cemetery and one proceeds to enter the cemetery, one is acting courageously, if the purpose of the act is for the good.

When a negative consequence is desirable, there is no courage. When one is not fully aware of the possible consequences, there is no courage. In ambivalence, the choices have inherent danger. An extreme example of facing dire consequences without courage occurs in the following example:

> A donkey is dying from thirst and dying from hunger. It is half way between hay and water. It believes that if it goes to the water, it will die of hunger and if it goes to the hay, it will die of thirst. Either choice is dire and it knows or believes in the consequences of a choice. If the donkey makes a choice, it is not expressing bravery, since both will result in death.

Nevertheless, courage is required in most cases of responding to ambivalence. Usually there is a mixture of positive and negative consequences for any choice made. A person can be helped to make a choice if that person is helped to understand the negative consequences of each choice. Then, the person is able to select the lesser of the negatives. The focus on the negative is necessary because the negative immobilized the person.

Medals given for military courage are really given for acts that go beyond the normal. Being a lone machine gunner, firing at an enemy, may not be courageous unless the person is aware that the process of firing makes him known to the enemy and he will thereby increase his chances of being killed. Thus, Rachman (1990) distinguishes between "fearlessness" and "courage" in that the latter implies action in the face of fear. The Congressional Medal of Honor is not given for courage, because no one asks the person what he/she felt. In fact, some people may be awarded a medal without their awareness of the potential consequences.

However, the awareness of consequences in courage is quite different from acting on *faith,* and no understanding of courage would be complete without an understanding of what constitutes faith.

An act of courage is the opposite of an act of faith, although faith is an important ingredient of hope. An act of courage is independent behavior, while an act of faith is dependent behavior. When there is an act of courage, the individual is fully aware of the possible negative consequences. Despite this recognition, the person acts. When there is an act based on faith, the individual believes that some external force will make the outcome good, or protect the person from harm, or will reward the person for doing the act. Martyrdom, which is usually based on faith, often assumes that in the end one will be rewarded. Sacrificing one's life to protect another or an ideal becomes an act based on faith if one believes that in the end he or she will be rewarded for the good deed. When there are nine people in a row boat that can carry only eight people and one person decides to sacrifice his or her life by jumping into shark-infested water, it is because the logic of the situation tells him or her what needs to be done, and it is an act of courage. If that same person believes that he or she will be protected from the sharks and rewarded in after-life, then it is an act of faith. When a person goes along with someone whom he/she trusts, it is an act of faith because the person believes that the trusted person will be a protector. It is dependent behavior because the person has placed the power to decide into the hands of the trusted person. The person acquiesces to this superior being. The person who acts on such faithful expectation is submerging oneself to an external power. Submerging oneself is not courageous. It may be valid, admirable, or desirable, but it is not courageous.

Many persons who abuse substances or who succumb to disabling illness or injury and who therefore indulge in self-destructive behavior, see the future as having only devastation and calamity. They have to avoid thinking about the future. It is like the belief, before Columbus' time, that if one sailed too far one would fall off a precipice and land in Hell. If the person's feelings are that only negatives will happen, the only choice available is to do nothing or erase from the mind the entire idea of a future. The ultimate way of doing this is to eradicate the mind and the self via suicide. Instead of looking for courage, it may be best to lead the person toward positive consequences, i.e., show the person that the fears of direness are not self-evident. This is one of the ways we treat phobias. If the person has a fear of heights one can try to reduce the fear by gradually having the person stand on higher and higher platforms. It is probably a very slow process, because the person needs to repeat prior successes before going on to a slightly higher level.

Rather than building on success, courage is related to punishment. Since the consequences to an act of courage are the potential for hurt, punishment is also a consequential act that involves hurt. Thus courage can have nonpersonal consequences as well as personal ones. When the negative consequence is punishment, it usually refers to the administration of the hurt by another person.

Courage relates to at least three different areas of behavior. It can be physical or motoric, emotional, and/or intellectual. In physical or motoric courage, the potential dire consequences are physical. The person might be physically hurt. In emotional courage, the consequences may be via other people or through self. The possible negative consequences are that others may disfavor the person, or it may result in an attack upon one's own integrity. The major concern is in the social area. Bill Wilson, the famed co-founder of Alcoholics Anonymous, exhibited a lack of this type of courage when he used alcohol to reduce his fear of high-status persons with whom he had to deal in his career formation (Thomasen, 1975).

The third type of courage is intellectual. This probably touches on the emotional in that ideas that are scornfully rejected, are also social pains. Thus, a deficit in intellectual courage can explain aspects of denial, which is the refusal to consider perspectives of one's self that have the potential of inflicting emotional and social pain.

Courage Defined in the Existential Literature

Perhaps the greatest theorists on courage have been Tillich (1952) and his protege, May (1967, 1969, 1975, & 1988). Tillich was a theologian-philosopher who dealt with courage on the philosophical level of existence and meaning, whereas May attempted to apply the construct of courage to psychological phenomena. Tillich and May viewed the human as having within him or her a directionality that exists from birth. As May (1988) stated in *Paulus: Tillich as Spiritual Teacher:* ". . . The Greek concept of entelechy has always impressed me: that the ultimate form is contained in the seed, and the tree or animal or human being grows toward this form, malformed though he may be in the process (p. 23)." This directionality is called by both men *intentionality,* or, as Tillich (1952) put it, "being related to meaningful contents of knowledge or will (p. 27)." Thus, intentionality is in contrast to meaninglessness, and May (1975) described the former as having the following elements: (a) conception, or to have in mind an intention or purpose; (b) a sense of self-confidence or self-efficacy; and (c) commitment, and the vitality to carry out that commitment. Thus, May's three elements in intentionality may be described as I conceive, I can, and I will. This motivational process, propelled forward with courage in difficult circumstances, results in the formation of identity—I am—in which the person perceives meaning in behavior. It is this last element that is inextricably bound up with courage, and the movement towards a purpose or intention is the measure of the person's courage.

Meaninglessness, or anomie as some have called it, results in a breakdown in intentionality, produced either through profound alienation from self and culture (through guilt, anger, or shame), or from fear of death. In this way, meaninglessness is related to despair, which Kierkegaard regarded as the wish to die but the knowledge that one is unable to do so. Kierkegaard (1954) calls despair "sickness unto death" and elaborates that when one becomes acquainted with an even more dreadful danger (than death), one hopes for death . . . (and) despair is the disconsolateness of not being able to die (p. 151). It is also related to anxiety, which is fear without an object. Anxiety is both neurotic and normal. Normal anxiety comes about as a result of fear of meaningless, fear of guilt, fear of condemnation, and fear of death. Tillich stated that "anxiety strives to become fear, because fear can be met by courage (p. 39)." Courage is self-affirmation in spite of the threat of nonbeing, or meaninglessness. Neurotic anxiety for Tillich (as well as for other existentialists such as May and Frank) is a surrendering of a part of the person's potentialities in order to save what is left, in other words, repression. Neurotic anxiety equals the inability to take existential anxiety upon oneself. Tillich stated that: "Pathological anxiety, in spite of its creative potentialities, is illness and danger and must be healed by being taken into a courage to be which is extensive as well as intensive" (p. 69).

May (1969) viewed neurotic anxiety as a lack of trust which is related to lack of courage and to lack of confidence, resulting in an inability to affirm life. He stated that the inability to affirm is merely another term for inability to trust. Not being able to trust, the neurotic lacks confidence and the related quality, courage. He must therefore endeavor to remain dependent in some situation of false security. Fear, also, has been related to self-confidence. Cox, Hallam, O'Connor, and Rachman (1983) confirmed a positive relationship between self-efficacy beliefs and low fear in a sample of parachute-jumper trainees.

Tillich's courage to be, to face one's destiny with freedom, takes the following forms: (a) the courage to be as part (or, the courage to be in community with others without loss of self); (b) the courage to be as oneself (or, the courage to be an individual, without living in isolation from others); and (c) the courage to accept acceptance (or, the courage to relinquish or make amends for guilt and shame). Thus, Tillich addressed the balancing act that is constantly being played by all of us in Western civilization, between the imperatives that we must endeavor to be ourselves without isolation (individuation) while at the same time living in community without giving up ourselves in mindless conformity. The courage to accept acceptance relates to May's concept of the ability to trust (Tillich, 1952).

ENCOURAGEMENT

It follows from the above discussion that our objectives in encouraging are to help individuals identify consequences of their decisions, define purpose, spur vitality, overcome free-floating anxiety, and try new ways of living, rather than those that would otherwise maintain dependency. That this is difficult is obvious, since the person is being asked to do something that goes against what that person has been doing and has found to be acceptable. Staying in one uncomfortable position or role is often far more comfortable than acting to get out of the rut into an unknown. The person may feel more comfortable with the known harshness than with the unknown. The unknown may appear to be more dangerous and devastating than the known. A person who is abused in a family situation may hang on to it, because the family and the behavior of its members may appear to be more desirable than moving away from family and its punishing members. The unknown has the potential for total annihilation.

When the situation is dire and extreme, one needs to recognize with the person, the potentially dangerous and negative consequences of acting. At the same time, one needs to point out that failure to act prolongs the current painful situation. The option to act involves courage to do something despite its potentially negative consequences. Here one needs to evaluate the degree of courage. Placing the decision on courage, when there is very little or none, can only result in depression, rejection of a desire to change, and even suicide. When asking a person to use courage, one must determine whether the person has even a tiny iota of courage. It may be extremely devastating to conclude that one does not have any courage. However, it is often difficult to determine beforehand whether there is any courage. In many cases it can only be determined by asking the person to express a courageous act, like doing something that the person is fearful to do, with full awareness of the possible negative consequences. If it is now determined that the person has too little courage to act, then whoever is in the helping position, needs to support or carry the person through the frightening act, in order to show the person that he/she has the potential for mastery. The counselor who is aware of the conditions of courage does not challenge or "confront" the person to act in new ways when the client has not yet been given the chance to demonstrate courage.

Therefore, one of the goals of treatment ought to be the assessment of courage and the conditions that underlie it. For example, a client who abuses substances because of the stresses of a demanding, unrelenting job is asked to take himself or herself to a career counselor to begin discussion of a job change. However, the prospect of changing jobs is too frightening to the client who suffers from low self-confidence and a lack of courage to make the overtures. A counselor in this situation could do several things. First, the counselor could support the client in his fear, and accept him for the ambivalence and difficulty that he is experiencing (Rogers, 1951).

Second, she/he could focus counseling efforts on low self-confidence ("I cannot") and low commitment ("will not"). Several forms of treatment could work in this regard. Reality therapy (Glasser, 1965) prescribes achievement in small steps towards a goal as a way of teaching a person independence through the formation and carrying-out of one's own goals. Behavioral management and social learning strategies do essentially the same thing, along with specific reinforcement, modeling, and vicarious learning techniques (Bandura, 1977). Attribution and expectancy approaches can be used by the counselor to model the counselor's belief that the client <u>can</u> do it, thus making it easier for the client to accept this belief (Bandura & Schunk, 1981). In addition, counselors can arrange for clients to meet other clients in similar situations who have successfully managed a desired change (if he/she can do it, so can I!).

Third, the counselor could work on reducing the fear of spiritual nothingness and finding the purpose that gives the person's life meaning. Existential counseling (May, 1967) is designed to accomplish exactly that end. This counseling approach has both confronting (e.g., breaking down nihilistic and melancholic tendencies) and encouraging components (e.g., elucidating the consequences of viewing destiny not with morbid resignation, but as an opportunity to test one's freedom). Dynamic, existentially oriented counseling approaches in general strive in their evaluative stage to uncover neurotic constrictions of experiencing (e.g, fear, anxiety, and guilt), to confront them, and to reduce their potential for blocking directionality and commitment. Behavioral medicine approaches have much to offer in the areas of relaxation training to teach the person a response incompatible with that of fear, as well as several cognitive approaches to dealing with asserting one's rights and reframing mental self-talk in the face of fear-inducing stressors (Turk, Meichenbaum, & Genest, 1983).

Fourth, the counselor could provide the client with an opportunity to join an appropriate group, which may establish a source of encouragement (i.e., Tillich's courage to be as part). Although there is the potential for the client's transferring his or her dependency to a group and the risk of further losing his or her self, the group experience may also provide models of behavior and success with which he or she can identify and emulate.

Finally, and most importantly, the counselor must see herself or himself as the *alter ego* of the client in the matter of courage. The counselor may help clarify matters, exhort the client to action, and lend the client strength, confidence, and expectation (I conceive, I can, I will, I am) at the crucial moment when the client is at a state of readiness to do something involving fear of anxiety. Rollo May (1967) stated: ". . . the counselor must give people courage to live . . ." (p. 193). She or he provides the vital empathetic link, that has been called "the encounter, involvement, and merger", upon which the client may rely while the client faces their difficulty or fear and takes the necessary first step forward.

CONCLUSION

This paper has attempted to define courage, its conditions, its blocks, and some of its facilitators, including some ways in which counselors might approach creating situations in which it may emerge. It also distinguished between confrontation and encouragement, which the author sees as complimentary processes—one breaking down of defenses and the other facilitating the emergence of intentionality.

This paper has also tried to distinguish between support and encouragement so that, in those cases in which persons are so devastated by experience that they no longer have any courage, active support can be applied until they have gained strength.

Courage is a concept that is elusive, metaphysical, and somewhat vague. However, if clients are to become "empowered", meaning that they are able to rely on a positively functioning motivational system, then the process of encouragement must be understood. Empowerment (or "self-empowerment" as it is sometimes called) is an objective in counseling, not a process. Thus, empowerment as process implies a stronger person directing a weaker client. Empowerment as objective where encouragement is the fuel for the process implies creatively erecting conditions in counseling in which empowerment is the result. Empowerment is the result of "rehabilitating the will," in the midst of medical-model passivity. Counseling involves affirming life, which in its part involves creation, and creation implies satisfying the requirements of intentionality. Intentionality is driven by and is a measure of courage. Where courage is lacking due to either a deficit in the conceiving process—I conceive; or to a lack of self-confidence—I can; or to a lack of commitment—I will; or to an immobilizing fear or anxiety, guilt, shame, or feeling of non-acceptance or trust; the counselor may give courage by addressing the particular lack and by being the client's partner in his or her struggle. The counselor may, indeed, encourage.

REFERENCES

Adler, A. (1955). *The practice and theory of individual psychology.* New York: Humanities Press.

Beck, R. & Lustig, P. (1990). Counseling the chronic pain patient. In Miller, T. (ed.) *Chronic Pain (Vol. 2).* Madison, CT: International Universities Press, Inc.

Bandura, A. (1977). Self-efficacy: Toward a unifying theory of behavior change. *Psychological Review, 84,* 191–215.

Bandura, A. & Schunk, D. (1981). Cultivating competence, self-efficacy, and intrinsic interest through proximal self-motivation. *Journal of Personality and Social Psychology, 41,* 586–598.

Bratter, T. (1985). Special psychotherapeutic concerns for alcoholic and drug-addicted individuals. In Bratter, T. & Forrest, G. (Eds) *Alcoholism and substance abuse: Strategies for clinical intervention* (pp. 523–574). New York: The Free Press.

Cox, D., Hallam, R., O'Connor, K. & Rachman, S. (1983). An experimental analysis of fear and courage. *British Journal of Psychology, 74,* 107–117.

Emener, W. (1991). An empowerment philosophy for rehabilitation in the 20th Century. *Journal of Rehabilitation, 57*(4), 7–12.

Glasser, W. (1965). *Reality therapy.* New York: Harper & Row.

Hahn, H. (1989). Theories and values: Ethics and contrasting perspectives on disability. In Duncan B. and Woods, D. (eds.) *Ethical issues in disability and rehabilitation: Report of a 1989 international conference.* New York: World Rehabilitation Fund.

Kierkegaard, S. (1954). *Fear and trembling: The sickness unto death.* Garden City, NY: Doubleday/Anchor Books.

Lustig, P. (1991). Letter to Richard Beck dated January 15, 1991.

May, R. (1967). *The art of counseling.* New York: Abingdon Press.

May, R. (1969). *Love and will.* New York: W.W. Norton & Co., inc.

May, R. (1975). *The courage to create.* New York: Bantam Books, Inc.

May, R. (1988). *Paulus: A personal portrait of Paul Tillich.* Dallas: Saybrook Publishing Co.

Rachman, S. (1990). *Fear and courage, 2nd Edition.* New York: W.H. Freeman and Company.

Rogers, C. (1951). *Client-centered therapy.* Boston: Houghton Mifflin.

Simon, D. (1986). Alienation and alcohol abuse. The untested dimensions. *The Journal of Drug Issues, 16*(3), 339–356.

Thomsen, R. (1975). *Bill W.* New York: Harper & Row.

Tillich, P. (1952). *The courage to be.* Binghamton, NY: Vail-Ballou Press, Inc.

Turk, D., Meichenbaum, D., & Genest, M. (1983) *Pain and behavioral medicine.* New York: The Guilford Press.

Vash, C. (1991). More thoughts on empowerment. *Journal of Rehabilitation, 57*(4), 13–16.

Walton, D. (1986). *Courage, a philosophical investigation.* Berkeley, CA: University of California Press, Ltd.

Wright, B. (1983). *Physical disability: A psychosocial approach (2nd ed.)* New York: Harper & Row.

Yalom, I. (1980). *Existential psychotherapy.* New York: Basic Books.

24

The Family Experience of Mental Illness: Implications for Intervention

Diane T. Marsh and Dale L. Johnson

T he serious mental illness of a close relative is a catastrophic event for families. In the words of one family member: "This terrible illness colors everything—a family cannot escape." Because mental illness is often severe and persistent, psychologists are likely to have many opportunities to meet the needs of family members themselves and to assist them in supporting their relative's treatment, rehabilitation, and recovery. In fact, with their broad biopsychosocial perspective and wide range of expertise, psychologists are uniquely suited for meeting the needs of this highly stressed population.

In this article, we assist practitioners to build on their existing competencies, to acquire new knowledge and skills, and to develop more effective intervention strategies. We begin with a discussion of the family experience of mental illness, sharing vignettes from our research with family members (vignettes without citations are from Marsh & Dickens, 1997). We then present a number of family interventions that can be modified to meet the needs of individual families and can be offered in a variety of settings.

THE FAMILY EXPERIENCE OF MENTAL ILLNESS

Mental illness has a profound effect on all members of the family, as the following woman asserts:

> All family members are affected by a loved one's mental illness. The entire family system needs to be addressed. To assure us that we are not to blame and the situation is not hopeless. To point us to people and places that can help our loved one. The impact still lingers on.

From *Professional Psychology: Research and Practice, 28*(3) (1997), 229–237. Reprinted with permission.

Indeed, the current system of care is as much family-based as community-based, and families generally serve as the first and last resort for their relatives, often with little professional guidance. In the present era, families fulfill crucial roles as primary caregivers for relatives who reside at home, as informal case managers who advocate for their relatives with service providers, and as crisis intervention specialists who handle relapses and emergencies. Whether the relative who has a serious mental illness lives at home or in another community setting, most families remain involved.

Researchers have consistently documented the devastating impact of mental illness on other members of the family. The family experience of mental illness has frequently been defined in terms of family burden, which consists of subjective and objective aspects (see Lefley, 1996). Subjective burden is the personal suffering experienced by family members in response to their relative's illness; objective burden refers to the daily problems and challenges associated with the illness.

Family burden increases the risk that other important dimensions of the family experience may be ignored, including the family's potential for a resilient response to this devastating event. Resilience is the ability to rebound from adversity and prevail over the circumstances of one's life. As with any catastrophic event, mental illness may serve as a catalyst for family members to change in constructive ways, as a sibling affirms: "When a family experiences something like this, it makes for very compassionate people—people of substance. My brother has created a bond among us all that we will not allow to be broken."

Professionals are now developing a more balanced view of the family experience of mental illness, one that incorporates family resilience as well as family burden. Following our discussion of family burden, we share results of recent research concerned with family resilience.

Subjective Burden

In response to their relative's mental illness, most family members experience a powerful grieving process as well as numerous intense emotions, including shock, disbelief, anger, despair, guilt, anxiety, and shame. This mother conveys the anguish that family members may undergo in response to the mental illness of a close relative:

> The problems with my daughter were like a black hole inside of me into which everything else had been drawn. My grief and pain were so intense sometimes that I barely got through the day. It felt like a mourning process, as if I were dealing with the loss of the daughter I had loved for 18 years, for whom there was so much potential. (Marsh, 1992, p. 10).

In this article, we discuss several components of the subjective burden: grief, symbolic loss, chronic sorrow, the emotional roller coaster, and empathic pain.

Grief

At the core of the family experience of mental illness is a grieving process. Family members may mourn for the relative they have known and loved before the onset of the illness, for the anguish of their family, and for their own losses. Reflecting this grieving process, an adult offspring wrote about "my loss of a healthy mother, a normal childhood, and a stable home."

Symbolic Loss

In addition to their grieving process, family members experience many symbolic losses that pertain to hopes, dreams, and expectations and to individual and family myths and identity. A father spoke of the symbolic losses that accompanied his son's mental illness: "You felt there was no limit to the possibility of his success. The possibility of him being President of the United States. And that dream is shattered" (Marsh, 1992, p. 94).

Chronic Sorrow

Although many family members experience a grieving process in response to their relative's mental illness, rarely do they move through a series of stages that culminate in a final state of peaceful acceptance. They are far more likely to experience continuing feelings of grief and loss that wax and wane in response to the course of their relative's illness or to events in their own lives. These intense emotions are woven into the familial fabric on a continuing basis, with the potential for periodic emotional firestorms. One family member talked about her experience of chronic sorrow: "It's like someone close died, but there's no closure. It's never over."

Emotional Roller Coaster

Family members sometimes feel as if they are riding an emotional roller coaster, their ride punctuated by the alternating periods of relapse and remission that often characterize the course of mental illness. These cycles create considerable turmoil for family members, who often experience intense distress when renewed hope is shattered by yet another relapse, as the following mother conveyed: "When things are going well, you begin to hope and dream again about a better future. And when things fall apart, it is like a small death. You are more vulnerable for having dared to hope again" (Marsh, 1992, p. 74).

Empathic Pain

With time, most family members largely resolve their emotional burden. However, they often continue to experience empathic pain for the losses experienced by their relative, their family, and themselves. Empathic pain may remain insistent over time, as family members share in their relative's anguish over an impoverished life and in his or her struggle against the forces of psychosis. Speaking for legions of parents, one mother told of her devastation at seeing her daughter "so crushed and destroyed and broken" (Marsh, 1992, p. 79).

Objective Burden

In addition to this powerful subjective burden, family members are confronted with the reality demands that comprise the objective burden. Here is one man's account of the objective burden that accompanied his father's mental illness during his own childhood and adolescence:

> My father's paranoid schizophrenia meant we moved frequently, because he felt the conspiracy was closing in on him. He battered my mother, because he felt she was part of the conspiracy. I was too frightened to go to her aid. I couldn't have friendships with peers because my father felt they might "poison" my mind against him.

Components of the objective burden include the symptoms of mental illness, caregiving responsibilities, family disruption and stress, limitations of the service delivery system, and social stigma.

Symptomatic Behavior

Family members often experience significant distress in response to their affected relative's symptoms of mental illness. These symptoms may include (a) positive symptoms (the *presence* of certain unusual experiences, thoughts, and feelings), such as hallucinations, delusions, disorganized thought and speech, and bizarre behavior; (b) negative symptoms (an *absence* or decline of certain normal functions), such as apathy, inability to follow through on tasks, inability to experience pleasure and to enjoy relationships, and impoverished thought and speech; (c) disturbances of mood, including severely depressed mood, unusually elevated mood, or extreme mood swings; (d) potentially harmful or self-destructive behavior; (e) socially inappropriate or disruptive behavior; and (f) poor daily living habits.

Undoubtedly, people with mental illness are the greatest victims of these symptoms, which can adversely affect all aspects of their lives. However, family members are also victimized by the symptoms of the illness, either directly, when they are the target of symptomatic behavior, or indirectly, when they are helpless observers of their relative's aberrant behavior. In addition, the specter of harm is very real for these families because their relative faces a death rate from suicide and other causes of death that is significantly higher than the rate for the general population (see Torrey, 1995). Reflecting this risk, one family member portrayed his "overwhelming sense of loss and tragedy" following the death of three relatives with mental illness, including a brother who committed suicide.

Caregiving

As Lefley (1996) discussed, family members must assume roles for which they are unprepared and untrained. They must gradually learn (a) to cope with the challenges of daily life with someone who has mental illness; (b) to obtain services from the mental health, welfare, and medical systems; and perhaps (c) to negotiate with the legal and criminal justice systems.

Practitioners are most likely to have contact with parents who serve as primary caregivers for their adult children with mental illness. The lives of these parents are often profoundly affected, as the following mother indicated: "My daughter's mental illness . . . pushed us back into parenting of the most demanding kind, probably for the rest of our lives" (Marsh, 1992, p. 64). Spouses, siblings, and offspring may also assume caregiving responsibilities for their relative. An adult offspring described the impact of her mother's mental illness on her own life: "When I was 18, I became my mother's caretaker. My mother lived with me until she died. I married, had children, and took care of Mother throughout my whole life."

Family Disruption and Stress

Most families do survive the catastrophic event of mental illness. None does so without experiencing family disruption and stress, as one family member indicated: "Mental illness is a ravaging, devastating disease that disrupts a family." Specific problems may include household disarray, financial difficulties, employment problems, strained marital and family relationships, impaired physical and mental health, and diminished social life. Most families experience some of these problems, at least occasionally. Others experience many of them on a long-term basis, with little opportunity for respite. Under these circumstances, exhaustion and burnout are almost inevitable.

The Service Delivery System

People with mental illness often require a wide spectrum of mental health, physical health, social, rehabilitative, vocational, and residential services. Unfortunately, these services are not always available, and they are not always satisfactory when they are available. Researchers have documented many problems with the service delivery system, including the absence of treatment for large numbers of people with serious mental illness, the relative neglect of people with the most severe and persistent problems, inadequate funding for the full range of community-based services, and fragmentation of existing services (see Torrey, 1995). These problems may increase in our current era of managed care, which sometimes emphasizes the cost of services at the expense of their quality.

The consequences of these shortcomings are considerable for people with mental illness, whose lives may be marked by poverty, isolation, and abuse.

There are as many people with mental illness residing in our jails and prisons as in all of our hospitals, and at least one third of the homeless are estimated to have a mental illness. Families pay the price for the absence of treatment in the criminal justice system and for the people with mental illness who have joined the ranks of the homeless. Indeed, the specter of homelessness haunts many family members, as this sibling conveyed: "I see my brother in every disheveled and disoriented homeless person."

Another problem is the absence of services for family members, who often find the system insensitive to their anguish and unresponsive to their needs. In numerous studies, family members have reported unsatisfactory handling of crises and emergencies, insufficient communication and availability on the part of professionals, an absence of programs and services for families, and minimal involvement of families in treatment planning. In addition, many family members have been adversely affected by earlier and unsupported theories that held families accountable for the mental illness (see Marsh, 1992). Thus, during a period of intense distress, family members may find that the system not only fails to address their expressed needs but also intensifies their anguish. In the words of one family member, "Caring families get socked with most of the responsibility and blame but little legal or therapeutic support. We must change the system."

Stigma

The most debilitating handicap surrounding mental illness is stigma. Stigmatization in the larger society results in the marginalization and ostracism of people with mental illness; discrimination in insurance, housing, and employment; an adverse effect on all aspects of their functioning; and decreased likelihood that they will receive effective treatment. Accordingly, we practitioners need to counter the negative attitudes and expectations that are often internalized by patients and to foster feelings of hopefulness rather than helplessness.

In recent years, there have been many encouraging developments, including the enactment in 1990 of the Americans with Disabilities Act. Nevertheless, stigmatization remains a pervasive problem for people with serious mental illness, for their families, and even for the professionals who work with this population. The adverse effects of stigma for family members may include lowered self-esteem and damaged family relationships, risk of self-stigmatization, and feelings of isolation and shame (see Lefley, 1996). Reflecting the risks of self-stigmatization and isolation, one family member remarked that the stigma had "translated into an internalized feeling that something is wrong with me"; another family member wrote of feeling like a "perpetual outsider."

Family Resilience

In the past, researchers focused almost exclusively on family burden, which is the most salient aspect of the family experience of serious mental illness. As with any catastrophic event, however, the illness offers families an opportunity to change in constructive ways, an important consideration for practitioners.

In recent research, for example, we found evidence for family resilience (Marsh et al., 1996). When asked specifically about any family strengths that had developed as a result of the mental illness, survey participants told us about their family bonds and commitments, their expanded knowledge and skills, their advocacy activities, and their role in their relative's recovery. Our participants also affirmed their potential for personal resilience, noting that they had become better, stronger, and more compassionate people. They cited their contributions to their family, their enhanced coping effectiveness, and their healthier perspectives and priorities. Here are the words of one family member:

> I have become much more tolerant of imperfection in myself and others . . . I have learned to appreciate the strengths of other people who appear to be different or are handicapped in some way. Our daughter's younger siblings accept her and make special efforts to help her feel a part of the family. I can face adversity with courage. My husband and I are closer and more honest with each other as a result of our shared grief and stress . . . We are proud that our family has remained intact and strong. (Marsh et al., 1996, p. 10)

In addition, family members commented on the resilience of their relative with mental illness. Describing her adult son, a mother commented, "It is gratifying to witness our son's courage as he deals with his illness" (Marsh et al., 1996, p. 9).

It is essential to consider these research findings in light of the compelling evidence for family burden. In fact, in responding to open-ended questions designed to elicit positive responses, almost two-fifths of participants offered negative comments, such as the following: "I was and am devastated by her illness and discouraged by the system" (Marsh et al., 1996, p. 7). Even when respondents answered in a more positive manner, their answers were often infused with a sense of anguish and grief: "I thought that my son's tragedy would completely ruin our lives because it broke our hearts. But we've learned—finally, painfully—not to let this tragedy totally dominate our lives" (Marsh et al., 1996, p. 7). These family members never lost sight of the terrible price paid for any family and personal strengths that had developed. As one family member noted in a separate study of adult siblings and offspring (Marsh & Dickens, 1997), "Any increased sensitivity to others or any other 'side effects' would be traded in an eyeblink for a healthy relative."

Nevertheless, the potential for resilience is also part of the family experience. When practitioners work with families, one goal of intervention is to maximize the family's potential for resilience and to assist them in coping effectively with the mental illness. In fact, three fourths of our participants reported they had undergone a process of adaptation as they acquired the competencies and skills needed to cope with the mental illness. In addition to understanding family burden and resilience, practitioners need to understand the unique experiences and concerns of parents, spouses, siblings, and offspring so that they can address the needs of individual family members.

FAMILY ROLES

The impact of mental illness on family members depends partly on its timing in their life span and on their roles and responsibilities within the family. As a result, individual members of the family have special experiences, needs, and concerns in their role as parent, spouse, sibling, or offspring (see Wasow, 1995). Thus in addition to addressing the needs of the family as a unit, psychologists can offer services to individual family members. We briefly mention each of these family roles.

When a child develops a mental illness, his or her parents generally experience a range of intense losses, both real and symbolic. Moreover, it is parents who are most likely to assume responsibilities as primary caregivers or informal case managers, sometimes for a lifetime. They are also prone to feelings of guilt and responsibility, which may be intensified by professionals who espouse earlier conceptual models that incorporate unsupported assumptions of family pathogenesis or dysfunction. At the time of his son's initial hospitalization, this father felt as if professionals were holding him and his wife responsible for the mental illness: "They seemed to be trying to find out how we caused it. It was just devastating" (Marsh, 1992, p. 14).

Spouses often experience emotional, social, and financial losses similar to those that accompany the death of a spouse. Husbands and wives may face increased responsibility for parenting and other aspects of family life as well as substantial conflict if they consider separation or divorce. One spouse who decided to seek a divorce in response to her husband's mental illness talked about his angry accusation: "I was the one who was at fault with this divorce because we married for better, for worse, in sickness and health.' He says I'm the one that didn't live up to our marriage vows" (Marsh, 1992, p. 133).

Because of their developmental status, young siblings and offspring share a special vulnerability to the mental illness in their families (see Marsh & Dickens, 1997). It would be expected, for instance, that the mental illness of a close relative might undermine the acquisition of basic trust during infancy, the development of peer relationships and academic skills during childhood, and the establishment of a secure sense of identity during adolescence. A child who is confronted from birth with the mental illness of a parent or older sibling may be vulnerable to all of these risks. Some of these concerns were described by the following adult offspring:

> Very much of my young life was affected. I had trouble concentrating in school, was afraid Dad would appear at the school grounds when he was sick. I could not bring any school friends home for fear that they would not understand. Mom was busy working full time to make ends meet. Not much time was spent helping me get prepared for school.

Siblings may experience the dual losses of their brother or sister and of their parents, whose energy may be consumed by the mental illness. One sibling told us: "I lost out in my childhood." In the wake of the turmoil in their family, they may feel their needs are neglected or may try to compensate their anguished parents (the replacement child syndrome). Siblings may lose sight of their own needs, as the following sibling affirmed: "For many years I looked for reasons for my brother's problems, never realizing I had to find myself first." Almost inevitably, these siblings feel alienated from the world of their peers.

Offspring also have unique issues and concerns. Because of the significance of the parent–child bond, the losses of these family members may be profound. Especially if the offspring are exposed to mental illness when they are very young, they may become enveloped in the psychotic system, with an adverse impact on their own lives: "My mother has been sick practically my whole life. It is hard for me to decipher which of my experiences are 'normal' and which are not." Moreover, they may move into a parentified role before the have finished being children or may attempt to become perfect children to spare their beleaguered family additional problems, as this adult offspring attested: "As a child I tried desperately never to have a problem because our family had so many. So I became perfectionistic and his my fears, concerns, and needs from everyone."

FAMILY AND PERSONAL VARIABLES

Like families in general, families of people with mental illness are characterized by diversity and vary along a continuum of competence. Some of these families demonstrate mastery in fulfilling all of their functions, whereas others experience difficulty in solving even minor problems. Most families fall someplace in the middle of the continuum. Thus practitioners need to avoid making general assumptions about families and need to evaluate each family on its own terms.

Many personal and family variables influence the impact of mental illness. For example, the family environment is affected by other stressful events confronting the family, such as unemployment or serious medical problems, as well as the overall quality of family life and relationships. Likewise, the impact of a relative's mental illness on individual family members is mediated by those family members' ages, genders, and roles in the family; by their personal strengths, limitations, and resources; and by their living arrangements, which are likely to determine their level of involvement in their relative's life.

The meaning of mental illness is also important for the family, who may view the illness as a challenge or an overwhelming burden. In a similar manner, they may view themselves as helpless victims or active agents. Practitioners can enhance the family's sense of hopefulness and mastery by sharing current research regarding mental illness and its prognosis and by assisting them in supporting their relative's recovery.

Thus, psychologists need to view the mental illness within the context of the larger family life space. The illness is simply one experience shared by family members, whose lives are part of an intricate family tapestry woven of common bonds, memories, celebrations, and losses. Reflecting this sense of a larger family life space, one sibling remarked that her brother's mental illness had only been a part of her family life, adding: "My parents were there for me too, and I felt loved and valued."

MEETING FAMILY NEEDS

Families who are coping with a relative's mental illness have a number of essential needs, including the need for a truly comprehensive and humane system of care that can support their relative in living a meaningful and productive life in the community. If such a system were available, it would transform the lives of these families. In the meantime, there are many ways in which psychologists can meet the needs of these highly stressed families. For example, when working with individual families, practitioners can assist families in the following:

1. Understanding and normalizing the family experience of mental illness;
2. Focusing on the strengths and competencies of their family and their relative;
3. Learning about mental illness, the mental health system, and community resources;
4. Developing skills in stress management, problem solving, and communication;
5. Resolving their feelings of grief and loss;
6. Coping with the symptoms of mental illness and its repercussions for their family;
7. Identifying and responding to the signs of impending relapse;
8. Creating a supportive family environment;
9. Developing realistic expectations for all members of the family;
10. Playing a meaningful role in their relative's treatment, rehabilitation, and recovery; and
11. Maintaining a balance that meets the needs of all members of the family.

A number of intervention strategies can facilitate the accomplishment of these objectives and address the concerns of particular families.

FAMILY INTERVENTIONS

The family interventions we describe reflect an historical shift in perspective from the family as a cause of mental illness to the family as a source of support. Acknowledging families' supportive role, practitioners can intervene to assist families in carrying out their caregiving functions, which will in turn enhance the recovery of the person with mental illness. In addition to their need for effective caregiving, families have needs of their own. For example, they need to resolve their emotional burden, preserve the integrity of their own lives, and fulfill their personal hopes and dreams. Family interventions that focus largely on the family's supportive functions may ignore other important needs. Thus, practitioners need familiarity with a variety of interventions that can be tailored to address the needs of specific families and family members.

We discuss several effective interventions, including family support and advocacy groups, family consultation, family education, family psychoeducation, and psychotherapy. Each of these interventions has particular strengths and calls for different skills and resources. Only family psychoeducation has been extensively evaluated, although families generally find the other interventions very helpful.

Family Support and Advocacy Groups

One of the most important things a psychologist can do when working with people who have serious mental illnesses and with their families is to refer them to the National Alliance for the Mentally Ill (NAMI) or one of its local affiliates. With over 1,000 local affiliates in all 50 states, no family is far from a NAMI affiliate. Families are burdened and distressed, at a loss for information, and greatly in need of supportive resources. NAMI was created by families to respond to these problems. Members tend to be relatives of people with serious mental illnesses, but large numbers of consumers also belong, and today NAMI is the largest single mental health consumer organization. Referral to other support and advocacy organizations may also be warranted, such as the National Depressive and Manic Depressive Association (*see Appendix* in this chapter).

Family support and advocacy groups serve three essential functions. First, they provide vital support to families through member-facilitated group sessions and informal networking. Second, they offer a variety of educational programs through local NAMI affiliates and at state and national NAMI conventions. In many communities, local NAMI chapters offer the Journey of Hope program, a comprehensive family education program presented by trained family members. Third, these groups encourage advocacy, as members join forces to work for expanded research and improved services throughout the country.

Psychologists should learn about these organizations and support them. Most groups need speakers for monthly meetings and welcome presentations by professionals. By participating in meetings, practitioners develop an intimate acquaintance with the group; equally important, group members become acquainted with the psychologist and feel comfortable calling on him or her when needed. Practitioners can also benefit from attending local meetings as well as state and national conventions. They will gain knowledge about serious mental illness and innovative treatments, about family experiences and needs, and about effective coping strategies. This knowledge is essential for clinicians who use any of the intervention strategies we describe.

Psychologists can assist families by encouraging them to join local NAMI groups, offering information about the groups, explaining the benefits of participation, and providing telephone contact numbers. In affirming the value of support groups, one family member wrote: "The group has been like a beacon, providing me with information, support, and understanding."

Family Consultation

A promising form of family intervention is the consultation model described by Bernheim (1989) and by Wynne and associates (1987). Family consultants offer expert knowledge and advice to family members, who are responsible for determining their own goals and deciding whether to accept professional recommendations. There are a broad range of problems a family consultant can deal with, such as helping the family to manage a psychotic family member at home or helping the family to make decisions about living arrangements.

Family consultants can also assist families in making an informed choice regarding their use of other available services. Families may decide (a) to decline services or defer their use of services, (b) to receive a single service offered in a provider setting or in the community, or (c) to pursue complementary services, such as an educational or psychoeducational program led by professionals and a family-facilitated support group in the community. Families can often benefit from consultation on an ongoing and as-needed basis, especially during crises or periods of inpatient treatment for their relative.

Although the efficacy of the consultation model has not been evaluated, it offers a flexible and collaborative approach to working directly with families and to assisting them in accessing other services. Practitioners should be clear about the distinction between consultation and therapy in working with families and should make sure the distinction is clear to family members.

Family Education

Families have a need for information about mental illness and its treatment, about caregiving and management issues, about the mental health system and community resources, and about family coping and adaptation. Practitioners can meet this need by offering a formal educational program to groups of families, either in a 1-day workshop or in a series of sessions. For example, Anderson, Reiss, and Hogarty (1986) designed a day-long Survival Skills Workshop that includes information on the nature of serious mental illness (prevalence, course, personal experience, and biological etiology), treatment (both pharmacological and psychosocial), the family and mental illness (needs of the patient and the family and family reactions to the illness), and family coping skills and strategies.

In an educational workshop for families, one of us (Dale L. Johnson) adapted this format to place more emphasis on NAMI and to include bipolar disorder and major depression along with schizophrenia. Other elements of the workshop include education about the neurobiological substrate of serious mental illness, information about the importance of stress and its management, and opportunities for families to ask questions and interact with each other. The medication portion is presented by a psychiatrist, who is invited for that purpose and is briefed with an outline of recommended topics and procedures. Family members and patients participate in separate sessions, which allows both groups to be open about their concerns. Professionals who have taken part in the program have commented that they enjoyed participating and gained increased understanding of families.

Numerous studies have shown the beneficial effects of family education (e.g, Solomon, Draine, Mannion, & Meisel, 1996). The benefits may include increased knowledge about serious mental illness, greater acceptance of the illness among families, enhanced family relationships, and improved coping ability. As one family member remarked, "Family education enabled us to be a help rather than a hindrance" (Marsh et al., 1996, p. 9). A psychologist who has worked with families individually and in groups shared the following vignette:

> The parents came into my office with frustrated, angry looks on their faces, escorting their decompensating son. "It's been hell living with him these past 20 years," his mother exclaimed, as if it were his fault. I acknowledged how horrible it is for the patient and the family to live with this brain disorder and educated them about schizophrenia. The mother looked stunned by the realization that it is an illness, not a volitional behavior. In later months, I learned that their family relationships had improved significantly and that their son was now included in family dinners and celebrations.

Family Psychoeducation

Family psychoeducation differs from family education in that family and patient are included together, and coping skills and stress management skills training are provided to the entire family over a longer period of time (Lam, 1991). Family education is also provided. Because family psychoeducation is complex and generally takes place over many months, this intervention is typically carried out by a group of professionals who work together as a team.

Research in England in the 1970s led to the discovery that certain family behaviors were related to increased relapse rates for people with schizophrenia. These behaviors (criticism, hostility, and overinvolvement) were termed *expressed emotion*. Family sessions were found to be successful in reducing relapse rates. Subsequent controlled studies with variations on the family psychoeducation model confirmed the earlier findings, and a substantial body of literature is now available regarding this form of intervention (see Dixon & Lehman, 1995).

The following conclusions about the effectiveness of family psychoeducation seem warranted: (a) The programs have been successful in reducing the rate of relapse beyond the effects of medication; (b) relapse rates are reduced by including coping skills training for families; (c) the addition of social skills training for patients further reduce the risk of relapse; (d) programs that decrease the expression of criticism and hostility between family members are more effective than those that do not; (e) specifically targeted, in vivo problem-solving training may be an essential component; and (f) two family psychoeducation projects based on psychodynamic principles and procedures were not effective.

The strength of the research model and its replication in diverse settings argue strongly for the availability of family psychoeducation for families who are coping with mental illness. If the goal of intervention is the reduction of relapse rates, researchers have demonstrated that family psychoeducation is without doubt the preferred mode. There is also some evidence that this approach alleviates family burden. In settings where professionals offer services as a team, as in community mental health centers or many hospitals, these programs should certainly be made available to interested families.

Psychotherapy

The family interventions we have discussed thus far are largely educational and supportive. These are the initial interventions of choice for family members, whose central needs are for information, skills, and support. If these interventions are not sufficient, other services may also be appropriate, including individual, marital, or family therapy. For example, individual therapy may be beneficial for family members who desire the privacy and intimacy of a dyadic relationship, are having difficulty resolving their emotional burden, are experiencing intrapsychic conflict, or are dealing with issues of separation and autonomy. Some siblings and offspring appear to be good candidates for individual therapy (*see* Marsh & Dickens, 1997). One adult offspring told us she learned in therapy to feel like "a healthy human for the first time." Long after her initial encounter with parental mental illness, another family member found personal therapy beneficial: "It wasn't until I sought therapy for anxiety upon my divorce that I began to understand some of the dynamics of my family and myself. Therapy opened doors to my self and answered many puzzling questions."

Family or marital therapy may be helpful when there are preexisting problems in communication or conflict management. Traditional family therapy may also be appropriate when the family is unable to cope adequately with the mental illness of their relative or when successful treatment of an individual requires the involvement of other family members. Both family and marital therapy carry potential risks, including loss of privacy and increased family disruption (in family therapy) and deflection from personal problems and concerns (in marital therapy). Additional risks are associated with general prescriptions of family therapy that are based on assumptions of family dysfunction or pathogenesis or that do not take into account the needs, desires, and resources of specific families (see Marsh, 1992).

CONFIDENTIALITY

One potential barrier to working with families is confidentiality. In fact, a rigid barrier of confidentially is rarely in the best interest of patients, family members, or professionals. Effective treatment of serious mental illness often requires a partnership that builds on the strengths, resources, and expert knowledge of all parties. Thus, psychologists need to understand potential conflicts regarding confidentially and the ways in which these conflicts can be resolved. The American Psychological Association (APA) Ethical Principles of Psychologists and Code of Conduct (APA, 1991) protects the right of patients to a confidential therapeutic relationship (Standard 5: Privacy and Confidentiality). At the same time, family members also have rights. For example, parents who are serving as primary caregivers should not be expected to assume responsibility in the absence of meaningful involvement in decisions that affect them.

First, we need to distinguish between confidential and nonconfidential information. Much information regarding serious mental illness in general is available to the public and can be shared with families, including information about diagnostic categories, prognosis, symptoms, medication, and treatment. Such information is essential for family members, who can benefit from handouts and suggestions for reading materials (*see Appendix* in this chapter) as well as educational programs.

When confidentiality does pertain, potential conflicts can be resolved in a number of ways (see Zipple, Langle, Spaniol, & Fisher, 1990). Practitioners can use a release of information form designed specifically for families (for a sample form, see Marsh, Lefley, & Husted, 1995, or contact Diane T. Marsh). If the release form is presented at the right time (when the patient is able to provide informed consent) and in the right manner (as something that will enhance treatment), most patients are willing to authorize the release of relevant information to their families. In the Pittsburgh, Pennsylvania, area, for instance, where there are county-wide procedures concerned with confidentiality, 90% of patents approached in this manner choose to sign the release form.

Practitioners can also function as mediators, negotiating the boundaries of confidentiality to meet the needs of particular patents and families. Psychologists can discuss with patients the importance of keeping their families informed and can work with both parties in deciding what specific information will be shared. In group practice or institutional settings, separate staff members can be designated as family advocates. Family advocates can provide relevant information to families and consult with the therapist to enhance treatment planning and coordination. In many settings, with the consent of their relative, families can be actively involved in treatment (e.g., as members of the treatment team). As active participants, family members can offer their insights and observations; they can also play a meaningful role in decisions that affect them.

There are a number of additional considerations regarding confidentiality. Patients can always reveal information to their families. By signing a release form, they can also assign that role to their therapists. Thus, patients should be encouraged as early as possible to make an informed choice about the information that will be shared with family members and the ways in which information will be shared. Moreover, consent requires competence: A decision should be deferred if the patient is experiencing psychotic symptoms. Other ethical principles may conflict with (and take precedence over) confidentiality. For instance, if there is the risk of imminent harm, practitioners may be required to take action to avoid that risk, including contacting family members.

SUGGESTIONS FOR PRACTITIONERS

We offer a number of suggestions that can enhance the effectiveness of psychologists who work with families of people who have a serious mental illness. First, practitioners should offer services to families in a manner that acknowledges their contributions, provides opportunities for them to enhance family functioning, and promotes a sense of intrafamilial mastery and control. The ascendant mode is a collaborative one that build on the strengths of clients, families, and practitioners.

Second, psychologists need to learn about the family experience of mental illness; the unique issues and concerns of parents, spouses, siblings, and offspring; and effective intervention strategies. Many helpful publications are available (*see References* section and *Appendix* in this chapter).

Third, practitioners should strive to meet the needs of all members of the family for information about mental illness and its treatment, for skills to cope with the illness and its consequences for their family, and for support for themselves. Practitioners can reach out to family members, listen to their stories, answer their questions, and offer individual assistance. A single informed and caring professional can make a significant difference in the lives of family members.

Fourth, psychologists can offer immediate and long-term assistance by referring families to NAMI or its local affiliates. The educational and supportive services offered by NAMI will meet the needs of families themselves and enable them to work more effectively with professionals in improving the well-being of their relative who has a mental illness. Psychologists also benefit from their participation in these organizations.

Fifth, family consultation offers a flexible and collaborative approach that practitioners can use in all settings. Family consultants can offer direct services to families for a wide range of illness-related concerns and can also assist families in making an informed choice regarding their use of other available services. The objective of professional intervention is to provide an optimal match between the needs, desires, and resources of individual families and the available services. Practitioners should consider the potential benefits, risks, and costs of all services as well as the research support for their effectiveness.

Sixth, family education and psychoeducation both offer useful approaches to professional practice with families. Family education is designed to meet the informational and supportive needs of families themselves through a 1-day workshop or a series of sessions. Family psychoeducation is a more intensive and long-term intervention that includes family education, skills training, and support. Although the latter intervention is demanding of time and energy for both families and professionals, there is impressive evidence that family psychoeducation can reduce the risk of relapse for patients with serious mental illness.

Seventh, some family members may also benefit from traditional clinical intervention, including individual, marital, or family therapy. Family members who pursue psychotherapy will also profit from complementary nonclinical services, such as support groups and educational programs.

Eighth, consistent with the general psychotherapy literature, the central consideration is the quality of the working alliance that is formed with family members. A constructive alliance is likely to be promoted by a respectful and empathic attitude toward families, an understanding of their phenomenological reality, an effort to meet their expressed needs, and a goal of family empowerment.

Finally, there are a number of steps practitioners can take immediately:

1. Attend continuing education programs concerned with serious mental illness and family concerns.
2. Contact us or other members of the APA Task Force on Serious Mental Illness and Serious Emotional Disturbance to learn about current initiatives.
3. Refer families to their local NAMI affiliate and offer to provide consultation and programs to the group.
4. Develop family-focused services in professional settings.
5. Ask family members to speak to professional groups about their experiences and to offer suggestions.
6. Invite families to serve as members of the treatment team.

REFERENCES

American Psychological Association (1992). Ethical principles of psychologists and code of conduct. *American Psychologist, 47,* 1597–1611.

Anderson, C. M., Reiss, D. J., & Hogarty, G. E. (1986). *Schizophrenia and the family.* New York: Guilford Press.

Bernheim, K. F. (1989). Psychologists and families of the severely mentally ill: The role of family consultation. *American Psychologist, 44,* 561–564.

Dixon, L. B., & Lehman, A. F. (1995). Family interventions for schizophrenia. *Schizophrenia Bulletin, 21,* 631–643.

Lam, D. H. (1991). Psychosocial family intervention in schizophrenia: A review of empirical studies. *Psychological Medicine, 21,* 423–441.

Lefley, H. P. (1996). *Family caregiving in mental illness* (Family caregiver applications series, Vol. 7). Thousand Oaks, CA: Sage.

Marsh, D. T. (1992). *Families and mental illness: New directions in professional practice.* New York: Praeger.

Marsh, D. T., & Dickens, R. M. (1997). *Troubled journey: Coming to terms with the mental illness of a sibling or parent.* New York: Tarcher/Putnam.

Marsh, D. T., Lefley, H. P., Evans-Rhodes, D., Ansell, V. I,. Doerzbacher, B. M.,

LaBarbera, L., & Paluzzi, J. E. (1996). The family experience of mental illness: Evidence for resilience. *Psychiatric Rehabilitation Journal, 20*(2), 3–12.

Marsh, D. T., Lefley, H. P., & Husted, J. R. (1995). Families of people with mental illness. In M. Harway (Ed.), *Treating the changing family: Handling normative and unusual events* (pp. 171–203). New York: Wiley.

Solomon, P., Draine, J., Mannion, E., & Meisel, M. (1996). Impact of brief family psychoeducation on self-efficacy. *Schizophrenia Bulletin, 22,* 41–50.

Torrey, E. F. (1995). *Surviving schizophrenia: A manual for families, consumers, and providers* (3rd ed.). New York: HarperCollins.

Wasow, M. (1995). *The skipping stone: Ripple effects of mental illness on the family.* Palo Alto, CA: Science & Behavior Books.

Wynne, L. C., McDaniel, S. H., & Weber, T. T. (1987). Professional politics and the concepts of family therapy, family consultation, and systems consultation. *Family Therapy, 26,* 153–166.

Zipple, A. M., Langle, S., Spaniol, L., & Fisher, H. (1990). Client confidentially and the family's need to know: Strategies for resolving the conflict. *Community Mental Health Journal, 26,* 533–545.

APPENDIX

Resources

Additional Relevant Publications

Backlar, P. (1994). *The family face of schizophrenia.* New York: Tarcher/Putnam.

Bernheim, K. F., & Lehman, A. F. (1985). *Working with families of the mentally ill.* New York: Norton.

Dickens, R. M., & Marsh, D. T. (Eds.). (1994). *Anguished voices: Personal accounts of siblings and children.* Boston: Boston University Center for Psychiatric Rehabilitation.

Falloon, I. R. H., Boyd, J. L., & McGill, C. W. (1984). *Family care of schizophrenia.* New York: Guilford Press.

Lefley, H. P., & Johnson, D. L. (Eds.). (1990). *Families as allies in treatment of the mentally ill.* Washington, DC: American Psychiatric Press.

Lefley, H. P., & Wasow, M. (Eds.). (1994). *Helping families cope with mental illness.* Newark, NJ: Harwood Academic.

Mueser, K. T., & Gingerich, S. (1994). *Coping with schizophrenia: A guide for families.* Oakland, CA: New Harbinger.

Petrila, J. P., & Sadoff, R. L. (1992). Confidentiality and the family as caregiver. *Hospital and Community Psychiatry, 43,* 136–139.

Family Support and Advocacy Groups

National Alliance for the Mentally Ill, 200 North Glebe Road, Suite 1015, Arlington, Virginia 22203. Phone: (703) 524-7600.

National Depressive and Manic Depressive Association, 730 North Franklin Street, Suite 501, Chicago, Illinois 60010. Phone: (312) 642-0049.

25

Using Rational Emotive Behavior Therapy Techniques to Cope with Disability

Albert Ellis

I have had multiple disabilities for a long number of years and have always used Rational Emotive Behavior Therapy (REBT) to help me cope with these disabilities. That is one of the saving graces of having a serious disability—if you really accept it, and stop whining about having it, you can turn some of its lemons into quite tasty lemonade.

I started doing this with my first major disability soon after I became a practicing psychologist in 1943, at the age of 30. At age 19 I began to have trouble reading and was fitted for glasses, which worked well enough for sight purposes but left me with easily tired eyes. After I read or even looked steadily at people for no more than 20 minutes, my eyes began to feel quite fatigued, and often as if they had sand in them. Why? Probably because of my prediabetic condition of renal glycosuria.

Anyway, from 19 years onward I was clearly handicapped by my chronically tired eyes and could find no steady release from it. Today, over a half-century later, it is still with me, sometimes a little better, sometimes a little worse, but generally unrelieved. So I stoically accepted my tired eyes and still live with them. And what an annoyance it is! I rarely read, especially scientific material, for more than 20 minutes at a time—and I almost always keep my eyes closed when I am not reading, working, or otherwise so active that it would be unwise for me to shut them.

My main sight limitation is during my work as a therapist in the world. For at our clinic at the Institute for Rational Emotive Behavior Therapy in New York, I usually see individual and group clients from 9:30 am to 11:00 pm—with a

From *Professional Psychology: Research and Practice, 28*(1) (1997), 17–22. Reprinted with permission.

couple of half hour breaks for meals, and mostly for half hour sessions with my individual clients. So during each week I may easily see over 80 individual and 40 more group clients.

Do I get tired during these long days of working? Strangely enough, I rarely do. I was fortunate enough to pick high-energy parents and other ancestors. My mother and father were both exceptionally active, on-the-go people until a short time before she died of a stroke at the age of 93 and he died, also of a stroke, at the age of 80.

Anyway, for more than a half century I have conducted many more sessions with my eyes almost completely shut than I have with them open. This includes thousands of sessions I have done on the phone without ever seeing my clients. In doing so, I have experienced some real limitations but also several useful advantages. Advantages? Yes, such as these:

1. With my eyes shut, I can focus unusually well on what my clients are telling me and can listen nicely to their tones of voice, speech hesitations and speed-ups, and other aspects of their verbal communications.
2. With my eyes closed, I can focus better, I think, on what my clients are telling themselves to make themselves disturbed: on their basic irrational meanings and philosophies that are crucial to most of their symptoms.
3. When I am not looking at my clients I am quite relaxed and can easily avoid bothering myself about how well I am doing. I avoid rating myself and producing ego problems about what a great therapist and noble person I am—or am not!
4. My closed eyes and relaxed attitude seem to help a number of my clients relax during the session themselves, to open up to concentrating on and revealing their worst problems.
5. Some of my clients recognize my personal disabilities. They see that I refuse to whine about my adversities, work my ass off in spite of them, and have the courage to accept what I cannot change. They therefore often use me as a healthy model and see that they, too, can happily work and live in spite of their misfortunes.

Do not think, now, that I am recommending that all therapists, including those who have no ocular problems, should often shut their eyes during their individual therapy sessions. No. But some might experiment in this respect to see what advantages closing their eyes may have, especially at certain times.

Despite the fact that I could only read for about 20 minutes at a time, I started graduate school in clinical psychology in 1942, when I was 28, finished with honors, and have now been at the same delightful stand for well over a half century—still with my eyes often shut and my ears widely open. I am handicapped and partially disabled, yes—but never whining and screaming about my disabilities, and always forging on in spite of them.

In my late sixties my hearing began to deteriorate, and in my mid-seventies I got two hearing aids. Even when working in good order, they have their distinct limitations and have to be adjusted for various conditions, and even for the voice loudness and quality of the voices of the people I am listening to. So I use them regularly, especially with my clients, but I am still forced to ask people to repeat themselves or to make themselves clearer.

So I put up with all these limitations and use rational emotive behavior therapy to convince myself that they are not awful, horrible, and terrible but only a pain in the ass. Once in awhile I get overly irritated about my hearing problem—which my audiologist, incidentally, tells me will definitely get a little worse as each year goes by. But usually I live very well with my poor auditory reception and even manage to do my usual large number of public talks and workshops every year, in the course of which I have some trouble in hearing questions and comments from my audiences but still manage to get by. Too bad that I have much more difficulty than I had in my younger years.

I was diagnosed as having full-blown diabetes at the age of 40, so that has added to my disabilities. Diabetes, of course, does not cause much direct pain and anguish, but it certainly does lead to severe restrictions. I was quickly put on insulin injections twice a day and on a seriously restricted diet. I, who used to take four spoons of sugar in my coffee in my prediabetic days, plus half cream, was suddenly deprived of both. Moreover, when I stuck with my insulin injections and dietary restrictions, I at first kept my blood sugar regularly low but actually lost 10 pounds off my usually all-too-thin body. After my first year of insulin taking, I became a near-skeleton!

I soon figured out that by eating 12 small meals a day, literally around the clock, I could keep my blood sugar low, ward off insulin shock reactions, and maintain a healthy weight. So for over 40 years I have been doing this and managing to survive pretty well. But what a bother! I am continually, day and night, making myself peanut butter sandwiches, pricking my fingers for blood samples, using my blood metering machines, carefully watching my diet, exercising regularly, and doing many other things that insulin-dependent diabetics have to do to keep their bodies and minds in good order.

When I fail to follow this annoying regimen, which I rarely do, I naturally suffer. Over the many years that I have been diabetic, I have ended up with a number of hypoglycemic reactions, including being carried off three times in an ambulance to hospital emergency wards. And, in spite of my keeping my blood sugar and my blood pressure healthfully low over these many years, I have suffered from various sequelae of diabetes and have to keep regularly checking with my physicians to make sure that they do not get worse or that new complications do not develop. So, although I manage to keep my health rather good, I have several physicians whom I regularly see, including a diabetologist; an internist; an ear, nose, and throat specialist; a urologist; an orthopedist; and a dermatologist. Who knows what will be next? Oh, yes: Because diabetes affects the mouth and the feet, my visits to the dentist and podiatrist every year are a hell of a lot more often than I enjoy making them. But, whether I like it or not, I go.

Finally, as a result of my advancing age, perhaps my diabetic condition, and who knows what else, I have suffered for the last few years from a bladder that is easily filled and slow to empty. So I run to the toilet more than I used to do, which I do not particularly mind. But I do mind the fact that it often takes me much longer to urinate than it did in my youth and early adulthood. That is really annoying!

Why? Because for as long as I can remember, I have been something of a time watcher. I figured out, I think when I was still in my teens and was writing away like a demon, even though I had a full schedule of courses and other events at college, that the most important thing in my life, and perhaps in almost everyone else's life, is time. Money, of course, has its distinct value; so does love. But if you lose money or get rejected in your sex–love affairs, you always have other chances to make up for your losses, as long as you are alive and energetic. If you are poor, you can focus on getting a better income; if you are unloved and umated, you can theoretically get a new partner up until your dying day. Not so, exactly, with time. Once you lose a few seconds, hours, or years, there is no manner in which you can get them back. Once gone, you can in no way retrieve them. Tempus fugit—and time lost, wasted, or ignored is distinctly irretrievable.

Ever since my teens, then, I have made myself allergic to procrastination and to hundreds of other ways of wasting time, and of letting it idly and unthinkingly go by. I assume that my days on earth are numbered and that I will not live a second more than I actually do live. So, unless I am really sick or otherwise out of commission, I do my best to make the most of my 16 daily hours; and I frequently manage to accomplish this by doing two or more things at a time. For example, I very frequently listen to music while reading and have an interesting conversation with people while preparing a meal or eating.

This is all to the good, and I am delighted to be able to do two things at once, to stop my procrastinating and my occasional day dreaming and, instead, to do something that I would much rather get done in the limited time that I have to be active each day and the all too few years I will have in my entire lifetime. Consequently, when I was afflicted by the problem of slow urination in my late seventies, I distinctly regretted the 5 to 15 minutes of extra time it began to take me to go to the toilet several times each day and night. What a waste! What could I effectively do about saving this time?

Well, I soon worked out that problem. Instead of standing up to urinate as I had normally done for all my earlier life, I deliberately arranged for most of the times I went to the john to do so sitting down. While doing so, I first settled on doing some interesting reading for the several minutes that it took me to finish urinating. But then I soon figured out that I could do other kinds of things as well to use this time.

For example, when I am alone in the apartment that I share with my mate, Janet Wolfe, I usually take a few minutes to heat up my regular hot meal in our microwave oven. While it is cooking, I often prepare my next hot meal as well as put it in a microwave dish in the refrigerator, so that when I come up from my office to our apartment again, I will have it quickly ready to put in the oven again. I therefore am usually cooking and preparing two meals at a time. As the old saying goes, two meals for the price of one!

Once the microwave oven rings its bell and tells me that my cooked meal is finished, I take it out of the oven, and instead of putting it on our kitchen table to eat, I take it into the bathroom and put it on a shelf by the side of the toilet, together with my eating utensils. Then, while I spend the next 5 or 10 minutes urinating, I simultaneously eat my meal out of the microwave dish that it is in and thereby accomplish my eating and urinating a the same time. Now some of you may think that this is inelegant or even boorish. My main goal is to get two important things—eating and urinating—promptly done, to polish them off as it were, and then to get back to the rest of my interesting life. As you may well imagine, I am delighted with this efficient arrangement and am highly pleased with having efficiently worked it out!

Sometimes I actually can arrange to do tasks while I am also doing therapy. My clients, for example, know that I am diabetic and that I have to eat regularly, especially when my blood sugar is low. So, with their permission, I actually eat my peanut butter and sugarless jelly sandwiches while I am conducting my individual and group sessions, and everyone seems to be happy.

However, I still have to spend a considerable amount of time taking care of my physical needs and dealing with my diabetes and other disabilities. I hate doing this, but I accept the fact that I have little other choice. So I use rational emotive behavior therapy (REBT) to overcome my tendencies toward low frustration tolerance that I may still have. I tell myself whenever I feel that I am getting impatient or angry about my various limitations,

> Too damned bad! I really do not like taking all this time and effort to deal with my impairments and wish to hell that I didn't have to do so. But alas, I do. It is hard doing so many things to keep myself in a relatively healthy condition, but it is much harder, and in the long run much more painful and deadly, if I do not keep doing this. There is no reason whatsoever why I absolutely must have it easier than I do. Yes, it is unfair for me to be more afflicted than many other people are. But, damn it, I should be just as afflicted as I am! Unfairness should exist in the world—to me, and to whomever else it does exist—because it does exist! Too bad that it does—but it DOES! (Ellis, 1979, 1980)

So, using my REBT training, I work on my low frustration tolerance and accept—yes, really accept—what I cannot change. And, of course, barring a medical miracle, I cannot right now change any of my major disabilities. I can live with them, and I do. I can even reduce them to some extent, and I do. But I still cannot get rid of them. Tough! But it is not awful.

REBT, as you may or may not know, posits that there are two main instigators of human neurosis: First, low frustration tolerance (e.g., I absolutely must have what I want when I want it and must never, never be deprived of anything that I really, really desire). Second, self-denigration (e.g., when I do not perform well and win others' approval, as at all times I should, ought, and must, I am an inadequate person, a retard, a nogoodnik!).

Many disabled people in our culture, in addition to suffering from the first of these disturbances, suffer even more seriously from the second. People with serious disabilities often have more performance limitations in many areas (e.g., at school, at work, and at sports) than those who have no disabilities. To make matters worse, they are frequently criticized, scorned, and put down by others for having their deficiencies. From early childhood to old age, they may be ridiculed and reviled, shown that they really are not as capable and as "good" as are others. So not only do they suffer from decreased competence in various areas but also from much less approval than more proficient members of our society often receive. For both these reasons, because they notice their own ineptness and because many of their relatives and associates ignore or condemn them for it, they falsely tend to conclude, "My deficiencies make me a deficient, inadequate individual."

I largely taught myself to forgo this kind of self-deprecation long before I developed most of my present disabilities. From my early interest in philosophy during my teens, I saw that I did not have to rate myself as a person when I rated my efficacy and my lovability. I began to teach myself, before I reached my mid-twenties, that I could give up most of my feelings of shame and could unconditionally accept myself as a human even when I did poorly, especially at sports. As I grew older, I increasingly worked at accepting myself unconditionally. So when I started to practice REBT in 1955, I made the concept of unconditional self-acceptance (USA) one of its key elements (Balter, 1995; Dryden, 1995; Ellis, 1973, 1988, 1991, 1994, 1996; Hauck, 1991).

As you can imagine by what I stated previously in this article, I use my REBT-oriented high frustration tolerance to stop myself from whining about disabilities and rarely inwardly or outwardly complain about this. But I also use my self-accepting philosophy to refrain from ever putting myself down about these handicaps. For in REBT one of the most important things we do is to teach most of our clients to rate or evaluate only their thoughts, feelings, and actions and not rate their self, essence, or being. So for many years I have followed this principle and fully acknowledged that many of my behaviors are unfortunate, bad, and inadequate, because they do not fulfill my goals and desires. But I strongly philosophize, of course, that I am not a bad or inadequate person for having these flaws and failings.

I must admit that I really hate growing old. Because, in addition to my diabetes, my easily tired eyes, and my poor hearing, old age definitely increases my list of disabilities. Every year that goes by I creak more in my joints, have extra physical pains to deal with, slow down in my pace, and otherwise am able to do somewhat less than previously. So old age is hardly a blessing!

However, as I approach the age of 82, I am damned glad to be alive and to be quite active, productive, and enjoying. My brother and sister, who were a few years younger than I, both died almost a decade ago, and just about all my close relatives are also fairly long gone. A great many of my psychological friends and associates, most of whom were younger than I, unfortunately have died, too. I grieve for some of them, especially for my brother, Paul, who was my best friend. But I also remind myself that it is great that I am still very much alive, as is my beloved mate, Janet, after more than 30 years of our living together. So, really, I am very lucky!

Do my own physical disabilities actually add to my therapeutic effectiveness? I would say, yes—definitely. In fact, they do in several ways, including the following.

1. With my regular clients, most of whom have only minor disabilities or none at all, I often use myself as a model and show them that, in spite of my 82 years and my physical problems, I fully accept myself with these impediments and give myself the same unconditional self-acceptance (USA) that I try to help these clients achieve. I also often show them, directly and indirectly, that I rarely whine about my physical defects but have taught myself to have high frustration tolerance (HFT) about them. This kind of modeling helps teach many of my clients that they, too, can face real adversities and achieve USA and HFT.

2. I particularly work at teaching my disabled clients to have unconditional self-acceptance by fully acknowledging that their deficiencies are unfortunate, bad, and sometimes very noxious but that they are never, except by their own self-sabotaging definition, shameful, disgraceful or contemptible. Yes, other people may often view them as horrid, hateful people, because our culture and many other cultures often encourage such unfair prejudice. But I show my clients that they never have to agree with this kind of bigotry and can actively fight against it in their own lives as well as help other people with disabilities to be fully self-accepting.

I often get this point across to my own clients by using self-disclosure and other kinds of modeling. Thus, I saw a 45-year-old brittle, diabetic man, Michael, who had great trouble maintaining a healthy blood sugar level, as his own diabetic brother and sister were able to do. He incessantly put himself down for his inability to work steadily, to maintain a firm erection, to participate in sports, and to achieve a good relationship with an attractive woman who would mate with him in spite of his severe disabilities.

When I revealed to Michael several of my own physical defects and limitations, such as those I mentioned previously in this article, and when I showed him how I felt sad and disappointed about them but stubbornly refused to feel at all ashamed or embarrassed for having these difficulties, he strongly worked at full self-acceptance, stopped denigrating himself for his inefficacies, shamelessly informed prospective partners about his disabilities, and was able to mate with a woman who cared for him deeply in spite of them.

In this case, I also used REBT skill training. As almost everyone, I hope, knows by now, REBT is unusually multimodal. It shows people with physical problems how to stop needlessly upsetting themselves about their drawbacks. But it also teaches them various social, professional, and other skills to help them minimize and compensate for their hindrances (Ellis, 1957/1975, 1988, 1996; Gandy, 1995). In Michael's case, in addition to teaching him unconditional self-acceptance, I showed him how to socialize more effectively; how to satisfy female partners without having perfect erections; and how to participate in some sports, such as swimming, despite his physical limitations. So he was able, although still disabled, to feel better and to perform better as a result of his REBT sessions. This is the two-sided or duplex kind of therapy that I try to arrange with many of my clients with disabilities.

3. Partly as a result of my own physical restrictions, I am also able to help clients, whether or not they have disabilities, with their low frustration tolerance (LFT). As I noted earlier, people with physical restrictions and pains usually are more frustrated than those without such impediments. Consequently, they may well develop a high degree of LFT. Consider Denise, for example. A psychologist, she became insulin dependent at the age of 30 and felt horrified about her newly acquired restrictions. According to her physicians, she now had to take two injections of insulin and several blood tests every day, give up most of her favorite fat-loaded and salt-saturated foods, spend a half-hour a day exercising, and take several other health-related precautions. She viewed all of these chores and limitations as "revolting and horrible," and became phobic about regularly carrying them out. She especially kept up her life-long gourmet diet and gained 20 extra pounds within a year of becoming diabetic. Her doctors' and her husband's severe criticism helped her feel guilty, but it hardly stopped her in her foolish self-indulgence.

I first worked with Denise on the LFT and did my best to convince her, as REBT practitioners often do, that she did not need the eating and other pleasures that she wanted. It was indeed hard for her to impose the restrictions her physical condition now required, but it was much harder, I pointed out, if she did not follow them. Her increased limitations were indeed unfortunate, but they were hardly revolting and horrible; I insisted that she could stand them, though never necessarily like them.

I at first had little success in helping Denise to raise her LFT because, as a bright psychologist, she irrationally but quite cleverly parried my rational arguments. However, using my own case for an example, I was able to show her how, at my older age and with my disabilities greater than hers, I had little choice but to give up my former indulgences or die. So, rather than die, I gave up putting four spoons of sugar and half cream in my coffee, threw away my salt shaker, stopped frying my vegetables in sugar and butter, surrendered my allergy to exercise, and started tapping my fingers seven or eight times a day for blood tests. When Denise heard how I forced my frustration tolerance up as my pancreatic secretion of insulin went down, and how for over 40 years I have thereby staved off the serious complications of diabetes that probably would have followed from my previous habits, and from her present ones, she worked on her own LFT and considerably reduced it.

Simultaneously, I also helped Denise with her secondary symptoms of neurosis. As a bright person and as a psychologist who often helped her clients with their self-sabotaging thoughts, feelings, and behaviors, she knew how destructive her own indulgences were, and she self-lambasted and made herself feel very ashamed of them, thereby creating a symptom about a symptom: self-downing about her LFT. So I used general REBT with her to help her give herself unconditional self-acceptance (USA) in spite of her indulging in her LFT. I also specifically showed her how, when I personally slip back to my predisability ways and fail to continue my antidiabetic exercise and other prophylactic routines, I only castigate my behavior and not my self or personhood. I therefore see myself as a goodnik who can change my no-goodnik actions, and this USA attitude helps me correct those actions. By forcefully showing this to Denise, and using myself and my handling of my disabilities as notable examples, I was able to help her give up her secondary symptoms—self-deprecation—and go back to working more effectively to decrease her primary symptom—low frustration tolerance.

I have mainly tried to show in this article how I have personally coped with some of my major disabilities for over 60 years. But let me say that I have found it relatively easy to do so because, first, I seem to be a natural born survivor and coper, which many disabled (and nondisabled) people are not. This may well be my innate predisposition but also may have been aided by my having to cope with nephritis from my 5th to my 8th years and my consequent training myself to live with physical adversity. Second, as noted earlier, I derived an epicurean and stoic philosophy from reading and reasoning about many philosophers' and writers' views from my 16th year onward. Third, I originated REBT in January 1955 and have spent the great majority of my waking life teaching it to clients, therapists, and members of the public for over 40 years.

For these and other reasons, I fairly easily and naturally use REBT methods in my own life and am not the kind of difficult customer (DC) that I often find my clients to be. With them, and especially with DCs who have disabilities and who keep complaining about them and not working too hard to overcome and cope with them, I often use a number of cognitive, emotive, and behavioral techniques for which REBT is famous and which I have described in my book, *How to Cope With a Fatal Illness* (Ellis & Abrams, 1994) and in many of my other writings (Ellis, 1957/1975, 1985, 1988, 1994, 1996).

Several other writers have also applied REBT and cognitive behavior therapy (CBT) to people with disabilities, including Rochelle Balter (1995), Warren Johnson (1981), Rose Oliver and Fran Bock (1987), and J. Sweetland (1991). Louis Calabro (1991) has written a particularly helpful article showing how the anti-awfulizing philosophy of REBT can be used with individuals suffering from severe disabilities, such as those following a stroke, and Gerald Gandy (1995) has published an unusual book, *Mental Health Rehabilitation: Disputing Irrational Beliefs*.

The aforementioned writings include a great many cognitive, emotive, and behavioral therapy techniques that are particularly useful with people who have disabilities. Because, as REBT theorizes, human thinking, feeling, and acting significantly interact with each other, and because emotional disturbance affects one's body as well as one's physical condition affects one's kind and degree of disturbance, people who are upset about their disabilities often require a multi-faceted therapy to deal with their upset state. REBT, like Arnold Lazarus' (1989) multimodal therapy, provides this kind of approach and therefore often is helpful to people with disability-related problems.

Let me briefly describe a few of the cognitive REBT methods that I frequently use with my clients who have disabilities and who are quite anxious, depressed, and self-pitying about having these handicaps. I bring out and help them dispute their irrational beliefs (IBs). Thus, I show these clients that there is no reason why they must not be disabled, although that would be distinctly desirable. No matter how ineffectual some of their behaviors are, they are never inadequate persons for having a disability. They can always accept themselves while acknowledging and deploring some of their physical and mental deficiencies. When other people treat them unkindly and unfairly because of their disabilities, they can deplore this unfairness but not damn their detractors. When the conditions under which they live are unfortunate and unfair, they can acknowledge this unfairness while not unduly focusing on and indulging in self-pity and horror about it.

Preferably, I try to show my disabled clients how to make a profound philosophical change and thereby not only minimize their anxiety, depression, rage, and self-pity for being disadvantaged but to become considerably less disturbable about future adversities. I try to teach them that they have the ability to consistently and strongly convince themselves that nothing is absolutely awful, that no human is worthless, and that they can practically always find some real enjoyment in living (Ellis, 1994, 1996; Ellis & Abrams, 1994). I also try to help them accept the challenge of being productive, self-actualizing, and happy in spite of the unusual handicaps with which they may unfortunately be innately endowed or may have acquired during their lifetime. Also, I point out the desirability of their creating for themselves a vital absorbing interest, that is, a long-range devotion to some cause, project, or other interest that will give them a real meaning and purpose in life, distract them from their disability, and give them ongoing value and pleasure (Ellis, 1994, 1996; Ellis & Harper, 1975).

To aid these goals of REBT, I use a number of other cognitive methods as well as many emotive and behavioral methods with my disabled clients. I have described these in many articles and books, so I shall not repeat them here. Details can be found in *How to Cope With a Fatal Illness* (Ellis & Abrams, 1994).

Do I use myself and my own ways of coping with my handicaps to help my clients cope with them? I often do. I first show them that I can unconditionally accept them with their disabilities, even when they have partly caused these handicaps themselves. I accept them with their self-imposed emphysema from smoking or with their 100 extra pounds of fat from indulging in ice cream and candy. I show them how I bear up quite well with my various physical difficulties and still manage to be energetic and relatively healthy. I reveal some of my time-saving, self-management, and other discipline methods that I frequently use in my own life. I indicate that I have not only devised some sensible philosophies for people with disabilities but that I actually apply them in my own work and play, and I show them how. I have survived my handicaps for many years and damned well intend to keep doing so for perhaps a good number of years to come.

CONCLUSION

I might never have been that much interested in rational or sensible ways of coping with emotional problems had I not had to cope with a number of fairly serious physical problems from the age of 5 years onward. But rather than plague myself about my physical restrictions, I devoted myself to the philosophy of remaining happy in spite of my disabilities, and out of this philosophy I ultimately originated REBT in January 1955 (Ellis, 1962, 1994; Wiener, 1988; Yankura & Dryden, 1994). As I was developing REBT, I used some of its main principles on myself, and I have often used them with other people with disabilities. When I and these others have worked to acquire an anti-awfulizing, unconditional self-accepting philosophy, we have often been able to lead considerably happier and more productive lives than many other handicapped individuals lead. This hardly proves that REBT is a panacea for all physical and mental ills. It is not. But it is a form of psychotherapy and self-therapy especially designed for people who suffer from uncommon adversities. It points out to clients in general and to physically disadvantaged ones in particular that however much they dislike the harsh realities of their lives, they can manage to make themselves feel the healthy negative emotions of sorrow, regret, frustration, and grief while stubbornly refusing to create and dwell on the unhealthy emotions of panic, depression, despair, rage, self-pity, and personal worthlessness. To help in this respect, it uses a number of cognitive, emotive–evocative, and behavioral methods. Its results with disabled individuals has not yet been well researched with controlled studies. Having used it successfully on myself and with many other individuals, I am of course prejudiced in its favor. But controlled investigations of its effectiveness are an important next step.

REFERENCES

Balter, R. (1995. Spring). Disabilities update: What role can REBT play? *IRETletter,* pp. 1–4.
Calabro, L. E. (1991). *Living with disability.* New York: Institute for Rational–Emotive Therapy.

Dryden, W. (1995). *Brief rational emotive behavior therapy.* London: Wiley.

Ellis, A. (1962). *Reason and emotion in psychotherapy.* Secaucus, NJ: Citadel.

Ellis, A. (1973). *Humanistic psychotherapy: The rational–emotive approach.* New York McGraw-Hill.

Ellis, A. (1975). *How to live with a neurotic: At home and at work* (rev. ed.). Hollywood, CA: Wilshire Books. (Original work published 1957)

Ellis, A. (1979). Discomfort anxiety: A new cognitive behavioral construct. Part 1. *Rational Living, 14*(2), 3–8.

Ellis, A. (1980). Discomfort anxiety: A new cognitive behavioral construct. Part 2. *Rational Living, 15*(1), 25–30.

Ellis, A. (1985). *Overcoming resistance: Rational–emotive therapy with difficult clients.* New York: Springer.

Ellis, A. (1988). *How to stubbornly refuse to make yourself miserable about anything—yes, anything!* Secaucus, NJ: Lyle Stuart.

Ellis, A. (1991). Using RET effectively: Reflections and interview. In M. D. Bernard (Ed.), *Using rational–emotive therapy effectively* (pp. 1–33). New York: Plenum Press.

Ellis, A. (1994). *Reason and emotion in psychotherapy* (revised and updated). New York: Birch Lane Press.

Ellis, A. (1996). *Better, deeper and more enduring brief therapy.* New York: Brunner/Mazel.

Ellis, A., & Abrams, M. (1994). *How to cope with a fatal illness.* New York: Barricade Books.

Ellis, A., & Harper, R. A. (1975). *A new guide to rational living.* North Hollywood, CA: Wilshire Books.

Gandy, G. L. (1995). *Mental health rehabilitation: Disputing irrational beliefs.* Springfield, IL: Thomas.

Hauck, P. A. (1991). *Overcoming the rating game: Beyond self-love—beyond self-esteem.* Louisville, KY: Westminster/John Knox.

Johnson, W. R. (1981). *So desperate the fight.* New York: Institute for Rational–Emotive Therapy.

Lazarus, A. A. (1989). *The practice of multimodal therapy.* Baltimore, MD: Johns Hopkins University Press.

Oliver, R., & Bock, F. A. (1987). *Coping with Alzheimer's.* North Hollywood, CA: Melvin Powers.

Sweetland, J. (1991). *Cognitive behavior therapy and physical disability.* Point Lookout, NY: Author.

Wiener, D. (1988). *Albert Ellis: Passionate skeptic.* New York: Praeger.

Yankura, J., & Dryden, W. (1994). *Albert Ellis.* Thousand Oaks, CA: Sage.

Part VI: *Study Questions and Disability Awareness Exercise*

1. Discuss the disabilities that create the greatest challenge for intervention strategies.
2. Can traditional psychotherapeutic strategies be extended to all people with disabilities or must some modification take place?
3. Explain how a person's role and identity can affect the disability experience.
4. How are the cognitive interventions presented different from or similar to "the power of positive thinking?"
5. How can cognitive therapy facilitate the adaptation to disability?
6. What are the assets and limitations of Livneh's model as well as the CT model?
7. Discuss how the disability experience can challenge a person's assumption about life and living.
8. How can disability impact and alter coping mechanisms?
9. Explore and discuss the factors in treating depression in persons with disabilities and without disabilities.
10. What role does denial have in the loss process?
11. Why is it important to address grief in the treatment and rehabilitation process?
12. Discuss the potential impact of empowerment on rehabilitation theory and practice.
13. What role does the concept of courage have in the counseling and rehabilitation process?
14. Are there problems or limitations related to the implementation of courage in the treatment or rehabilitation process?
15. How does subjective and objective burden relate to the family experience of mental illness?
16. Discuss family resilience as it relates to coping.
17. What persons with disabilities would you believe to be most responsive to REBT? What individuals would be least responsive?
18. What do you view as deficits in REBT?
19. Do you believe Ellis would have developed REBT if he had not grown up with a disability?

TOO MUCH TO HANDLE

Frequently, treatment and rehabilitation systems and personnel are faced with very complex issues that challenge both the resources of the system and present a variety of complex economic, proceedural, and ethical issues.

Goals

1. To present the complex issues faced by agencies providing services to people with very complex needs.
2. To explore the limitations and assets of systems limited by funds, policy and resources.

Procedure

You have just been appointed a counselor in an agency that has as its mission the provision of humane, comprehensive, and long-term care for underserved people with disabilities.

Your first client is a 24-year-old person with a history of mental illness. He acquired a spinal cord injury that resulted in quadriplegia when he attempted suicide. In addition, he sustained a head injury. Recently, he was diagnosed as having AIDS, which resulted from his activities while under the influence of drugs and alcohol.

1. Discuss the multiple issues generated by this client.
2. Develop the mission statement for the agency.
3. Resolve if any public agency can meet the needs of this person.
4. What interventions and resources might you use to be of help to this client?
5. Where should the resources come from? How much money should be spent?

Part VII

New Directions

Rehabilitation is changing dramatically. Some would call it evolution, others upheaval or even revolution. The most significant symbol of this dramatic change is the passage of the Americans with Disabilities Act by the U.S. Congress in 1990. This legislation, which goes further than any other in ensuring civil rights and accessibility for millions of American citizens with disabilities, is seen by many as the culmination of significant positive changes in the 1990s and a symbol of hope for the 21st century.

The new directions of the 1990s have resulted in individuals being served in greater numbers who were underserved in the past. These include persons with head injuries, older persons, and persons with AIDS. Consequently, new moral and ethical concerns have arisen related to changing and emerging clients' needs. Part VII addresses many of these significant concerns from a futuristic perspective.

Rehabilitation has been greatly impacted by the medical model, economic factors, and our technocratic society. McCarthy, in chapter 26, presents a model for integrating spirituality perspectives and practices with the goal of improving the physical and mental health of both rehabilitation consumers and providers.

AIDS and other HIV-related disorders have created multidimensional problems for persons infected, their significant others, and the human service system aiding them. With advances in treatment persons with AIDS are living 10–15 years or longer past diagnosis. Feist-Prince, in chapter 27, provides information related to HIV and AIDS including biological implications, psychosocial issues impacting both the persons with HIV and the rehabilitation service system, and future practice implications.

Dual diagnosis, which is defined as a cooccurring mental health and substance abuse disorder, results in complex problems and multifaceted rehabilitation needs for persons with this diagnosis. Chapter 28 is intended to inform the reader about the characteristics of dually diagnosed clients and their assessment, treatment, and rehabilitation.

Recovery from mental illness as a process, outcome, and a vision is discussed by Spaniol and his associates in chapter 29. They focus on a series of questions and responses regarding topics such as "What is recovery?"; "What are people recovering from?"; "How are people impacted by what they are recovering from?" and "What is helpful to people in their recovery process?" They emphasize close collaboration and shared decision making between those recovering and those assisting in the recovery process.

With the increase in complexity of health care and rehabilitation systems in the 1970s, surviving the system is a critical issue for people with disabilities. In chapter 30, Buchanan describes her personal experience as a survivor of this system. She discusses the importance of "taking charge" and developing a plan with several strategies for dealing with the system; a number of these are presented in the chapter.

26

Integrating Spirituality into Rehabilitation in a Technocratic Society

Henry McCarthy

S ome societies emphasize the development of technology and the implementation of meritocracy through corporations, professional organizations,
and governmental bureaucracies. For many people throughout the world,
the U.S. is a shining example of the success of these principles, which I will refer
to as "technocratic." Figure 26.1 lists several of these priorities maintained by
technocratic societies and their institutions. Next to each of these priorities are
listed the principles of an alternative "spiritual" perspective. The latter represents
my own amalgamation of beliefs and guidelines that I have observed to be professed and popularly perceived as spiritual values. Although each of them can be
associated with various cultures, philosophies or religions, together they transcend any single tradition or worldview that I am aware of.

TECHNOCRATIC PRIORITIES
VERSUS SPIRITUAL VALUES

In the technocratic domain, power is conceived in two ways, both of which contrast with how it is seen spiritually. Power is either knowledge—technical expertise—obtained through education and/or experience that is limited to select
groups and then purchased from them by all others; or it is demonstrated by
physical properties such as speed, size and force. Power in the spiritual realm is
derived from metaphysical sources through personal consciousness and practices
such as verbal affirmation and visual imagery. The emerging field of psychoneuroimmunology (e.g., Ader, Felten, & Cohen, 1991; Borysenko, 1993;
Chopra, 1989) has investigated and demonstrated, through traditional scientific

From *Rehabilitation Education,* 9(2) (1995), 87–95. Reprinted with permission.

methods, some amazing influences of these metaphysical practices and energy on a variety of physical phenomena, such as tumor growth and immune system function, not just on mental states. Although these metaphysical processes may require practice and guidance to perfect, it is important to acknowledge that these methods are: (a) often useful even in their uncultivated state, (b) always available, and (c) independently accessible to each person, regardless of physical limitations, socio-economic status, or other potentially restricting characteristics. Along with this greater opportunity to harness power within the spiritual realm, there comes ongoing and ultimate responsibility for personal assessment, development and sharing of oneself and one's gifts. Where technical knowledge is the defined source of power, however, responsibility for outcomes is shifted to the recognized expert, who is professionally sanctioned and legally accountable. A relevant application of this technocratic expertise is captured by the expression, "waging war on disease" such as cancer or AIDS. While institutions devote themselves to this effort with teams of specialists, spiritualists encourage each of us to discern the life lessons that adversity brings, to engage our natural powers of healing, and to create wellness through internal balance and peace.

Unity in thought, perception and action is a common spiritual value. It is symbolized by the circle or mandala, complete and unbroken, an image that is utilized in many religions. In contrast to the simplicity of a circle's unity is the complex maze of categories, distinctions and specializations that technocratic society generates and validates. One consequence of this is that people in our society often feel and act as if they are being fragmented, compared, and pigeonholed rather than supported by a circle of acceptance. Being in harmony with the moment and with the rest of the natural world is taken by some as a spiritual duty. In contrast, a major goal of technocracies is productivity. Therefore, they focus on prediction or alteration of the future rather than appreciation of the here-and-now; they invest in exploiting or controlling nature rather than respecting Mother Earth, Father Sky, Brother Sun, Sister Moon.

Another spiritual value is a belief in the inherent beauty and sacredness of all creation, of which we have been given temporary stewardship. Ever since our forefathers declared in the founding documents of this nation that "all men are created equal," we have publicly endorsed the premise of equality in patriotic pledges and songs. Nevertheless, the daily reality is one in which status is achieved, bestowed or denied on the basis of societal criteria. This thinking leads to the common assumption that selective policies—like determining eligibility for essential life-sustaining resources—are inevitable or desirable, rather than leading to the acceptance of universal access as a given, upon which we must organize our human development strategies and service programs. A related contrast is seen in the typical technocratic reaction to crisis, which is often protectionist and punitive, whereas the spiritual response would be grounded in hopeful, healing outreach.

Rehabilitation practice is an enterprise and product of contemporary American society. Hence, it is hardly surprising that the technocratic priorities described apply to the field of rehabilitation to a significant degree, especially the characteristic extolling of professional specialization (Thomas, 1982) and expertise. Ideologically, nevertheless, the spiritual perspective also resonates with some fundamental values of rehabilitation as a profession, such as our attention to maximizing client self-responsibility and espousal of a holistic orientation (Andrews, 1981; Jaques, 1970).

Intended primarily for parsimonious presentation of the material, the format of Figure 26.1 and its discussion juxtaposes the spiritual and technocratic in a way that may make them appear to be locked in open, dramatic conflict. I do not wish to convey that. Indeed, as implied by the following quote, those devoted to the spiritual perspective tend to be immersed in the elevation of the consciousness of individuals and the cosmos, and not worried about the institutional workings and technocratic business in between the individual and cosmic levels; ". . . the holistic health movement does not appear nearly as concerned with changing the way medicine is practiced as it is with changing the fundamental orientation of people toward themselves, the universe and especially the supernatural realm" (Reisser, Reisser & Weldon, 1986, p. 17). Although it tends to have concerns about "competitors" (particularly ones that offer alternative interventions that may be more appealing in terms of lower cost, or greater comfort, convenience and credibility), the technocratic world is also very likely to be interested in what they could borrow from the spiritual movement to make their own efforts more effective or accepted.

Technocratic Priorities	Spiritual Values
expertise and planning	intuition and vision
reductionistic specialization	holistic integration
control and productivity	being in harmony
focus on the future	living in the moment
external selection	internal choice
legal accountability	self-responsibility
rugged individualism	creation of community
achieved status	inborn sacredness
material ownership	resource stewardship
competition and conquest	acceptance and embracing
curing disease	illness as a lesson and path
power, speed, strength	peace, balance, wellness

FIGURE 26.1 Comparison of technocratic priorities and spiritual values.

SPIRITUAL FOUNDATIONS OF HEALTH CARE

Etymologically, there is a direct connection between holistic thinking and concerns about medical matters. The term holistic (sometimes spelled wholistic) originated from the Greek word *holos,* which means whole and is a relative of the Greek root for heal and health. We also get our word "holy" from this root (Khan, 1982, p. 6). Historically, up through the Middle Ages, the religious community had as much of a monopoly in defining and delivering health care as the scientific community has today.

> During the early Christian era, physicians were clergy members, and the church was the first to grant a medical license. Priests were custodians of public health and were interested in the whole person. It was the development of a scientific basis for medicine that made it necessary to separate it from religion. (McKee & Chappel, 1992, p. 205)

The scientific model has quite recently been modified to incorporate consideration of a broader ideology for physicians and additional (non-scientific) sets of factors. Fonder of logotherapy, an existential and spiritual approach to psychotherapy, Viktor Frankl (1965) insisted in his book *The Doctor and the Soul* that every physician (not just his fellow psychiatrists) be engaged in "medical ministry." Engel (1980) argued for the profession's acceptance of a biopsychosocial model, which is now widely taught in medical schools. A few years later, Hiatt (1986) suggested that the model be broadened to biopsychosocialspiritual, but his proposal has not enjoyed anywhere near the same level of adoption. These and related changes, too slow for many clients and critics of the health care industry, have been introduced as physicians recognized (often with considerable resistance) that these non-scientific components of the health equation had a substantial impact on patients' sense of well-being and response to treatment.

There are two excellent articles particularly targeted to counselors that contribute, with respect to spirituality, a comparable level of conceptual model-building and clinical innovation to what the Engel and Hiatt articles did for the field of medicine. These articles—by Chandler, Holden and Kolander (1992) on counseling for spiritual wellness and by Goodwin (1986) on holistic rehabilitation counseling—deserve a thorough reading. The nursing literature also offers some well-developed conceptual and didactic material on integrating spirituality into the practice (e.g., Burhardt, 1989; Burnard, 1987; Labun, 1988) and the education (e.g., Carson, Winkelstein, Soeken & Brunins, 1987; Piles, 1990) of nurses that could readily be utilized by rehabilitation counselors and educators.

ASSESSING THE BLESSINGS AND BURDENS OF SPIRITUALLY-BASED THERAPIES

In terms of both values and practice, the way in which rehabilitation is most likely to be affected by spirituality will be determined by the field's acceptance or rejection of the host of spiritually-based therapeutic interventions (and their practitioners) that have emerged or been imported from non-Western cultures. Although many of them are ancient, they have become collectively perceived and referred to as the lifestyle choices and therapeutic tools of the New Age movement. They include: acupuncture (Brumbaugh, 1993); herbal medicine (Duke, 1995); hypnosis (Rossi, 1993); meditation (Benson & Klipper, 1976; Kabat-Zinn, 1993), prayer (Ashby & Lenhart, 1994; Bearson & Koenig, 1990; Dossey, 1993; Poloma & Pendeleton, 1991; Stern, Canda & Doershuk, 1992); therapeutic touch (Baldwin, 1986); and transactional psychophysiology (Thomas, 1989).

Current and Potential Contributions

In several ways already stated or suggested, adoption and integration of spiritual perspectives and practices could make rehabilitation more in keeping with its professed ethos. It would reinforce the profession's expressed commitments to: (a) treating the client holistically; (b) maximizing consumer choice and self-responsibility; (c) upholding the dignity and worth of all individuals; and (d) responding to client values. Particularly for the client, spiritually-based therapeutic interventions usually possess certain characteristics that make treatment more accessible in the broadest meaning of that term. Specifically, compared to traditional physical medicine and rehabilitation, such interventions typically are: (a) considerably cheaper, although to date seldom reimbursed by medical insurance; (b) not dependent on physician prescription or other professional gate-keeping; (c) simpler in their presentation and, therefore, more easily understood; (d) more diverse in style and substance; and (e) more directly affirming of clients' search for meaning in their disordered lives. Unlike invasive procedures that require intimidating equipment, they are not depersonalizing and risk-ridden. To the extent that they are self-administered (e.g., meditation), they can be accessed whenever needed and are not constrained by the time schedules imposed by providers. They are applicable to a range of handicapping conditions (e.g., cancer, chronic pain, hypertension, substance abuse). Although they offer a genuinely "alternative" experience, most spiritually-based therapies are non-exclusive in that they allow concurrent patronage of other, more "orthodox" treatments. Indeed, there has always been much more rejection of spiritually-based health practitioners by the allopathic medical community than vice versa. However, a growing group of physicians and medical schools is taking the initiative to learn from and work collaboratively with these modalities, which are referred to collectively as "alterative and complementary medicine" (see, e.g., Daly, 1995; Micozzi, 1995; Siegel, 1989).

Caveats and Concerns

Misinterpretation or misuse of well-meant and worthwhile resources is always a possibility. Spiritually-based therapies and perspectives are vulnerable to some of the conditions that can increase the danger of this occurring. Because many holistic health disciplines have not been accepted by the medical or insurance establishments, their practitioners have not been brought under the same level of peer and public scrutiny as other professionals. This provides the opportunity for inadequately trained or unscrupulous individuals to practice with less monitoring and for clients to be exploited or harmed with less or no redress. Also, because their outcomes are much less subjected to formal critique by peers and objective review panels, the effectiveness of results from spiritually-based therapies can be overzealously reported and yet substantially untested. To the extent that spiritually-based therapies are distanced from mainstream sources of information exchange, it makes it more difficult, both for lay consumers and professionals who are in a position to make referrals, to distinguish sound modalities and appropriate practices from senseless or irresponsible ones.

Aside from the above caveats about the parameters within which these interventions are conducted, there have been concerns expressed about the potentially deleterious impact when some spiritual principles get misinterpreted or unduly extrapolated. One of these is the tenet of self-responsibility, that some people translate as "you create your own reality." In the typology of Brickman et al. (1982), this combination of responsibility for both the cause of and the solution to one's problem is referred to as the "moral model" of helping and coping. Cancer cell biologist and psychotherapist, Joan Borysenko recognizes the empowering potential of taking responsibility for oneself; but she is also outspoken in her concern that this often results in blaming the person for illnesses or even accidental injuries. In her book, *Guilt is the Teacher, Love is the Lesson* (1990) she explained:

> Pessimistic people, because of their underlying helplessness, are at great risk. They are prone to confusing responsibility for learning to live well with an illness, with blame for having caused it. Illness is seen as a failure, and the illusion of power is purchased by the attitude that we can cure what we have caused. Sometimes we can cure our bodies, but sometimes we can't. The idea that the bodily state is a simple reflection of our psychological or spiritual state is a dangerous and prevalent misunderstanding. (pp. 151–152)

Such thinking could lead clients to guilt and self-denigration, and counselors to blaming the victim, particularly when the results of attempted healing interventions turn out to be less than desired or expected. Clients are likewise prone to feeling guilt about having abandoned orthodox treatments for a "fraudulent" one, or for not having tried hard enough, otherwise the intervention would have been successful.

CONCLUSION

Rehabilitation counseling and other allied health professions grew up in the shadow of the medical model. Thus, early on, the profession accepted implicitly a role delimited by that model's mechanistic, pathology-oriented conception of disability within the body and assumptions about repairing and controlling clients as the appropriate interventions. Gradually, the profession became drawn to the benefits of attending to the influences that the constellation of dynamic, ecological factors of the psychosocial paradigm can have not only on clients but indeed on the determination of disability itself. Recent demographic and political changes have prompted all health-related professions to focus their attention and decisions on dealing with the economic demands of corporate managed care. To this melange of forces that are shaping rehabilitation, we should seek and add harmony and vision through openness to and reflection on the metaphysical and spiritual around us. In particular, we need to engage in unembarrassed exploration and sensitive utilization of the potentially significant impact that spiritual perspectives and practices can have on the physical and mental health of rehabilitation consumers and providers alike.

REFERENCES

Ader, R., Felten, D., & Cohen, N. (1991). *Psychoneuroimmunology* (2nd ed.). New York: Academic Press.

Andrews, II. B. (1981). Holistic approach to rehabilitation. *Journal of Rehabilitation, 47,*(2), 28–31.

Ashby, J., & Lenhart, R. S. (1994). Prayer as a coping strategy for chronic pain patients. *Rehabilitation Psychology, 39*(3), 205–209.

Baldwin, L. (1986). The therapeutic use of touch with the elderly. *Physical & Occupational Therapy in Geriatrics, 4*(5), 45–50.

Bearon, L., & Koenig, H. (1990). Religious cognitions and use of prayer in health and illness. *Gerontologist, 30,* 249–253.

Benson, H., & Klipper, M. (1976). *The relaxation response.* New York: Avon Books.

Borysenko, J. (1990). *Guilt is the teacher, love is the lesson.* New York: Warner Books.

Borysenko, J. (1993). *Fire in the soul: A new psychology of spiritual optimism.* New York: Warner Books.

Brickman, P., Rabinowitz, V., Karuza, J., Coates, D., Cohn, E., & Kidder, L. (1982). Models of helping and coping. *American Psychologist, 37*(4), 368–384.

Brumbaugh, A. (1993). Acupuncture: New perspectives in chemical dependency treatment. *Journal of Substance Abuse Treatment, 10,* 35–43.

Burkhardt, M. (189). Spirituality: An analysis of the concept. *Holistic Nursing Practice, 3*(3), 69–77.

Burnard, P. (1987). Spiritual distress and the nursing response: Theoretical considerations and counseling skills. *Journal of Advanced Nursing, 12,* 377–382.

Carson, V., Winkelstein, M., Soeken, K., & Brunins, M. (1986). The effects of didactic teaching on spiritual attitudes. *Image: Journal of Nursing Scholarship, 18*(3), 161–164.

Chandler, C., Holden, J., & Kolander, C. (1992). Counseling for spiritual wellness: Theory and practice. *Journal of Counseling and Development, 71*(2), 168–175.

Chopra, D. (1989). *Quantum healing: Exploring the frontiers of mind/body medicine.* New York: Bantam Books.

Daly, D. (1995). Alternative medicine courses taught at U.S. medical schools: An ongoing list. *Journal of Alternative and Complementary Medicine, 1*(1), 111–113.

Dossey, L. (1993). *Healing words: The power of prayer and the practice of medicine.* New York: Harper-Collins.

Duke, J. (1995). Assessment of plants as medicines. *Journal of Alternative and Complementary Medicine, 1*(1), 9–14.

Engel, G. L. (1980). The clinical application of the biopsychosocial model. *American Journal of Psychiatry, 137,* 535–544.

Frankl, V. (1965). *The doctor and the soul.* New York: Borzoi

Labun, E. (1988). Spiritual care: An element in nursing care planning. *Journal of Advanced Nursing, 13,* 314–320.

Goodwin, L. R. (1986). A holistic perspective for the provision of rehabilitation counseling services. *Journal of Applied Rehabilitation Counseling, 17*(2), 29–36.

Hiatt, J. F. (1986). Spirituality, medicine, and healing. *Southern Medical Journal, 79,* 736–743.

Jaques, M. E. (1970). *Rehabilitation Counseling: Scope and services.* Boston: Houghton Mifflin.

Kabat-Zinn, J. (1993). Meditation. In B. Moyers & B. Flowers (Eds.), *Healing and the mind* (pp. 115–144). New York: Doubleday.

Khan, P. V. I. (1982). *Introducing spirituality into counseling and therapy.* New Lebanon, NY: Omega Publications.

McKee, D., & Chappel, J. (1992). Spirituality and medical practice. *Journal of Family Practice, 35*(2), 201, 205–206, 108.

Micozzi, M. (1995). Alternative and complementary medicine: Part of human heritage. *Journal of Alternative and Complementary Medicine, 1*(1), 1–4.

Piles, C. (1990). Providing spiritual care. *Nurse Educator, 15*(1), 36–41.

Poloma, M., & Pendleton, B. (1991). The effects of prayer and prayer experiences on measures of general well-being. *Journal of Psychology and Theology, 19*(1), 71–83.

Reisser, P., Reisser, T., & Weldon, J. (1986, Winter). What holistic healers believe. *Journal of Christian Nursing,* pp. 16–21.

Rossi, E. (1993). *The psychobiology of mind/body healing: New concepts of therapeutic hypnosis.* New York: Norton.

Siegel, B. (1989). *Peace, love & healing: Bodymind communication and the path to self-healing.* New York: Harper & Row.

Stern, R., Canda, E., & Doershuk, C. (1992). Use of nonmedical treatment by cystic fibrosis patients. *Journal of Adolescent Health, 13*(7), 612–615.

Thomas, K. (1982). A critique of trends in rehabilitation counselor education toward specialization. *Journal of Rehabilitation 48*(1), 49–51.

Thomas, S. (1989). Spirituality: An essential dimension in the treatment of hypertension. *Holistic Nursing Practice, 3*(3), 47–55.

27

The Biopsychosocial Approach to HIV and AIDS: Implications for Instruction

Sonja Feist-Price

As the number of persons infected with the Human Immunodeficiency Virus (HIV) continues to grow and the life expectancy increases for persons with the Acquired Immune Deficiency Syndrome (AIDS), rehabilitation professionals are more likely to be called upon to provide services that will significantly impact the lives of persons living with HIV/AIDS. Beck, Carlton, Allen, Rosenkoetter, and Hardy (1993) stated that persons infected with HIV will likely constitute a growing number of rehabilitation clients in the coming years as their life spans have risen to 10-15 years post diagnosis. Wong, Allen, and Moore (1988) indicated that as the disease is brought under better medical care and as the prognosis improves for persons with HIV/AIDS, rehabilitation professionals will be required to provide rehabilitation and restorative services for infected individuals.

Given the myriad of issues surrounding HIV/AIDS, and the likelihood that almost every rehabilitation practitioner will inevitably provide services to persons living with HIV/AIDS, it is incumbent upon rehabilitation educators to prepare students adequately for the biopsychosocial implications involved. Therefore this paper will provide information that is crucial to preparing present and future rehabilitation service providers to assist effectively persons with HIV/AIDS. This objective will be accomplished by discussing HIV/AIDS from the following perspectives: Biological implications, psychosocial issues, and factors that may impede rehabilitation professionals.

BIOLOGICAL IMPLICATIONS OF HIV/AIDS

HIV is a chronic, progressive, immunologic deficiency disease that is manifested in various ways (Howard, 1991). Mulder (1994) stated that HIV is associated with a gradual decline in the function of the body's immune system, and has a

From *Rehabilitation Education, 11*(1–2) (1997), 39–53. Reprinted with permission.

wide variety of disease manifestations. The course that this disease takes is very identifiable and predictable, and can be divided into several stages. The Centers of Disease Control (CDC) (1993) have developed three clinical stages of the course of HIV. These stages are based upon the duration of the illness, a specific set of symptoms and diseases, and ordered according to type, site, and severity of the illness. The progression of HIV through the various stages is consistent with one's progression from a state of asymptomatic HIV infection to symptomatic HIV disease (Atkins & Hancock, 1993).

HIV is transmitted to an uninfected individual by two means, sexual or blood contact (Cohen, 1990). Unless an individual experiences a condition called *acute HIV infection,* he or she may remain asymptomatic for up to 15 years (Beck et al., 1993; Howard, 1992). According to Howard (1992), "[a]cute HIV infection manifests itself as a flu-like illness, characterized by fever, body aches, swollen lymph nodes, and a faint rash" (p. 94). The presence of acute HIV infection lasts only a few days and usually goes undetected. Most individuals attribute this illness to the flu, and HIV is detected only after a blood test for the presence of HIV antibodies (Mulder, 1994). The presence of HIV antibodies in the blood is the body's way of attempting to eliminate the noxious virus. As persons move from the status of HIV to AIDS, the number of HIV antibodies declines (Howard, 1992).

HIV destroys the body's immune system, and this destruction begins soon after HIV transmission occurs (CDC, 1993). Although infected persons may remain asymptomatic for long periods of time, soon after transmission occurs the virus begins to attack a vital, infection-fighting white blood cell. This white blood cell is called the CD4+ lymphocyte (Howard, 1992). Mulder (1994) stated that the number of CD4+ cells is important because HIV infects and kills them, and these cells play a vital role in the immune system by allowing the body to fight off infections. The destruction of CD4+ cells leaves the person prone to many infections and tumors. These infections and tumors are the hallmark of HIV infection (Howard, 1992). HIV gradually depletes the body's supply of CD4+ cells, resulting in a progressively worsening state of immunodeficiency. Therefore, it becomes extremely important to maintain a count of the body's CD4+ cells in persons with HIV an AIDS. A declining number of cells indicates evidence of the virus' progression to a more advanced state of immunodeficiency and the development of *early symptomatic HIV infection,* the next inevitable stage.

According to Howard (1992) early symptomatic HIV disease is characterized by relatively nonspecific signs and symptoms. These may include swollen glands or lymph nodes, mild fevers, and a state of fatigue or low energy. In a limited time, these signs and symptoms become worse and additional complications appear. These additional signs and symptoms progress from moderate to severe HIV disease, also known as *AIDS-Related Complex* or *ARC* (Howard, 1992). While there are no universally accepted signs and symptoms identified as benchmarks for ARC, a myriad of signs and symptoms typically manifest. Included are daily fevers, night sweats, fatigue and weakness, weight loss of more than 10 pounds, intermittent diarrhea, oral thrush (yeast growing in the mouth), swollen lymph nodes, various skin conditions such as fungal rashes and herpes zoster infection or "shingles," and memory and concentration problems. (Howard, 1992, p. 95)

As HIV progresses, infections and tumors are very prevalent. The most commonly seen infection among persons with HIV is a pneumonia called Pneumocystis carinii (Howard, 1992). This pneumonia is caused by a protozoa that is common in small amounts, however, in humans. With a normal functioning immune system, this protozoa is destroyed and problems never occur. In addition to protozoa, bacterial, viral, or fungal organisms also exist in a low level of virulence or ability to harm persons with an intact immune system. Thus, Pneumocystis carinii is called an *opportunistic infection* because it takes advantage of the body's somewhat defenseless posture caused by HIV and causes an infection (Howard, 1992).

Kaposi's sarcoma, the most common tumor, usually affects the skin and results in a violet-colored skin tumor (Howard, 1992). Unlike Pneumocystis carinii, the development of Kaposi's sarcoma is not necessarily related to the level of immunodeficiency present. Cancers such as non-Hodgkin's lymphoma also qualify as an AIDS-defining tumor. This tumor, however, occurs less frequently than Kaposi's sarcoma.

The progression from early HIV disease to ARC and eventually to AIDS is inevitable. According to the CDC (1993), regardless of the presence of infections, tumors, or both, a person has progressed from HIV to AIDS when their CD4+ cell count is 200 or fewer per cubic millimeter.

In addition to infections and tumors, neurological dysfunctions occur frequently among persons with HIV and AIDS. Howard (1992) reports that as many as 20% of patients with AIDS have some type of neurological dysfunction as their presenting manifestation of AIDS. Often neurological symptoms occur prior to any other manifestations of the HIV disease. In addition, approximately 60% of persons with AIDS have various neurological symptoms. Neurological problems are caused by both opportunistic infections and tumors of the central nervous system. *Subacute encephalitis,* also known as *AIDS encephalopathy* or *AIDS dementia complex,* is the most insidious neurological problem seen in persons with AIDS (Howard, 1992). This problem can be very complex because of its affects on one's ability to process information accurately, as well as cope with one's condition. In addition, AIDS dementia complex affects one's memory, verbal, and motor skills, and causes affective and behavioral changes.

In addition to the many medical complications specific to HIV and AIDS, persons infected must also deal with a host of psychosocial issues that sometimes exacerbate their physical condition. The following section will identify pertinent psychosocial issues specific to persons with HIV and AIDS, as well as their family members.

PSYCHOSOCIAL IMPLICATIONS

The medical ramifications for persons with HIV/AIDS have far reaching implications, especially because of its terminal nature. Not only is HIV/AIDS a health
issue, but it touches all major facets involved in one's quality of life (Atkins &
Hancock, 1993). According to Cohen (1986), persons living with HIV/AIDS are
overwhelmed with severe and multiple illnesses, decreased cognitive functioning, devastating weaknesses and limitations, weight loss, fevers, cancers, opportunistic infections, disfigurement, blindness, pain, and psychiatric disorders.
Persons with HIV/AIDS face the losses of health, fitness, attractiveness, strength,
independence, family, friends, lovers, jobs, homes, money, health insurance, and
ultimately life itself (Cohen, 1990). These stressors and losses are compounded
further by societal stigmatization, resulting in a sense of alienation and expend-
ability. Therefore, it is incumbent upon present and future rehabilitation professionals not only to be aware of how psychosocial issues impact persons with
HIV/AIDS, but also to identify how they can assist persons in a process that is
terminal.

The overwhelming issues of HIV/AIDS cause persons to explore their values, beliefs, sexual behaviors, views of death and dying, relationship development, fears, hopes, dreams, religion, and more (Atkins & Hancock, 1993).
Individuals that are members of high-risk groups sometimes experience the multiple losses of those closest to them. For example, a person with hemophilia may
encounter the loss of family members and friends who were hemophiliac and
were infected with the HIV virus. Also, a gay male may experience the loss of
close friends from HIV-related diseases. Nichols (1985) recognized four categories of psychosocial reactions for persons with HIV/AIDS: initial crisis-cata-
strophic effect, transitional state, deficiency state, and preparation for death. As
with other reactions to catastrophe or stages of adjustment, these phases do not
occur in any specific order, or exist in a particular time frame. Additionally, persons may move back and forth among stages.

Initial Crisis-Catastrophic Effect

As with other life threatening diseases, persons infected with HIV progress
through various stages of the adjustment. One's initial reaction to HIV status is
that of shock and denial (Nichols, 1985). From these initial responses, persons
then experience feelings of guilt, fear, sadness, anger, bargaining, and acceptance
(Kubler-Ross, 1969; Nichols, 1983). According to Cohen (1990), it is at the
period of initial crisis that information should be provided regarding education,
support, and therapy, as well as assistance with legal and financial issues.

Transitional State

Feelings of anxiety, guilt, self-pity, and anger are commonly experienced emotions by persons with HIV/AIDS. Given the terminal nature of this disease, indi-

viduals usually experience a review of life experiences (Atkins & Hancock, 1993). This review may lead to feelings of confusion, distress, and self-devaluation. In addition, persons usually experience lowered self-esteem, shifts in identity and values, as well as estrangement and isolation from families and loved ones (Cohen, 1990). The culmination of these emotions may lead to either the internalizing or projecting of feelings. Internalized feelings lead to withdrawal, depression, and sometimes suicide attempts. Projecting one's feelings on others may lead to anger at family members, loved ones, and caretakers. Additionally, the overwhelming emotional affects of an HIV-positive diagnosis may lead to acting out sexually, or an increase in intravenous drug use. Hence, as individuals make a mental transition from a state of health to the acceptance of an HIV-positive status, the adjustment phase is very erratic.

Deficiency State

This stage deals with the acceptance and resolution of the inevitable, death. Persons usually experience a resurgence of spirituality, a redefined sense of self, and a renewed sense of purpose (Cohen, 1990). Nichols (1985) described this stage as one in which persons have a new stable identity characterized by the acceptance of HIV/AIDS and the limitations associated with this illness. Persons cope with this disease by living one day at a time, and with a reassessment of the values of courage, commitment, concern for others, and an appreciation for quality rather than quantity of life. In addition, "individuals begin to feel less victimized by life and less egocentric, deriving satisfaction from altruistic and community activities" (Cohen, 1990, p. 100). It is within this stage that people embrace the concept of public speaking and educating others regarding the behavioral risks of HIV/AIDS. Additionally, persons in this stage begin to see themselves as survivors rather than victims.

Preparation for Death

From the day of diagnosis, persons with HIV/AIDS are confronted with the terminal nature of their illness. Persons with AIDS may require assistance in completing unfinished business, tying together loose ends, writing a will, and making plans for their funeral. Parents infected with HIV/AIDS may need to identify or designate persons to care for their children. Preparation for death among some parents may involve developing video or audiotapes, letters, or poems. As persons prepare for death, they should be encouraged to discuss openly their thoughts and feelings regarding death and dying, and regarding becoming dependent on others for care.

Just as persons infected with HIV/AIDS must cope with psychosocial issues associated with their illness, so must family members. In addition to being informed of one's HIV-positive status, family members must also cope with the terminal effects of this virus, and the possibility of having to meet health care demands of their loved one. Regarding disclosure to family members by persons that are gay or bisexual, Bonuck (1993) stated that

> The disclosure of HIV infection may be how spouses and partners first learn of the infected partner's bisexual, drug using, or commercial sex activities. Thus, along with the prospect of being infected themselves, the partner's previous image of family life and/or pattern of denial is shattered (p. 80).

Disclosure of one's HIV-positive status by individuals with hemophilia entail different implications for wives. In addition to accepting the fact that their husbands are infected with a virus that is ultimately fatal, wives must cope with the reality that due to safe sexual precautions they are unable to have additional (or perhaps any) children parented by their husbands (Dew, Ragni, & Nimorwicz, 1991). Additionally, this HIV-positive status means that the wives will ultimately be single parents.

Disclosure may also mean informing parents, children, siblings, extended family members, and friends about one's HIV status. Responses to and feelings of families of persons with the HIV illness vary tremendously. Cohen (1990) stated that while families and loved ones experience feelings that are very similar to persons infected with HIV/AIDS, their responses are not as intense. However, Mason, Olson, Myers, Huszti, and Kenning (1989) conducted a study on the perceptions of HIV/AIDS infected men with hemophilia, their spouses, and their parents. The results of their study indicated that parents are more concerned, angry, and unhappy about the HIV/AIDS status than the persons infected or their spouses. Nevertheless, the psychosocial implications of family members can be very intense. Bonuck (1993) identified six possible reactions of family members to someone with HIV/AIDS. Among them are social stigma and isolation, fear of contagion, fear of infection, fear of abandonment, guilt, and psychological and physical fatigue.

Social stigma and isolation is an issue that sometimes plagues family members and persons infected with HIV/AIDS. Persons with hemophilia and their families are less likely to seek out information from relatives and friends who may typically serve as information sources for other parenting and lifestyle issues because of the stigma associated with HIV/AIDS (Mason, Olson, Myers, Huszti, & Kenning, 1989). Some families strive to maintain secrecy of a person's infected status. This secrecy may be due to any number of issues; however, when it occurs family members are cut off from potential sources of physical, moral, financial, and spiritual support. Thus, families are left to bear the burden of caregiving alone.

Although *fear of contagion* is often unfounded, it can result in persons infected being isolated. Bonuck (1993) stated that fear of contagion may preclude intimacy and caretaking involvement of wives, lovers, parents, and siblings. A sense of increased personal vulnerability on the part of family members may precipitate disengagement and cause alienation to the person infected with the virus. Mason et al. (1989) found that parents of persons with hemophilia reported that they were reluctant to be physically close to their sons because of fear of transmission of AIDS. Usually, when family members are provided with accurate information and are reassured that AIDS is not transmitted by casual contact, they are able to provide the care and emotional support required (Cohen, 1990).

Fear of infection commonly involves fears on the part of family members as well as the person infected. Because those with HIV/AIDS have a lowered immune system, persons infected may be afraid that they will be contaminated by the germs and bacteria of others. Education, reassurance, and safety precautions are very important with this reaction. Family members must be encouraged to take the necessary safeguards to ensure that germs and bacteria do not further tax the person's immune system. After all of the necessary safety measures are utilized, family members must be made aware of the importance of support during a time that is frightening, lonely, and uncertain for persons infected.

Fear of abandonment usually occurs in many ways. Because HIV and AIDS are medical diagnoses that never have happy endings, family members fear the inevitable. That fear is often exacerbated due to the demands of caring for someone with AIDS. Family members sometimes find themselves in a situation that is too painful to watch and thus pull away at a time when the most critical care is required.

Guilt is a frequently pervasive reaction among family members of persons who are infected with HIV/AIDS. Mothers of sons who have hemophilia often times feel intense guilt for being the genetic cause of hemophilia which resulted in their child's HIV-positive status. Parents and family members may feel guilt for their estranged relationship with their family member due to their gay or drug-using lifestyle. Parents, lovers, or spouses may feel guilt from having been spared from the infection. Partners, spouses, or mothers who have transmitted the disease are usually overwhelmed with guilt.

Lastly, *psychological and physical fatigue* are common reactions among family members with caregiving responsibilities. The manifestations of HIV/AIDS present a myriad of physical and psychological challenges. As a result, family members will spend a significant amount of time visiting different social service agencies, medical specialists, and health care facilities for assistance with treatment and medication. In addition, family members who are caretakers will have to assist with the activities of daily living of the person infected. These day-to-day demands are overwhelming if respite is not available from other family members of community resources. Each of the reactions noted above have underlying commonalities and may overlap. Many of the perceptions and reactions of family members are contingent upon the way in which the person contracted the disease.

Family members are usually placed in the role of caregivers for persons infected with HIV/AIDS. There are times when family members are required to provide health care and psychological support to persons that are gravely ill. Lewert (1988) stated that the psychological trauma of one's HIV-positive status is experienced primarily by their caregivers. In order to provide optimal assistance and sustain the support structure of persons infected, support services within the community are required to assist caregivers. Financial assistance programs, family or individual therapy, support groups, and housekeeping services or in-home care are only a few resources that are essential to meeting the health and physical care needs of persons with HIV/AIDS. These resources help to alleviate stress on caregivers and contribute to optimal family structuring (Lewert, 1988).

FACTORS THAT MAY IMPEDE
REHABILITATION PRACTITIONERS

The rise in the number of persons infected with HIV/AIDS, and their increased life expectancy, indicate the likelihood that rehabilitation professionals will be required to provide services that will enhance the lives of persons infected. Carlton, Beck, and Allen (1993) stated that rehabilitation counselors will increasingly encounter clients who have HIV and AIDS. Rehabilitation professionals are mandated not only to participate in implementing strategies, but also to function as leaders for the nation as it responds to the problems associated with HIV and AIDS (Atkins & Hancock, 1993).

Presently, many agencies (e.g., the Department of Vocational Rehabilitation) have services and resources that can readily enhance the lives of persons infected with HIV/AIDS. These services can be provided with little, if any, changes to existing programs. However, additional elements sometimes preclude present and future rehabilitation professionals from providing services to the fullest extent possible. Therefore, the following section will address factors that may impede rehabilitation service provisions, as well as ways to overcome these issues.

HIV and AIDS elicit negative responses from many people in society. These responses are based on types of behavior that directly result in HIV transmission. With the exception of persons infected due to blood transfusions or heterosexual involvement, the transmission of HIV is due to behaviors that are either illegal or socially taboo in most places in the United States (Howard, 1992). Gay men and intravenous drug users are still at greater risk for contracting HIV/AIDS. Both of these groups have been the subject of social stigma, legal sanctions, or both. Still further, because HIV/AIDS affects a disproportionate number of ethnic minorities, the members of which are already the subject of various social imitations and prejudice in American society, they are viewed as undesirable in both respects (Atkins & Hancock, 1993; Howard, 1992).

Rehabilitation professionals are not exempt from the attitudes and perceptions that are held by society at large regarding persons infected with HIV/AIDS. Wong, Allen, and Moore (1988) maintained that the major hurdles faced by rehabilitation personnel who provide services to persons with HIV and AIDS include overcoming the social, personal, and institutional barriers that exist. Green and Bobele (1994) asserted that before counselors can begin to meet the needs of persons with HIV/AIDS they must examine their own values and beliefs regarding sexuality and religious issues, death and dying, prejudice and fear, and culturally and ethnically diverse people. Hence, rehabilitation professionals must examine their own inherent values and attitudes, understand how they arrived at their values and perceptions, and learn to accept and respect the lifestyles of persons who are culturally and technically different. Only when rehabilitation professionals examine their values and perceptions can they work to enhance the lives of persons with HIV/AIDS and avoid unconsciously projecting an insensitivity for the needs and rights of people with HIV/AIDS.

One of the variables that leads to negative attitudes and perceptions regarding persons with HIV/AIDS is a lack of knowledge or a limited knowledge base. Many rehabilitation professionals lack accurate knowledge regarding HIV/AIDS. One of the mitigating factors of attitudinal barriers is having a current and accurate knowledge base regarding medical and psychosocial issues involving HIV and AIDS. Only when assertive action is taken to acquire such knowledge can rehabilitation professionals be equipped to assist persons with HIV/AIDS.

Atkins and Hancock (1993) identified areas where assertive action is needed by rehabilitation professionals and educators to prepare them adequately to work with clients living with HIV/AIDS. First, in an effort to enhance the knowledge base of rehabilitation professionals, there is a need for development of training materials specific to persons with HIV/AIDS. These materials may include brochures, tapes, films, and other community resources. Second, professionals in related disciplines need to exchange accurate and up-to-date information regarding biopsychosocial issues specific to HIV/AIDS. While this information must be provided, rehabilitation professionals must avail themselves of these resources once they are in place. Sharing of information may include continuing education and training through workshops, seminars, presentations, etc. Third, rehabilitation educators must expose students to field placement sites where they will encounter persons living with HIV/AIDS, and service provisions must be considered. This helps to educate future professionals about the myriad of issues that confront persons living with this disease, as well as ways in which rehabilitation practitioners can provide assistance. Fourth, valid and reliable research is needed regarding all facets of life for persons living with HIV/AIDS. This research can be done through master's theses and doctoral dissertations. Additionally, rehabilitation educators can conduct research projects that add to the existing knowledge base for the rehabilitation profession. Finally, professional ethics demand that rehabilitation educators and practitioners vigorously share knowledge and provide information to their students and communities that will positively impact the lives of persons with disabilities.

In addition to the actions noted above, rehabilitation professionals must network with other professionals. This sometimes involves educating other health and human service providers about rehabilitation resources and how they can enhance the lives of persons with HIV/AIDS. Hence, rehabilitation professionals should be included in the interdisciplinary team approach. Backer (1987) asserted that rehabilitation professionals can contribute their knowledge of effective rehabilitation techniques and various technologies that can help workers with AIDS cope with the demands of work. Knowledge of rehabilitation principles and programs can guide policies and practices in the work place regarding AIDS, including attitude-changing education for management and other workers. (p. 39)

Only when rehabilitation professionals possess accepting attitudes and an accurate knowledge base can they begin to impact positively the lives of persons living with HIV/AIDS. With these factors in place not only can rehabilitation assistance be provided, but practitioners can work to inspire and empower persons to regain power and control over their lives. Establishing a sense of power and control is an essential strategy in empowering persons with HIV/AIDS to live life fully. Atkins and Hancock (1993) summed it up best when they stated that "The acquisition of power by the individual is a cornerstone in the practice of rehabilitation and underscores the essence of the public vocational rehabilitation process" (p. 32). Empowerment may be accomplished by assisting persons in either maintaining employment or reentering the workforce. Persons must be encouraged to assert their innate rights and seek necessary forms of retribution when one's rights are violated.

In order to achieve empowerment, rehabilitation practitioners serve as advocates for the rights of persons infected with HIV/AIDS. This may include educating employers about the strengths and assets of employees who are infected with the virus. Additionally, as an advocate, rehabilitation professionals may have to inform employers of the rights of persons with HIV/AIDS as mandated by the Americans with Disabilities Act.

Serving as an advocate and empowering persons with HIV/AIDS are invaluable services that can be provided by rehabilitation professionals. However, practitioners may also be called upon to serve as liaisons. This may include referring persons with HIV/AIDS to the appropriate agencies and resources within the community in order to enhance their quality of life. Because the involvement and emotional support from family members are extremely crucial to the lives of persons infected, professionals may need to cultivate and facilitate their involvement.

Only when rehabilitation services are provided from a biopsychosocial approach can professionals assist persons living with HIV/AIDS to the fullest extent possible. A biopsychosocial model of rehabilitation intervention for professionals must confront specific objectives in order to meet the needs of persons with HIV/AIDS. This model includes the following:

1. An understanding of the medical and psychosocial issues confronting persons with HIV/AIDS.
2. Identifying and restructuring attitudes, values, and prejudices toward persons with HIV/AIDS.
3. Identifying overt and covert rehabilitation policy that would either hinder or preclude effective service provisions to persons with HIV/AIDS.

4. Sensitivity training to rehabilitation professionals on every level regarding issues that are specific to persons with HIV/AIDS.
5. A thorough understanding of ways in which persons with HIV/AIDS can benefit most from rehabilitation services.
6. An awareness of local, regional, and national resources that may benefit persons with HIV/AIDS.
7. Involvement in interdisciplinary networks regarding the needs and concerns of persons with HIV/AIDS.
8. Recognizing the importance of family, friends, and significant community leaders as part of the rehabilitation process.
9. Effectively communicating the attributes of persons with HIV/AIDS to employers to ensure employment, and
10. Providing sensitivity training in the workplace in an effort to minimize interpersonal and attitudinal barriers.

Rehabilitation professionals who are able to implement and utilize the above intervention strategies are the most qualified to begin effectively the rehabilitation process for persons with HIV/AIDS.

IMPLICATIONS FOR FUTURE PRACTICE

Once rehabilitation professionals and agency policy reflect a biopsychosocial understanding and sensitivity to issues regarding persons with HIV/AIDS, effectively carrying out the rehabilitation process becomes extremely important. Service provisions from a biopsychosocial approach require rehabilitation professionals to begin with a thorough assessment of the person's present medical condition. Wong, Allen, and Moore (1988) stated that rehabilitation professionals must possess knowledge, skills, and competencies to refer potential clients with HIV/AIDS to appropriate medical specialists and other allied health professionals for further diagnostic evaluations, treatment, and follow-up services. Thus, it is imperative that the rehabilitation professional assess the specific medical stability of each individual. Unlike some impairments that reach a level of permanence before the vocational rehabilitation process begins, individuals with HIV/AIDS have progressively and inherently unstable medical histories (Howard, 1992). Additionally, rehabilitation professionals must have an understanding of the positive and negative effects of prescribed medication, and of the client's CD4+ cell count. Both of these factors have direct implications on the immune system of clients and thus impact their employability.

Second, rehabilitation professionals must have an understanding of the client's psychological adjustment to HIV/AIDS, implications of the level of adjustment, and the impact this may have on job placement. Such emotional factors as depression and anxiety sometimes interfere with successful vocational outcomes and have grave implications on one's motivation to work (Howard, 1992). Hence, without a thorough understanding of these issues clients may be placed in employment settings prematurely, which may exacerbate psychosocial stress. Until rehabilitation professionals have an understanding of the client's emotional adjustment to his or her disability, clients should not be placed in a vocational situation. Wong, Allen, and Moore (1988) stated that

> professionals must be cognizant of psychosocial dynamics, especially regarding the adjustment process to a terminal illness, feelings of fear, grief, dying, as well as the attitudes of significant others and members of the community (e.g., family and employers) toward the client with AIDS. (p. 40)

A client's reluctance to reenter the labor force may also be due to external physical signs of HIV/AIDS that are at times a source of embarrassment. The presence of skin lesions on the face or other exposed surfaces of the body from Kaposi's sarcoma is an outward sign of HIV/AIDS and may impede the vocational rehabilitation process (Howard, 1992). "The application of cosmetics to cover such lesions may help clients overcome reluctance to enter the work environment" (Howard, 1992, p. 102).

Identifying the person's vocational potential is the third phase of the rehabilitation process. This issue is contingent on one's present medical condition and functional limitations. Matheson (1984) stated that three primary questions must be answered when determining vocational implications for persons with HIV/AIDS:

1. Is it possible for the person to return to a previous job or occupation?
2. Does the person have skills and abilities that are transferable to a new employment setting?
3. Taking into consideration the medical factors, what type of rehabilitation training needs to be conducted to facilitate reemployment?

The client's social support structure, the fourth part of the rehabilitation process, is also extremely important. A strong support system is essential in assisting and motivating persons with HIV/AIDS in participating in employment services to the fullest extent possible. The person's social support system can have profound medical, psychological, and vocational implications. Persons who possess a strong support network not only are more satisfied with life, but have an enhanced quality of life.

The fifth and final factor that may have vocational implication for persons with HIV/AIDS are the attitudes and perceptions of coworkers. Many people believe that individuals with HIV/AIDS pose a communicable disease risk in the workplace (Howard, 1992). The only possible risk of HIV transmission in the workplace is remote and may occur only as a result of an accident where noninfected persons come in direct contact with blood from an open wound. The possibility of this occurrence is highly unlikely; however, it can be anticipated, and appropriate safety steps can be planned (Howard, 1992).

Another attitudinal barrier of some coworkers toward persons with HIV/AIDS may have to do with prejudice based on personal judgments about their sexual behavior or drug use (Howard, 1992). This factor may also have severe limitations on the vocational rehabilitation process of persons with HIV/AIDS. Not only should the professional be aware of the reality of attitudinal barriers in the workplace, but they must be willing to be proactive in minimizing the potential for problems. Should the need arise, the counselor may want to consider the necessity of AIDS education and sensitivity training for employees. Additionally, employers should be encouraged to adopt policy and procedure that penalize or terminate persons that discriminate against those with HIV/AIDS.

As HIV progresses, clients will develop impairments that will preclude employment in all employment settings. Cognitive impairment secondary to the effect HIV can have on the central nervous system is such an impairment. Howard (1992) stated that "moderate to severe degrees of AIDS dementia complex manifested by memory deficits, lack of coordination, and poor concentration ability can be handicapping in all work environments" (p. 101). Thus, counselors must be aware that cognitive impairments may exist in persons with HIV/AIDS and neuropsychological testing should be included as a part of the evaluation.

Obviously, rehabilitation professionals can provide assistance in many areas that will positively impact the lives of persons living with HIV/AIDS. However, until attitudinal barriers and information regarding this disease are in place, efforts will be futile. In the words of Atkins and Hancock (1993), "If we do not accept the role demanded of us by the AIDS crisis, rehabilitation professionals and educators will become part of the problem rather than an important part of its solution" (p. 34).

REFERENCES

Atkins, B., & Hancock, A. (1993). AIDS: A continuing challenge for rehabilitation professionals. *American Rehabilitation, 19*(3), 30–34.

Backer, T. E. (1987). The future of rehabilitation in the work place: Drug abuse, AIDS & disability management. *Journal of Applied Rehabilitation Counseling, 19*(2), 38–41.

Batchelor, W. F. (1984). AIDS: A public health and psychological emergency. *American Psychologist, 39,* 1279–1284.

Beck, R., Carlton, T., Allen, H., Rosenkoetter, L., & Hardy, K. (1993). Understanding and counseling special populations with HIV seropositive disease. *American Rehabilitation, 19*(3), 20–29.

Bonuck, K. A. (1993). AIDS and families: Cultural, psychosocial and functional impacts. *Social Work in Health Care, 18*(2), 75–89.

Carlton, T., Beck, R., & Allen, H. (1993). Self-help groups for HIV seropositive people. *American Rehabilitation, 19*(3), 2–9.

Centers for Disease Control. (1993). Revised classification system for HIV infection and expanded surveillance case definition for AIDS among adolescents and adults. *Journal of American Medical Association, 269,* 729–730.

Cohen, M. A. A. (1990). Biopsychosocial approach to the human immunodeficiency virus epidemic. *General Hospital Psychiatry, 12,* 98–123.

Cohen, M. A. A. (1986). A biopsychosocial approach to AIDS. *Psychomatics, 27,* 245–249.

Dew, M. A., Ragni, M. V., & Nimorwicz, P. (1991). Correlates of psychiatric distress among wives of hemophiliac men with and without HIV infection. *American Journal of Psychiatry, 148*(8), 1016–1022.

Green, S. K., & Bobele, M. (1994). Family therapists' response of AIDS: An examination of attitudes, knowledge, and contact. *Journal of Marital and Family Therapy, 20*(4), 349–367.

Howard, J. J. (1992). The acquired immunodeficiency syndrome. In M. G. Brodwin, F. Teelez, & S. K. Brodwin (Eds.), *Medical, psychosocial and vocational aspects to disability* (pp. 912–105). Athens, Georgia: Elliott & Fitzpatrick.

Kubler-Ross, E. 91969). *On death and dying.* New York: Macmillan.

Lewert, G. (1988). Children and AIDS. *The Journal of Contemporary Social Work, 21,* 348–354.

Mason, P. J., Olson, R. A., Myers, J. G., Huszti, J. C., & Kenning, M. (1989). AIDS and hemophilia: Implications for interventions with families. *Journal of Pediatric Psychology, 14*(3), 341–355.

Matheson, L. (1984). *Work capacity evaluation: Interdisciplinary approach to industrial rehabilitation.* Anaheim: Employment and Rehabilitation Institute of California.

Mulder, C. L. (1994). Psychosocial correlates and the behavioral interventions on the course of human immunodeficiency virus infection in homosexual men. *Patient Education and Counseling, 24,* 237–247.

Nichols, S. E. (1985). Psychosocial reactions of persons with the acquired immunodeficiency syndrome. *Annals of Internal Medicine, 103,* 765–767.

Nichols, S. E. (1983). Psychiatric aspects of AIDS: *Psychomatics, 24,* 1083–1089.

Wong, H., Allen, H., & Moore, J. (1988). AIDS: Dynamics and rehabilitation concerns. *Journal of Applied Rehabilitation Counseling, 19*(3), 37–41.

28

Dual Diagnosis of Mental Illness and Substance Abuse: Contemporary Challenges for Rehabilitation

Susan D. M. Kelley and John J. Benshoff

D uring the past ten years, persons with coexisting substance use and mental health disorders have become the focus of attention for research studies and clinical seminars around the country. Despite increasing attention, however, dual disorders remain under-diagnosed. Persons with dual disorders are challenging to treat and have poorer outcomes than persons with single disorders. Treatment costs associated with dual disorders are substantial. Experts describe these persons as unmotivated and treatment noncompliant and suggest that their aggression, impulsivity, criminal and suicidal behavior, verbal hostility, and myriad social problems make them poor treatment candidates. Other experts point out that many of these individuals have been extruded from both mental health and substance abuse treatment systems, that treatment failure is as much the responsibility of inappropriate systems of care. There is growing professional concurrence that new integrated systems of treatment, rehabilitation, and recovery are needed for individuals with dual diagnosis (Jerrell, 1996; Minkoff & Drake, 1991; Oldham & Riba, 1995).

PREVALENCE OF DUAL DISORDERS

Rates of incidence and prevalence of dual disorders seem to be increasing. This is attributable in part to expanding awareness and better diagnostic skills of clinicians. It may also be attributable to unemployment, downward social drift, a pervasive sense of communal despair, and myriad factors that place vulnerable populations at risk. Deinstitutionalization and changing patterns of drug use in our culture have also contributed to real increases in prevalence. Prospective

From *Journal of Applied Rehabilitation Counseling,* 28(3) (Fall 1997), 43–49. Reprinted with permission.

research data regarding the onset and development of dual disorders are lacking; but recent epidemiologic studies (Kessler, McGonagle & Zhao, 1994; Regier, Farmer, & Rae, 1990) give us some useful information about clinical and nonclinical populations.

Regier et al. (1990) conducted two catchment area studies (ECA) of clinical populations. They found that, of 20,291 persons surveyed, 32.6% met **DSM III-R** criteria for at least one mental health disorder and a substance use disorder. Among persons in general psychiatric settings, over one-third had problems with substance use or dependence; 47% of individuals with a lifetime diagnosis of schizophrenia or schizophreniform disorder met criteria for some form of substance abuse or dependence.

Kessler et al. (1994) sampled 8,098 noninstitutionalized persons between the ages of 15 and 54, living in 48 states, in the National Comorbidity Study. Using the Composite International Diagnostic Interview, Kessler et al. found that 19.3% met criteria for lifetime affective disorder, 24.9% met criteria for anxiety disorder, and 26.6% experienced at some time a substance use disorder. Using their equations on observed rates of mental health disorders in the general population, Kessler and colleagues estimated that 10% or more of persons with substance use disorders have concurrent nonsubstance disorders.

In their study of alcohol use and abuse among people with disabilities, Moore and Li (1994a) found that individuals with disabilities used alcohol at rates approximating the general population. They noted that nearly half of their respondents who cited a history of mental illness reported using alcohol. In another study of individuals seeking rehabilitation services, Moore and Li (1994b) found that individuals with disabilities were much more likely to have abused illicit (e.g., cocaine, marijuana, etc.) psychoactive substances and tobacco than the general population.

A wide range of mental health disorders are more common among persons with substance use disorders than among their non-substance abusing peers. The odds ratios are especially telling: People with substance disorders have a 15.6 times greater rate of antisocial personality disorder, 5.8 times greater rate of mood disorders (bipolar disorder and depression), 5.0 times greater rate of anxiety disorders, and 10.9 times greater rate of other/ poly substance use disorders (Regier et al., 1990). Doweiko (1996) suggests there is an especially strong relationship between affective disorders and substance abuse among adolescents, and, according to Hanson and Venturelli (1995), adolescents who abuse psychoactive substances have suicide rates far in excess of national averages. The counterpart for antisocial personality disorder in adults is conduct disorder in adolescents. Adolescents diagnosed with conduct disorder are likely to demonstrate behaviors which impinge on the right of others, or which violate normative societal standards of conduct (American Psychiatric Association, 1994). Gang behaviors, sexual violence, relationship development, other acting out behaviors are closely linked to psychoactive substance abuse (Fishbein & Pease, 1996; Hanson & Venturelli, 1995).

The anxiety disorder classification embraces posttraumatic stress disorder and may be seen in Vietnam and Gulf War veterans who present for treatment with dual diagnoses. Opiate dependence has been strongly linked to conduct disorder and/or antisocial personality disorder while alcohol dependence has been strongly associated with bipolar illness and schizophrenia. Knowlton (1995) suggests that individuals with bi-polar disorders are 7 times as likely as members of the general population to develop alcoholism problems.

There appear to be connections between attention deficit disorder and stimulant dependence, although the literature on this issue is inconsistent at present. Literature on attention deficit disorder (ADD) lists drug taking or alcohol abuse as common behaviors among adolescents with ADD, without clear cut linkage or causality demonstrated in a consistent fashion.

Contrary to popular belief, there is no empirical support for the "addictive personality." Persons with substance use disorders often have dependent personality traits, which are probably secondary to the patterns and habits of substance use (Francis & Miller, 1991).

INFLUENCE OF PSYCHOPATHOLOGY ON OUTCOME

Two perspectives dominate the thinking about mental health disorders linked with substance use. The first view of secondary psychopathology is very much part of the tradition of self-help groups such as Alcoholics Anonymous which is supported by research data (Westermeyer, 1991; Woody, McLellan, Bedrick, 1995). This view postulates that the psychotoxic effects of substances like alcohol, cocaine, and benzodiazepines cause most of the psychopathology seen in substance abusing persons. Thus, the treatment implication is that treatment focuses on the substance abuse or dependence and successful intervention will reduce or eliminate the psychiatric symptoms. Those who adhere strongly to this view believe that attention to treating psychiatric symptoms such as dysphoria, depression, anxiety, and irritability diverts attention from the substance use disorder and introduces troublesome resistance to therapy. Moreover, individuals with dual diagnoses may perceive mixed messages. Professionals provide counseling and medication to treat psychiatric problems whereas the implicit and, at times, explicit message received at peer self help groups (Alcoholics Anonymous, Narcotics Anonymous, etc.) may be to discontinue all mind altering chemicals, including legitimately prescribed psychotropic medications (Aliesan & Firth, 1990). Carried to extremes, these messages can result in an individual with bipolar illness and alcohol abuse hearing in an AA meeting to discontinue psychotropic medications such as lithium or Depakote.

The second perspective, the *converse* of secondary psychopathology, is the self-medication hypothesis of addictive behaviors (Khantzian, 1985). It postulates that underlying psychological problems are significant contributors to the development and maintenance of substance use disorders. In this view, the underlying psychopathology is primary and the substance abuse or dependence is secondary and used as a means to cope with the painful psychological problems. Doweiko (1996) notes that opiate addicts may be drawn to the drug to deal with "powerful feelings of rage and anger" (p. 14). Glover, Janikowski and Benshoff (1995) have suggested that victims of incest may use drugs or alcohol to suppress the psychological pain of memories or to cope with ongoing events. The implication is that adequate treatment of the psychopathology is necessary for treatment of the substance use disorder. Proponents of this view believe that the substance use disorder will take care of itself provided the underlying psychopathology is treated; failure to do the latter will result in guaranteed treatment failure of the substance use disorder. Carried to extremes, some persons may be in therapy or analysis for years without efforts to address their substance use.

The truth probably lies between these two perspectives. Neither is wholly accurate. Some persons with abuse or dependence disorders report the onset of psychiatric symptoms before the inception of substance abuse problems, while others report that mental illness symptomatology occurred after the advent of substance abuse disorders (Tracy, Josiassen, & Bellack, 1995). For other individuals, the onset of psychiatric disability and psychoactive substance abuse or dependence are indistinguishable, a condition conceptualized as shared vulnerability (Tracy, Josiassen, & Bellack, 1995).

Questions of onset order aside, for nearly all individuals, the two disabilities have a mutually exacerbating, interactive effect (Raudenbush, 1996). By their nature, all psychoactive substances produce psychoactive effects; however the production of psychiatric symptoms is widely variable. For example, hallucinogens or inhalants are clearly psychotropic while caffeine or nicotine are less so. Paranoia and psychotic-like symptoms are associated with hallucinogens and stimulants like amphetamine and cocaine. Anxiety and depression are linked to alcohol.

There appears to be a gender relationship linkage issue with alcohol and depression. Jung (1994) reports that women are more likely than men to be dually diagnosed with alcoholism and depression. There are also gender differences, especially salient in neurocognitive status. There is some evidence that females have comparable or even more severe neurocognitive deficits with less severe drinking histories and may incur worse neurotoxic effects from alcohol at lower levels of ingestion.

An intriguing finding to emerge from longitudinal studies is that comorbid disorders, (i.e., dual disorders) may emerge from a common or shared vulnerability (Tracy, Josiassen, & Bellack, 1995) and the symptoms may be intrinsic to the illness of an as yet unnamed new disorder or classification of disorders. This is borne out in studies that focus on an atypical depression, a form that seems unique and specific in persons with coexisting substance use disorders. Researchers indicate that double depression, acute major depression layered on chronic ongoing depression, is such a form (Mirin & Weiss, 1991).

Other researchers have postulated models to explain the relationship between psychopathology and substance abuse. The sensitivity model suggests that, for some individuals, psychiatric disorders may alter the course of substance abuse. Anecdotal reports from treatment centers suggest that some clients may self-medicate depressive disorders with cocaine or amphetamine like substances while discontinuing prescribed psychiatric medications. Others may use cocaine or other stimulants to augment prescribed psychoactive medications. The early potentiation or exacerbation model suggests that substance abuse may alter the course of psychiatric disorders. This impact is readily seen in alcoholics who self-medicate depression with alcohol. Individuals with personality disorders who drink or use stimulant drugs (e.g., crack cocaine) may exacerbate their problems because of the disinhibiting effects of the drugs (Woody, McLellan, & Bedrick, 1995).

Individuals with dual disabilities may experience a variety of severe and frequently occurring medical problem⌐ (AIDS, diabetes, cirrhosis, gastrointestinal disorders, respiratory problems, etc.) which may be a consequence of, or exacerbate substance abuse and mental health problems (Mowbray et al., 1995). Treatment provision for these triply diagnosed (Knowlton, 1995) individuals is further compounded by their medical problems.

TREATMENT AND REHABILITATION

Traditional treatment outcomes and rehabilitation have focused on cure and/or stabilization of the disability process. Realistic and meaningful outcomes may be related more to the *reduction in severity of symptoms*, not to distinctions between abuse, dependence or psychiatric diagnosis alone, for individuals with mental illness and substance abuse problems. Consequently, the ability to remain abstinent from alcohol and drug consumption and to continue to function in the community are more meaningful and more important markers for success than the presence or absence of diagnostic labels. It is important to recognize and respond to the chronic, long term nature of dual diagnosis disabilities. Treatment for acute substance-induced mental health disorders is usually brief because of the relatively transient nature of the symptoms. Treatment of dual diagnoses, on the other hand, may involve periods of inpatient treatment and often include combining psychological and pharmacological therapies. The dosage, frequency of use, and addictive or abuse potential properties of any pharmacotherapy used with those dually diagnosed must be carefully considered and monitored to minimize the chances for abuse or misuse. This is especially true for the benzodiazepines (anti-anxiety drugs) which have addictive properties. The popular viewpoint contends that the abuse potential of low-potency, slow-onset benzodiazepines is much less than for high-potency, rapid-onset psychoactive pharmaceuticals. However, aside from anecdotal or case reports, empirical evidence on this issue is lacking.

Long-term pharmacotherapy is likely for persons with schizophrenia, mood, or anxiety disorders and paramount consideration must be given to stabilization, prolonged maintenance, and then rehabilitation/recovery. Axis I disorders such as schizophrenia, depression, or bipolar illness are more amenable to pharmacotherapy than Axis II disorders such as personality disorders. Symptoms that reflect primary disorders probably exert a stronger influence on outcome than those that are secondary because of the seeming relatively transient nature of the latter. Traditional treatment for individuals with substance abuse disorders have focused on short term and medically based interventions (e.g., detoxification) for acute treatment needs, followed by long term counseling support, usually emphasizing peer self help resources. Recently, cognitive behavioral strategies have gained increasing prominence in substance abuse treatment.

Drug counseling or pharmacotherapy alone is less effective than approaches that combine counseling, education, psychosocial intervention, pharmacotherapy, and the use of a variety of community based supports and services for persons with dual disorders.

Recent studies demonstrated that individuals with dual diagnoses who received a variety of substance abuse education and support services did significantly better than individuals who received little or nothing in the way of education and support (Crump & Milling, 1996; Jarrell, 1996). Treatment efficacy is optimized when therapeutic interventions are either integrated or administered concomitantly to ensure continuity of care.

STAFF DEVELOPMENT ISSUES

The rehabilitation and treatment of individuals with dual mental health and substance abuse disabilities present unique challenges for the training of rehabilitation specialists. Effective service delivery requires the development of knowledge, attitudes, and skills conducive to serving persons with dual disorders. This interplay of knowledge, skills, and attitudes, must then be augmented with adequate clinical supervision and role models to create successful programs. Rehabilitation counselors may encounter persons with dual disorders whose primary disability is either mental illness or substance abuse. Consequently, effective work in evolving integrated care systems requires knowledge of mental health and substance abuse service delivery systems plus complex, contemporary, relevant skills and attitudes.

In programs that structure services to meet integrated guidelines, counselors function both as direct services providers and case managers. They may co-lead groups consisting of active users (pretreatment or engagement/psychoeducation groups), those who are abstinent (active treatment), and those who are building repertoires of relapse prevention skills. They link clients to a variety of needed services. Hence, the functions and tasks of the professional encompass more complex clinical diagnosis, group facilitation, and teaching skills in addition to the usual and customary rehabilitation coordination, management, and counseling functions. In addition to being aware of traditional service delivery systems, rehabilitation counselors must come to grips with the continually emerging and changing demands of managed mental health care. Shortened stays in inpatient environments, increased use of psychotropic medication, greater scrutiny of treatment planning and delivery, and vigilant, external case management have become the norms of service delivery (Foos, Ottens, & Hill, 1991). In the past, the principal site of service delivery was dictated often by chance. If an individual with dual diagnosis walked into the mental health center, the primary disability became mental illness and vice-versa. Accurate diagnosis of dual disorders may be impeded by inadequate screening strategies and tools, under-reporting of substance abuse or mental health problems, concealment of co-morbid problems, or failure to provide accurate histories by the client because of acute intoxication or psychosis (Milling, Faulkner, & Craig, 1994).

Frequently in the past, initial referrals were to inpatient treatment followed by a lengthy course of outpatient treatment under the guise of the continuum of care. Now, managed care emphases require that rehabilitation professionals make quick and accurate distinctions about needed types of intervention such as engagement, persuasion, active treatment, and relapse prevention, and levels of care such as inpatient, outpatient, intensive outpatient, day treatment, supported employment, community living arrangements, and peer self-help programs. Case management goes beyond the typical internal agency practices of assessment, planning, linking, monitoring, and advocacy. Of special importance is the ability to consult with other agencies, especially managed care companies and their utilization reviewers.

Rehabilitation professionals who work with individuals with dual diagnoses will plan, work, and relate on multi-disciplinary teams comprised of professionals and recovering paraprofessional staff who provide direct and other services. The increased use of psychotropic medications and the emergence of medical-model behavioral management strategies may place psychiatrists and psychiatric nurses at the nexus of treatment delivery. Therefore, counselors must demonstrate a thorough understanding of medication uses in collaboration with medical staff with special regard to informed consent. Informed consent may be a particularly difficult issue. Can informed consent exist if the client is hallucinating or if judgment is clouded by continuing drug or alcohol abuse? Counselors, too, confer with colleagues whose principal credential may be recovery from addiction or mental illness to determine if a behavioral management strategy is effective.

Treatment planning with this population goes beyond the usual intervention, which is to emphasize very individualized alternative treatment strategies for more resistive and less compliant clients. Often these plans may be based on court mandated presentencing evaluations conducted under court rulings or state statues. An essential part of plans may be the establishment and consistent enforcement of reasonable and appropriate standards of community conduct to permit maximal level of client functioning (Luke et al., 1996). Individuals with troubling symptoms may experience difficulty in receiving and participating in basic services. Mowbray et al. (1995) note that staff in mental health facilities may respond with punitive measures to a client who presents resistant or acting-out drug or alcohol related behavior; staff in substance abuse facilities may respond negatively to individuals who present with delusions, hallucinations, or similar mental illness symptoms. Moreover, they note that Alcoholics and Narcotics Anonymous groups may reject individuals co-diagnosed with mental illness because of concerns about meeting disruption due to socially unacceptable behavior, drug (i.e., medication) use, and prejudices about the place of these individuals in the fellowship. Conversely, mental health peer recovery group members may see alcohol problems as moral issues and not amenable to their support interventions.

PROFESSIONAL ISSUES

Appropriate respect and sensitivity to the cultural, and psychosocial values of persons with dual disorders, their families or significant others, and other multi-disciplinary team members are vital counselor characteristics in working with this very heterogeneous population. Some individuals with dual disorders may be well acculturated to the mental health patient role (Aliesan & Firth, 1990), while others may be more acculturated into the drug culture, and many may be homeless, or living in marginal conditions. Long periods of institutionalization or separation from mainstream society may have resulted in life skill areas where maturation and development have been delayed or inhibited (Raudenbush, 1996).

Moreover, counselors should be comfortable in dealing with personally and emotionally charged situations including the counselor's own counter-transference reactions in the face of impulsive or disruptive behaviors and poor judgement. Counselors may find themselves in situations where they must demonstrate a willingness to attend to a variety of opinions, ideas, and attitudes set forth by persons with dual disorders or the community at large. Finally, developing a tolerance for slow progress and frustration is essential. Dually diagnosed substance abuse-mental illness disabilities are long term disorders with a high frequency of relapse (Aliesan & Firth, 1990; Raudenbush, 1996).

Current emphasis on short term, solution based therapies may be inconsistent with the long-term needs and complex problems presented by persons with dual diagnosis. Recent trends toward criminalization of homelessness and societally deviant behaviors may exacerbate these needs and problems. Professionals need to move beyond myopic perceptions of practice to embrace an understanding of the political and cultural values and realities of society and an understanding of the interplay of the diverse societal networks (mental health, substance abuse, criminal justice, health, etc.) which have an impact on the treatment of individuals with dual diagnoses. Client involvement with multiple systems of care and service increases the complexity and problem-potential of service delivery. Clients may be in various stages of treatment or recovery, depending upon the severity of problems, types of interventions, and client motivation towards recovery (Knowlton, 1995).

The individualization of treatment planning and the active involvement of individuals with dual diagnoses in the treatment planning and treatment implementation process are essential (Franco, et al., 1995). Research (Weinberg & Koegel, 1996) suggest that involvement of clients in the treatment process can do much to promote treatment efficacy. Rehabilitation educational strategies that focus on multi-disciplinary involvement, advocacy and team building would be helpful in this area of concern.

COUNSELOR TRAINING ISSUES

While the population of individuals with dual substance abuse and mental illness disorders is on the increase, there are few integrated treatment programs and even fewer training programs that cross train professional staff to meet the demands of this population (Minkoff & Drake, 1991). Moreover, few counselor educators have clinical experience with individuals with dual disorders and with emerging integrated treatment models. Nonetheless, the clear research message is that concomitant treatment is preferable to current non-integrated models (Jerrell, 1996).

In a substance use specialization in rehabilitation counselor education, dual disorders must be infused into relevant courses and presented in all their complexity. Dual disorders clearly fit into courses oriented toward psychopathology or medical aspects of disability. They also fit into courses such as assessment where students may develop analytical skills to better understand functional limitations imposed by dual disorders.

Because of their many problems, and often slow or limited progress, working with individuals with dual diagnosis is frequently seen as less valued and less prestigious in the eyes of educators, students and the behavioral health community. Moreover, numerous systems conflicts such as bureaucratic entanglements, professional elitism ("for psychologists or physicians only"), professional territoriality and weak links with academic training (rehabilitation, psychology, and social work) programs are continuing barriers.

SUMMARY

Persons with dual disorders of mental illness and substance abuse pose unique challenges to today's treatment and rehabilitation service providers. The increase in the number of individuals requiring treatment for concurrent mental illness and substance abuse problems may be attributable to a number of societal and professional factors. With continued emphases on deinstitutionalization and community based care, few individuals with mental illness are related to extensive confinement in large state-run institutions (Smith, 1996). Instead, they are being treated, appropriately, in smaller, community based facilities. Consequently, the upsurge in the prevalence of joint mental health-substance abuse disorders may be partially a function of increased client participation and visibility in a community treatment system ill-prepared and under-funded to meet the needs of this population.

The expanded availability of drugs and the expanded drug menu and differing side effects may be a factor, also. Twenty years ago principal drugs of abuse on the streets were alcohol and the opiates, both sedative hypnotic drugs. The emergence of crack-cocaine and synthetic amphetamine-type drugs has drastically altered both the context of drug abuse and its consequences. Violent, antisocial behavior is more frequently seen among abusers of stimulant drugs, a problem often compounded by the presence of a co-existing mental health problem which may include an acting out component. Unfortunately while drug availability and the negative behaviors associated with drug abuse have broadened, treatment continues to be predicated on paradigms reflecting a single, sedative-hypnotic drug type and a narrow range of behaviors.

Finally, the increased prevalence of concurrent disorders may be the result of increased attention to their existence. Rehabilitation Services Administration funding of the Substance Abuse Resources and Disability Issues (SARDI) Project of Wright State University has generated increased practitioner awareness and understanding of dual disorders. Additionally many rehabilitation counselor training programs (e.g., Southern Illinois University at Carbondale, University of North Texas, Virginia Commonwealth University, and others) offer specializations that prepare prospective rehabilitation counselors to work with individuals with psychoactive substance abuse disorders (Benshoff, Janikowski, Taricone, & Brenner, 1990). This increased knowledge among practitioners and students may result in heightened awareness of joint problems and increased willingness to serve this challenging population.

The question of treating psychopathology as either a component of continuing substance abuse or as a unique disability, or as a consequence of a mutually indistinguishable concurrent pathology exacerbates the challenges faced by the strategies which emphasize brief interventions. Specialized knowledge, understanding, and training will be required to serve individuals with dual disabilities effectively and flexibly in contemporary hybridized and integrated service delivery systems (Ridgely, 1992).

The efforts of rehabilitation counselor training programs to expand curricular offering are an important stride in developing integrated service delivery, and cross trained rehabilitation counselors will be uniquely positioned to serve individuals with dual disabilities. However, continued research is required to identify optimal rehabilitation strategies, and continued communication among professionals will be essential to overcome barriers crated by bureaucratic entanglements, parochial professional allegiances and narrow treatment paradigms.

REFERENCES

Aliesan, K., & Firth, R. C. (1990). A MICO program: Outpatient rehabilitation services for individuals with concurrent mental illness and chemical abuse disorders. *Journal of Applied Rehabilitation Counseling, 21*(3), 25–29.

American Psychiatric Association. (1994). *Diagnostic and statistical manual of mental disorders* (4th ed.). Washington, DC: Author.

Benshoff, J. J., Janikowski, T. P., Taricone, P. F., & Brenner, J. S. (1990). Alcohol and drug abuse: A content analysis of the rehabilitation literature. *Journal of Applied Rehabilitation Counseling, 21*(4), 9–12.

Crump, M. T., & Milling, R. N. (1996). The efficacy of substance abuse education among dual diagnosis patients. *Journal of Substance Abuse Treatment, 13,* 141–144.

Doweiko, H. E. (1996). *Concepts of chemical dependency* (3rd ed.). Pacific Grove, CA: Brooks/Cole.

Fishbein, D. H., & Pease, S. E. (1996). *The dynamics of drug abuse.* Boston: Allyn and Bacon.

Foos, J. A., Ottens, A. J., & Hill, L. K. (1991). Managed mental health: A Primer for counselors. *Journal of Counseling and Development, 69,* 3332–340.

Francis, R., & Miller, S. (Eds.) (1991). *Clinical textbook of addictive disorders.* New York: Guilford Press.

Franco, H., Galanter, M., Castaneda, R., & Patterson, J. (1995). Combining behavioral and self-help approaches in the inpatient management of dually diagnosed patients. *Journal of Substance Abuse Treatment, 12,* 227–232.

Glover, N. M., Janikowski, T. P., & Benshoff, J. J. (1995). The incidence of incest histories among clients receiving substance abuse treatment. *Journal of Counseling and Development, 73,* 475–480.

Hanson, G., & Venturelli, P. J. (1995). *Drugs and society* (4th ed.). Boston: Jones and Bartlett.

Jerrell, J. M. (1996). Toward cost-effective care for persons with dual diagnoses. *Journal of Mental Health Administration, 23,* 329–337.

Jung, J. (1994). *Under the influence: Alcohol and human behavior.* Pacific Grove, CA: Brooks/Cole.

Kessler, R., McGonagle, K., & Zhao, S. (1994). Lifetime and 12 month prevalence of DSM III-R psychiatric disorders in the United States: Results for the National Comorbidity Survey. *Archives of General Psychiatry, 51,* 8–19.

Khantzian, E. J. (1985). The self medication hypothesis of addictive disorders: Focus on heroin and cocaine dependence. *American Journal of Psychiatry, 142,* 1259–1264.

Knowlton, L. (1995). Public and research views of dual diagnosis explored. *MHI* (On-Line). Available : http://www.mhsource.com/edu/psytimes/p950536.html.

Luke, D. A., Mowbray, C. T., Klump, K., Herman, S. E., & Bootsmiller, B. (1996). Exploring the diversity of dual diagnosis: Utility of cluster analysis for program planning. *Journal of Mental Health Administration, 23,* 298–316.

Milling, R. N., Faulkner, L. R., & Craig, J. M. (1994). Problems in the recognition and treatment of patients with dual diagnoses. *Journal of Substance Abuse Treatment, 11,* 267–271.

Minkoff, K., & Drake, R. (Eds.) (1991). *Dual diagnosis of major mental illness and substance disorder.* (Number 50, Summer). San Francisco: Jossey Bass.

Mirin, S., & Weiss, R. (1991). Substance abuse and mental illness. In Frances, R. & Miller, S. (Eds.). *Clinical Textbook of Addictive Disorders* (pp. 271–298). New York: Guilford Press.

Mowbray, C. T., Solomon, M., Ribisl, K. M., Ebejer, M. A., Deiz, N., Brown, W., Bandla, H., Luke, D. S., Davidson, W. S., & Herman S. (1995). Treatment for mental illness and substance abuse in a public psychiatric hospital: Successful strategies and challenging problems. *Journal of Substance Abuse Treatment, 12,* 129–139.

Moore, D., & Li, L. (1994a). Alcohol use and drinking related consequences among consumers of disability services. *Rehabilitation Counseling Bulletin, 38,* 124–133.

Moore, D., & Li, L. (1994b). Substance use among applicants for vocational rehabilitation services. *Journal of Rehabilitation, 60*(4), 48–53.

Oldham, J. & Riba, M. (Eds.) (1995). *Review of Psychiatry, Volume 14.* Washington, DC: American Psychiatric Press.

Raudenbush, D. (1996). Substance abuse treatment for mental illness. *Proceedings of the First National Conference on Substance Abuse and Co-Existing Disabilities,* (pp. 58–60). Dayton, Ohio: Wright State University.

Regier, D., Farmer, M., & Rae, D. (1990). Co-morbidity of mental disorders with alcohol and other drug abuse: results from the Epidemiologic Catchment Area (ECA) Study. *Journal of the American Medical Association, 264,* 2511–2518.

Ridgely, M. (1992). Creating integrated programs for severely mentally ill persons with substance disorders. In Minkoff, K. & Drake, R. (Eds.). *Dual diagnosis of major mental illness and substance disorder.* (pp. 29–41). San Francisco: Jossey-Bass.

Smith, D. E. (1996). The 1995 distinguished lecturer in substance abuse. *Journal of Substance Abuse Treatment, 13,* 289–294.

Tracy, J., Josiassen, R., & Bellack, A. (1995). Neuropsychology of dual diagnosis: Understanding the combined effects of schizophrenia and substance use disorders. *Clinical Psychology Review, 15*(2), 67–97.

Weinberg, D., & Koegel, P. (1996). Social model treatment and individuals with dual diagnosis: An ethnographic analysis of therapeutic practice. *Journal of Mental Health Administration, 23,* 272–287.

Westermeyer, J. (1991). Historical and social context of psychoactive substance disorders. In Frances, R., & Miller, S. (Eds.), *Clinical Textbook of Addictive Disorders* (pp. 23–40). New York: Guilford Press.

Woody, G., McLellan, A., & Bedrick, J. (1995). Dual diagnosis. In Oldham, J. & Reba, M. (Eds.). *Review of Psychiatry, Volume 14.* (pp. 83–104). Washington, DC: American Psychiatric Press.

29

Recovery from Serious Mental Illness: What It Is and How to Support People in Their Recovery

LeRoy Spaniol, Cheryl Gagne,

and Martin Koehler

INTRODUCTION

There are four questions that we want to raise in this article. An understanding of these questions and our responses to them have been very helpful to us in working more effectively with people with serious mental illness. These four questions are:

1. What is recovery?
2. What are people recovering from?
3. What is the "impact" of "what" people are recovering from?
4. How can people be assisted by professionals in their recovery?

WHAT IS RECOVERY?

Recovery is a process, an outcome, and a vision. As a process, recovery is a common human experience. We all experience recovery at some point in our lives from injury, from illness, from loss, or from trauma. Recovery is a process of healing physically and emotionally, of adjusting one's attitudes, feelings, perceptions, beliefs, roles and goals in life. It is a painful process, yet often a process of self-discovery, self-renewal, and transformation. Recovery is a deeply emotional process. Recovery involves creating a new personal vision for oneself.

From *Developments in Ambulatory Health Care*, (in press). Arlington, VA: Association for Ambulatory Behavioral Health Care. Reprinted with permission.

As an outcome, recovery is the ability to return to work, to live in housing of one's choice, to have friends and an intimate relationship, and to become a contributing member of one's community. Yet, historically, schizophrenia has been viewed as an irreversible illness with increasing disability over time—hopeless and intractable. While the impact of severe mental illness is devastating to those who experience it and to their families, it does not appear that schizophrenia is a disease of slow and progressive deterioration as was once widely believed (Bleuler, 1950; Kraepelin, 1902). People with schizophrenia can achieve partial or full recovery from the illness at any point during its course, even in the later stages of their life (Harding, Strauss, Hafez, & Liberman, 1987; Huber, Gross, Schuttler, & Linz, 1980). As Harding has said:

> ". . . the course of severe psychiatric disorder is a complex, dynamic, and heterogeneous process which is non-linear in its patterns moving toward significant improvement over time and helped along by an active, developing person in interaction with his or her environment" (Harding, 1986).

Numerous current studies have demonstrated that one-half to two-thirds of people with severe mental illness significantly recover over time (Harding & Zahniser, 1994; Harding, Zubin, & Strauss, 1987, 1992). The evidence for a specific, inflexible natural history of every disorder is simply not there.

As a vision, recovery is the organizing construct that can guide the planning and implementation of mental health services because recovery is the purpose and the goal of all the programs and services that combine to assist the person with a psychiatric disability (Anthony, 1993). The goal of recovery is to become more deeply human, in all of our uniqueness. The goal of recovery is to become part of the human stream, in all of our individuality (Deegan, 1988; 1995).

One of the main benefits of utilizing recovery as the key organizing concept in our work with people with psychiatric disability is that it allows us to look at the whole person, in all of his or her humanity, instead of just at their illness (Deegan, 1995). If all human beings experience recovery, then people with serious mental illness, who are also human, also experience recovery.

WHAT ARE PEOPLE RECOVERING FROM?

It is important to be clear about "what" people are recovering from. From a psychosocial perspective people are recovering from the catastrophe of mental illness and from multiple and recurring traumas: trauma from the illness; the medical treatment of the illness, negative professional attitudes; lack of appropriate assisting skills of professionals; devaluing and disempowering programs, practices, and environments; lack of enriching opportunities; and stigma and discrimination in society. Professionals need to acknowledge the multiple sources of trauma experienced by people with mental illness. People with mental illness are well aware of these many sources of trauma. It is important that those who provide services validate these experiences and assist people with mental illness to cope with them. Because of the stereotypes prevalent in the training of many mental health professionals the "illness" has historically been the focal point of interventions (Minkoff, 1987). And the symptoms and behavior of the person have been primarily associated with the "illness," while the other sources of impact on the person have been rarely acknowledged. This has left many people with mental illness feeling devalued and ignored and has resulted in mistrust in and alienation from the mental health system.

WHAT IS THE IMPACT OF WHAT PEOPLE ARE RECOVERING FROM?

It is important to understand the "impact" of "what" people are recovering from, that is, "how" people are affected by the catastrophe of the illness and the multiple traumas they are recovering from. We know that multiple and recurring traumas have a devastating impact on the lives of people who experience them. The impact is devastating because people are left profoundly disconnected from themselves, from others, from their environments, and from meaning or purpose in life. While the illness itself causes people to feel disconnected, stigma and discrimination (negative personal, professional, and societal values, attitudes and practices) further disconnect people and represent serious barriers to building a new life. There are four types of impact that we would like to discuss in this paper.

Loss of Sense of Self

People with mental illness experience severe trauma to their sense of self. Although an enduring and developing core of meaning and knowing has been acquired over time by the person before the disorder, the illness and its treatment severely fragment and traumatize the self (Estroff, 1989). While the self is directly and deeply affected, it continues as an enduring, personal core that precedes, transcends, and outlasts the illness. Within every person with a mental illness there continues to be a persisting, healthy, trying-to-survive self and personhood, with a self-acknowledged history (Estroff, 1989).

As Estroff (1989) has reported, sickness in our culture alters the self (e.g., I am not myself today.) We reject the dysfunctional self of sickness as "not me." Yet if the illness persists, what is the implication for the self?

There are a number of dilemmas confronting the person as the illness persists (Estroff, 1989):

1. When being "not myself" is my self, that is, the illness persists.
2. When the most self-seeing, self-knowing, self-confirming others lose, alter, or put away the person's prior, not-sick self so it is unverifiable to and with them.
3. When the core self is no longer validated by others.

4. I "am" or I "have" an illness. How does the person integrate the illness, its treatment, and the self? What are the implications for the various options? For example, is there a continuum of joining versus separating from the illness? What is the experience of the person?

It is important to acknowledge the mediating function of the self. The self is a central and mediating factor among our various areas of functioning such as vocational, intellectual, emotional, social, and spiritual (Davidson & Strauss, 1992). When the self is less functional, our overall functioning will be impaired. When the self is functional, each area of functioning benefits synergistically. The self is the agent of recovery. Disconnection from the self results in an inability to move forward with one's life.

The self also has a social function. So when the self is not functioning well, the person becomes more easily isolated and alienated from others. The isolation that people with psychiatric disability feel has many other causes such as stigmatizing attitudes of some professionals and family members, unemployment and poverty, hypersensitivity to stimulation and affect, impairments in attention, concentration and communication, and disorientation and confusion (Davidson & Stayner, 1997). The inability to share these barriers with others further alienates and isolates people with mental illness.

Chronicity, as a characteristic of the self, and from a psychosocial perspective, is a transformation of a previous, enduring, known, and valued self into a less known and knowable, devalued, and dysfunctional self (Estroff, 1989). This occurs both within the person and in the eyes of family, peers, and professionals (Estroff, 1989). Chronicity, passivity, and dependence are fostered by an internal or external environment that undermines the functional self (Davidson & Strauss, 1992). Chronicity from this perspective is a form of learned hopelessness and helplessness that continues to be supported by uninformed knowledge, attitudes, and practices.

Loss of Power

This is a loss of one's ability to act in one's own interest. This is a loss of belief in oneself. This is the loss of one's sense of agency—oneself as an active agent. People with psychiatric disability experience themselves as having no power, no real choices. Power is lost through the severing of our connections. When our connections are broken, we feel powerless. There are a variety of forms of power (Mack, 1994). The power that is healing, that is more than oneself, that can move another person, is acquired through our relationships. It is power with people not over people. It is a power acquired through reconnecting with oneself, others, our larger environment, and larger meanings in life. It is a power acquired through a deepening of our capacity to experience life fully and directly without being overwhelmed or intimidated. It is a power acquired by coming alive.

Loss of Meaning

Meaning in life is intimately connected to the various roles we play. Unfortunately, the onset of mental illness frequently interrupts the valued roles of people, that is, wife, husband, mother, father, worker, student, son, daughter, or sibling. People with mental illness are still frequently assumed not to be capable of fulfilling these roles. And, people with mental illness often come to believe this themselves. One of the most frustrating experiences of people with mental illness is the awareness of the life course of friends and siblings they grew up with who have gone on to college, have acquired a career, have married, and children. People with mental illness have learned that these natural life events may never be available to them and they mourn them deeply.

Loss of Hope

The accumulation of traumatizing, devaluing experiences wears people down over time and leads to the giving up of hope. Hopelessness, apathy, and indifference are best seen not as problems but as learned solutions. They are strategies that desperate people adopt in order to stay alive (Deegan, 1995). They are strategies desperate people adopt in order to manage an inequality in the balance of power (Mack, 1994). Without hope it is hard to cope. People just barely survive. But they don't really feel alive or a part of life. We, also, certainly know of many examples where hope has been taken away; where someone has said there is no hope. This is especially devastating to people with a psychiatric disability. And, if it comes from a mental health professional, it is doubly disabling.

HOW CAN PEOPLE BE ASSISTED BY PROFESSIONALS IN THEIR RECOVERY?

It is important for professionals to understand "how" people can be assisted in their recovery, that is, in recovering from the impact of multiple and recurring traumas. Recovery is a process by which people with psychiatric disability rebuild and further develop their personal, social, environmental, and spiritual connections, and confront the devastating effects of stigma through personal empowerment. It is never too late to begin the recovery process. Understanding the recovery process and one's own recovery experience are important first steps in returning to a life that is personally fulfilling and a life that contributes to others. Recovery is ultimately a journey of the heart—a choice for life, a choice to live and to have a life (Deegan, 1996).

Reclaiming the Sense of Self

The onset of psychiatric disability and the stigma associated with it causes "self-shock." The sense of self is traumatized. It needs to heal and to recover. Recovery then, in one sense, is recovery from "self-shock."

The importance of rediscovering and reconstructing an enduring sense of the self as an active and responsible agent provides significant, and perhaps crucial, source of improvement for the person with mental illness. The sense of self provides a key theoretical construct in the understanding and treatment of the person (Davidson & Strauss, 1992).

Some authors have noted the way an enhanced sense of self, such as a sense of self-efficacy, self-esteem, and an internal locus of control, can help ameliorate various aspects of a disorder and encourage efforts at coping in the face of traumatic life events ((Davidson & Strauss, 1992). For example, there is a positive relationship between self-esteem, fitness, and recovery from depression. Yet the impact of these various life events on people with mental illness has not been carefully evaluated. (Davidson & Strauss, 1992; Skrinar, Hutchinson, & Williams, 1992).

Four key aspects of the recovery of a functional self are described by Strauss (1992) in the following ways.

Discovering a more active self. This is a process of gradually realizing that one can act in one's own interest, that one can do things that work, that make one's life work, that influence one's life. This is a critical awareness in the recovery process. How the person does this can seem quite simple to others (e.g., get up on time, keep an appointment, cook a meal), but the discovery that we *can* influence our life through our own incremental actions can have a profound impact on our self. This initial awareness will recur at different times and build up momentum. It is a fragile awareness and may be easily bruised by negative experiences. It is clear that others can be helpful in this process by being an occasion of this awareness or by supporting it.

Taking stock of self. Through additional positive experiences of acting in our own interest we begins to feel more grounded in our new self. Although it may continue to feel fragile, we deliberately test it and our newfound strengths. Confidence builds that our new functional self exists and is available when we need it. Feedback from others is important during this testing period.

Putting self into action. As our level of confidence in our new functional self grows we continues to build our self through personal action and feedback. This is a process of gradually enhancing and further grounding our new functional self. It is felt as real and available. Gradually reclaiming our living, learning, and working life and confronting negative personal, professional, and societal values, and attitudes and practices are important ways of "putting our self into action" and, thereby, further building our functional self.

Appealing to self. As our level of confidence grows we begins to acknowledge more deeply the presence of this stronger functional self and we can call upon it as needed. It becomes a readily available resource for us. While vulnerabilities may continue to exist, we are no longer so easily bruised by negative life experiences. We feel empowered.

Reclaiming Power

Power is reclaimed by rebuilding the broken connections. There are a number of strategies that people find helpful in reclaiming power.

Acceptance. Acceptance is one of the harder tasks in the recovery process. Acceptance means seeing and acknowledging all the various aspects of oneself without devaluing oneself. Negative judgments and evaluations are barriers to acceptance. They lead to disbelief or even denial because it is hard to accept what one devalues. Yet acceptance does not mean approval, or even disapproval. Acceptance means seeing and acknowledging what is.

Seeing and acknowledging what is seems like a simple task at first. Don't we all do this, all the time? Unfortunately, even an introductory exposure to psychology shows us that acceptance is not so easy at all. We all have a tendency to "color" our perceptions with our past learnings or to project feelings and meanings on what we see. Not surprisingly, certain meditative and focusing approaches require a lengthy practice in "seeing what is," because a person's personal history has often left his or her perceptions somewhat contaminated. People with mental illness can learn to be sensitive to their vulnerabilities in perceiving. They can learn to know themselves well enough to recognize when they are most likely to override "what is" with their own learned ideas, feelings, and sensations. They can learn how to be open to "what is" without being overwhelmed or intimidated by their history or their fears.

One of the problems with acceptance is that the mind can fool us. A frontal assault on someone's denial is usually not helpful. If a person with a mental illness knows that others view him or her as misperceiving reality— this can help, especially if he or she trusts the person. Acceptance is so hard when a person with a mental illness perceives as true what others see as a misperception. People with mental illness have to realize that their perception can be colored by the illness and by their history of stigma and discrimination.

Acceptance is a process and not an event. It involves both emotional as well as cognitive aspects of oneself. It is not simply a matter of making a decision. It involves working out this decision emotionally and through one's actions. The emotions tend to lag behind one's decisions. Yet actions help to deepen the emotional commitment to one's decision. A professional can help a person with a mental illness deepen his or her confidence in acceptance through assisting the person to face the feelings acceptance brings up and through supporting the actions that concretize acceptance in his or her life.

What people with mental illness need to accept are their strengths as well as their weaknesses. They need to accept all of themselves. Acceptance is difficult because it builds on hope. Without the foundation of hope, acceptance can be too terrifying. As Pat Deegan has said, "How can we accept the illness when we have no hope? Why should one pile despair on top of hopelessness? The combination could be fatal. So perhaps people are wise in not accepting the illness until they have the resources to deal with it" (Deegan, 1996). Professionals can learn to communicate realistic hope by becoming familiar with the literature supporting recovery and by actively collaborating with a person with a mental illness in rebuilding his or her life.

Acceptance also means dealing with loss: the dreams of what could have been, the loss of who the person was before the illness, and the knowledge that peers have gone on to have a life. This is very painful. Family members know this pain also. Dealing with loss is not an easy task. Yet acceptance means seeing oneself directly, without judging. One's bottom line. People with mental illness need to begin their recovery from where they are.

Effective coping builds on acceptance. It builds on reality. And that reality is not only the illness. The reality also includes stigma, abusive treatments, negative professional attitudes and practices, programs that are often unappealing, and lack of advancement in the community. Also, as people feel more confidence in themselves, they begin to acknowledge aspects of themselves that are also part of their reality. These include their many talents and strengths, their inner wisdom, and their relationships with family, friends, and helpers (Davidson & Strauss, 1992). They gradually begin to identify with these other aspects of themselves and to realize that they can call upon them as needed. Gradually, the illness then becomes less dominating and all-encompassing.

Acceptance reduces unnecessary pain and anguish. Acceptance can bring a sense of relief. People with mental illness can then stop struggling with what they don't want to see or acknowledge. Anguish is replaced with the ordinary suffering that comes with dealing directly with the often uncomfortable realities of one's life.

Acceptance for people with mental illness means acknowledging their own agency, their own ability to act in their own interest. It means moving from being acted upon to assuming responsibility for their life. Acceptance helps people find new solutions to replace the apathy, indifference, and hopelessness that have helped them survive up to now (Deegan, 1996). Acceptance is empowering. Acceptance helps people with mental illness to deal with the real barriers that exist within themselves and within their environment. The process of recovery is influenced by the person. People are active participants whose feelings, meanings, and interpretations of the illness impact on the course of the illness. The individual can call upon coping and regulatory mechanisms to modify, adapt, and adjust to the illness and to actively confront the many barriers in the environment (Strauss, 1992).

Acceptance is courageous. Courage can be defined as the ability to make a commitment to an imperfect or unknown process. This is what people with psychiatric disability do. Their commitment comes from their hope. They begin to believe hope is possible. As that hope takes root, they can make a commitment to themselves and to their recovery—and to do whatever is necessary to bring it about—knowing that it is not a perfect process. There are risks, there are dangers, there are failures, and there are successes. And this is OK. This is being courageous.

Acceptance requires support. When others accept one, it is easier to accept oneself. When others express hope for one, it is easier for one to have hope. People with mental illness are not an island. They live in relationship to people, places and events. They influence and they are influenced. Their self develops in relationship to others (Estroff, 1989). There is a partnership in this process with people and events. They are not alone in how they experience and respond to their life.

Acceptance can lead to compassion—compassion for oneself and compassion for others. People with mental illness become less judging of themselves and others. They become more focused on what they need to have a life and how to get those resources. They begin to be interested in how to help other people with psychiatric disability. People who are involved in their own recovery are important sources of support and mentoring to other consumers. It is helpful to see other people making it.

Acceptance is complex. It is a process that may take a long time. It involves all of a person, the mind, the body, the emotions, and behavior. It is a courageous process. It is a journey of the heart (Deegan, 1996).

Self-will/self-monitoring. Behind hopelessness is often helplessness. Doing things that are helpful to oneself creates hopefulness, often in small ways that are nevertheless very important, for example, exercising, reading something we like, spending time with a friend, completing a task that is valued. These incremental steps build a person's power and establish a new sense of who he or she is and what his or her world is all about. These steps empower people. They help people with mental illness to feel their "agency" and their ability to bring about change. They gradually build a new identity and new meanings. These steps also build an important relationship with another person—someone who believes in the person with a mental illness. This gives a person with a mental illness the mirroring, feedback, and validation he or she needs.

We often hear the expression, "If there is a will, there is a way." We sometimes think it is more helpful the other way around, that is, "If there is a way, there is a will." If people are given opportunities, they will be more likely to feel hopeful. If you want people to feel motivated, give them options that are appealing. The will and the motivation to have a life come out of a person's experience, often from a professional, a person, or program that is hopeful for him or her.

Mutual aid groups/supportive friends. Numerous authors have written about the profound importance that self-help and mutual aid groups can have in supporting individuals with disabilities (Gartner & Riessman, 1982; Killilea, 1976). Criticism and negative comments can undermine one's developing sense of self. Social support can facilitate a positive sense of self and a sense of empowerment (Davidson & Strauss, 1992). Professionals and families should encourage the person with a disability to join a self-help group. The risk is that the professional and family will lose a part of the person as he/she gains more independence and self-care. The benefit is that the person will find important parts of him/herself.

Spirituality. Spirituality provides solace, companionship, and meaning to a person's struggles. People with mental illness find belonging to a particular religion helpful both spiritually and socially. And if they can find ways to connect to the church or synagogue in a volunteer capacity they can also feel needed and valued.

A significant other. Relationships and biology are intimately related. If one's relationships are healthy and intimate, one's body will respond positively, and healing will be more likely. Intimacy is an important aspect of most people's lives. Intimacy is a state of closeness that can make a person feel authentic, whole, and intensely alive. Yet, at times, closeness brings up very intense feelings in people with mental illness. These feelings come from real experiences in one's past where the person was at risk or hurt—often by mental health professionals. Exploring these feelings can help to understand them and possibly even discover where they come from. The more people with mental illness become aware of their learned feelings, the less likely they will be to project them onto another person. And it is usually in an intimate relationship that people with mental illness learn about themselves, confront their learned images and feelings, and learn how to be open to the real "other person" they are connected with.

Temporal perspective. Understanding recovery as a process helps people with mental illness to cope more effectively with specific stressful events in their life. They come to know that the stressful events will not last forever. Although it often seems like a specific crisis will last forever, it will have a beginning, a middle and an end. The knowledge that the person is in this process can bring some relief. It can help her or him to focus on developing more effective coping strategies rather than "overdramatizing" a particular distressful event. The person can know that he or she has been through this before and survived, and can come to trust the increasing ability to deal with his or her symptoms, attitudes and perceptions, and the real barriers in his or her life.

One important aspect of the process of recovery is the tendency to be more symptomatic as a person becomes more active in his or her own behalf and to be more vulnerable to frustration as he or she copes more successfully. Recognizing this as a normal process and not as a sign of increasing illness can be calming and grounding as the person struggles to build a life for himself or herself.

Reclaiming Meaning

There is a great deal of evidence that rehabilitation works—that people can reclaim valued roles in life and enhance their personal sense of meaning (Harding & Zahniser, 1994; Harding, Strauss, Hafez, & Lieberman, 1987). Some of the strategies for helping people with mental illness reclaim valued roles include the following.

Vocational Training and Work. There is ample evidence from both consumer self-reports and from the research literature that work strengthens a person's self-esteem and helps that person to feel a part of the larger community. Work makes people with mental illness feel good about themselves and connects them socially to other people (Harding, Strauss, Hafez, & Lieberman, 1987; Rogers, 1995). Work builds on the competencies and strengths of people and builds up their pride in their accomplishments.

Supported Education. Supported education helps people to choose, get, and maintain themselves in an academic environment. For many people their illness began when they were in college or trade school. Returning to this environment is especially satisfying as people again begin to think in terms of a career for themselves (Sullivan, Nicolellis, Danley, & MacDonald-Wilson, 1993).

Mentors. The support of other people who are in recovery is a crucial aspect of the recovery process. Peer support provides a level and quality of support that can not be reproduced by professional or even family support. The support of someone who is in recovery and rebuilding his or her life can be especially helpful. He/she can provide the hope that is so often lacking to people who are beginning their recovery journey.

Models. The presence of people with psychiatric disability achieving in their chosen fields is another important aspect of recovery. The presence of people with psychiatric disability in all types of work and all levels of position is critically needed so that people with psychiatric disability can have models of people who are making it.

Reclaiming Hope

Deegan (1996) made perhaps the most useful distinction between optimism and hope. She describes optimism as like a cheerleader—there for a brief period of time, and then gone. Hope is the belief in one's self; a willingness to "hang in there" with one's self over the long haul—to pick oneself up again when one is knocked down and to persevere. Hope is helped by people in one's environment who have this same kind of hope for one. Hope is helped by an active and enduring presence of at least one other person.

Hope is an important aspect of recovery. Hopelessness is hard to deal with directly. Helping people to be helpful to themselves leads people to feel more hopeful. Knowing that they can act in their own interest, that they are not helpless, makes them feel more hopeful. So we deal with hopelessness by dealing with helplessness; by helping people to act in their own interest—initially by taking better care of themselves. And then by gradually helping them to acquire the knowledge, skills, and support to build a life for themselves.

Hope for people with mental illness frequently comes from the caring and concern of another person. Someone who has hope for you. Someone who gives you hope. Having someone believe in you helps you to believe in yourself.

Hope motivates. It makes you want to do what you should do. Hope transcends the illness. It has to do with the person, and how he or she feels about him or herself.

Restoring hope, or rejoining the human stream, is a risky journey of the heart for a person who has withdrawn and given up hope to protect himself or herself (Deegan, 1996). It should not be surprising that a person can be quite angry at professional efforts to help, can distrust the professional, or seem to sabotage our efforts at restoring hope. Giving up the learned solution and safety of hopelessness for the risk of trusting and building a life can be asking a lot. Professionals need to understand what they are asking people to do. Although people with a psychiatric disability sincerely want to reenter the human stream, they are also deeply aware of the potential for additional hurt and trauma (Deegan, 1996).

Medication

Medication is an important aspect of recovery and reclaiming hope for many people with psychiatric disability (Sullivan, 1994; Francell, 1994). Although many people struggle with medication because of its negative side effects and the profound meanings attached to medication, it can be an important resource in the recovery process and in the reclaiming of hope.

CONCLUSION

We have raised and responded to four basic questions about recovery. Because we are still uncovering this important process we need to acknowledge with sincere humility that there is still a long way to go and much to learn. It is through our connections with people who are experiencing this disability that we will continue to learn and to grow in our knowledge about recovery.

REFERENCES

Anthony, W. A. (1993). Recovery from mental illness: The guiding vision of the mental health service system in the 1990's. *Innovations and Research, 2*(3), 17–24.

Bleuler, E. (1950). Dementia praecox or the group of schizophrenias. Translated by J. Zinkin. New York: International Universities Press.

Davidson, L., & Stayner, D. (1997). Loss, loneliness, and the desire for love: Perspectives on the social lives of people with schizophrenia. *Psychiatric Rehabilitation Journal, 20*(3), 3–12.

Davidson, L., & Strauss, J. S. (1992). Sense of self in recovery from severe mental illness. *British Journal of Medical Psychology, 65*, 131–145.

Deegan, P. (1988). Recovery: The lived experience of rehabilitation. *Psychosocial Rehabilitation Journal, 11*(4), 11–19.

Deegan, P. (1995). Recovery from psychiatric disability. Presentation at AMI of Massachusetts Curriculum and Training Committee Conference, Boston State House, Boston, MA.

Deegan, P. (1996). Recovery as a journey of the heart. *Psychiatric Rehabilitation Journal, 19*(3), 91–98.

Estroff, S. E. (1989). Self, Identity, and Subjective Experiences of Schizophrenia: In Search of the Subject. *Schizophrenia Bulletin, 15*(2), 189–196.

Francell, Jr., E. G. (1994). Medication: The foundation of recovery. *Innovations and Research, 3*(4), 31–40.

Gartner, A. J., & Riessman, F. (1982). Self-help and mental health. *Hospital and Community Psychiatry, 33*(8), 631–635.

Harding, C. M. (1986). Speculations on the measurement of recovery from severe psychiatric disorder and the human condition. *Psychiatric Journal of the University of Ottawa, 11*(4), 19–204.

Harding, C. M., Strauss, J. S., Hafez, H.,, & Lieberman, P. (1987). Work and mental illness. I. Toward an integration of the rehabilitation process. *Journal of Nervous and Mental Disease, 175*(6), 317–327.

Harding, C. M., & Zahniser, J. H (1994). Empirical correction of seven myths about schizophrenia with implications for treatment. *Acta Scandinavica, 90*, 140–146.

Harding, C. M., Zubin, J., & Strauss, J. S. (1987). Chronicity in schizophrenia: Fact, partial fact, or artifact. *Hospital and Community Psychiatry, 38*(5), 477–486.

Harding, C. M., Zubin, J., & Strauss, J. S. (1992). Chronicity in schizophrenia: Revisited. *British Journal of Psychiatry, 161*(suppl. 18), 27–37)

Huber, G., Gross, G., Schuttler, R., & Linz, M. (1980). Longitudinal studies of schizophrenic patients. *Schizophrenia Bulletin, 6*, 592–605.

Killilea, M. (1976). Mutual help organizations: Interpretations in the literature. In G. Kapplan & M. Killilea (Eds.), *Support systems and mutual help*. New York: Grune & Stratton.

Kraeplin, E. (1902). *Dementia praecox, in clinical psychiatry: A textbook for students and physicians. 6th Edition*. New York: Macmillan.

Mack, J. E. (1994). Power, powerlessness, and empowerment in psychotherapy. *Psychiatry, 57*, 178–198.

Minkoff, K. (1987). Resistance of mental health professionals to working with the chronic mentally ill. In A.T. Meyerson (Ed.), *Barriers to treating the chronic mentally ill*. San Francisco: Jossey-Bass.

Rogers, J. (1995). Work is key to recovery. *Psychosocial Rehabilitation Journal, 18*(4), 5–10.

Skrinar, G. S., Hutchinson, D. S., & Williams, N. (1992). Exercise: An adjunct therapy for persons with psychiatric disabilities. *Med. Sci. Sports Exer., 24*(5), 536, supplement.

Strauss, J. S. (1992). The person—Key to understanding mental illness: Towards a new dynamic psychiatry, III. *British Journal of Psychiatry, 161*(suppl. 18), 19–26.

Sullivan, W. P. (1994). A long and winding road: The process of recovery from severe mental illness. *Innovations and Research, 3*(3), 11–19.

Sullivan, A., Nicolellis, D. L., Danley, K. S., & MacDonald-Wilson, K. (1993). Choose-get-keep: A psychiatric rehabilitation approach to supported education. *Psychosocial Rehabilitation Journal, 17*(1), 55–68.

30

Surviving a System: One Woman's Experience of Disability and Health Care

Susan Buchanan

When I first became disabled at sixteen, I had very little experience interacting with the health care system. In addition, my only knowledge about quadriplegia came from reading *The Other Side of the Mountain*. Over the years, I have learned that I am one of the lucky ones. I have never been institutionalized—except for short admissions to a rehabilitation centre. I am almost always healthy. I have strengthened and bolstered my self-confidence, believing that I have an emotional reserve that will see me through the worst and the best of times.

I say all this and yet, whenever I have to use the health care system, I begin to question my own confidence and competence. This is not an unusual experience. Many people do not look forward to the feelings of helplessness and the loss of control that come with hospitalization or interactions with health care providers. On one hand, we have elevated doctors and others to a position of godlike authority. On the other, we desperately want to interact with them on level ground. *They,* the doctors, nurses, therapists, x-ray technicians and others in the field, are not the enemy, at least not intentionally. However, many of us seek their care and expertise with the same trepidation we might feel when entering a war zone. By the time we leave hospitals, clinics, and doctors' offices we feel battered and victimized, our self-esteem wounded. We have been exposed to a subtle, almost subversive form of abuse.

My response to this has been to develop a plan and several strategies for dealing with the health care system. It isn't an offensive position; it's a position I take to protect myself.

From *Rehabilitation Digest, 26*(3) (1996), 7–10. Reprinted with permission.

Ironically, with swift and sometimes threatening changes in health care delivery, we are being asked to be more responsible for our own health, to strive for preventive health practises, and to be active participants in a healthy lifestyle. At the same time, the health care delivery system is not always responsive to our desire to play a more active role in it, especially if we are women with disabilities. In fact, women with disabilities are particularly vulnerable to all forms of violence and abuse.

DAWN Canada and other groups and individuals have researched the reality of being both female and disabled. The research has revealed a troubling picture. Women with disabilities are several times more likely to be physically, emotionally, and sexually abused than non-disabled women. However, although women who are disabled are not responsible for the abuse they experience, we can develop skills to counteract some of its more subtle effects.

If you are a woman with a disability, your experience within the health delivery system can be devastating. You can almost automatically assume that your experiences will be significantly different from those you would have if you were not female and disabled. You may leave it feeling destroyed and far less healthy than when you entered it. You may ask what you can do next time to leave with minimal wounds to your self-esteem. In addition, you may ask how you can avoid the institutionalized benevolence often directed toward women who are disabled and to become *healthy* in the broadest sense of the word.

These are tough questions and I do not have easy answers. I also do not presume that my experience reflects that of other women who are disabled. However, I do know many women with disabilities and when we talk, I know that we share common concerns when it comes to achieving and maintaining the grasp we have on our health.

The suggestions that follow come from my reflections of those times when my health was most challenged within the health care system. There are ways to leave a doctor's office or a health care institution healthy, there are ways to not only survive but to grow and learn from the experience.

The issue is complex. For many of us, our health and well-being is fragile although we may not be sick. We may rely on the skill and expertise of a wide range of health care providers. And we may live in places where our choices in health care providers are limited.

Linda Crabtree, a long-time activist in the disabled community, says, "Now that I know more about my rights as a patient and have quite a bit of experience refusing drugs and procedures that would make me worse, and with 53 years of living with this body, I stress that an informed and aware, as well as wary, patient, who thinks for herself and asks the doctor about the drugs and procedures he or she is prescribing, is a patient who is going to get well or at least well enough to survive hospital."

So, how do we become the kind of women who can survive the system? We need to begin looking at some of the issues that contribute to institutionalized benevolence.

DISPELLING THE MYTH OF THE INVALID

Many people with disabilities are healthy and strong and many non-disabled people are ill and weak.

The myths that disability means illness, that those who use the health care system are always sick, that people with disabilities are invalids, are based on stereotypes that continue to be all pervasive. Often these stereotypes can affect the treatment a woman with a disability will receive.

The simplest example of the above can be found in the use of the term "able-bodied." Able-bodied is meant to describe someone who is healthy and strong. It is not the opposite of disabled. Yet, when a woman with a disability seeks health care it is often assumed that any symptom of ill health has something to do with her disability. When this happens, a woman with a disability may not be given full consideration based on what she is describing as a health problem; the health care provider is relating all problems and complaints to the disability.

A DAWN Ontario publication, *Women with Disabilities: A Guide for Health Care Providers,* says:

> People with disabilities in our society face a host of stereotypes which have been perpetuated over the years and which do little to further positive images. These stereotypes include sentiments of pity, a belief that their lives must be unbearable or not worth living, that they cannot and should not function as full members of society, and that they are a drain on the health and social service system.

These beliefs can affect the care you receive. You have the right to the same good health care as the next person. You do not have to feel that yo are a "burden" to any system.

THE NON-WOMAN SYNDROME

If you need information on subjects such as sex or birth control, ask. Ask anyone you can think of who may have some answers. Your identity as a person is at stake. Don't allow anyone to rob you of part of yourself.

Perhaps the biggest challenge facing women with disabilities is that they are not seen as "real" women. They cannot or are unable to fulfil society's prescribed roles for women (wife, mother, lover, sexual partner). They are asexual or nonsexual. Health care providers frequently assume we do not need and are not interested in birth control or counselling on safe sex.

When I was sixteen, no one treating me seemed to feel it was important that I be educated when it came to sex. At an age when awakening sexuality is very much a part of a young girl's life, I was left feeling as though my questions were unimportant.

BECOME YOUR OWN EXPERT

You may well be the "expert" when it comes to your disability.

You need to be well informed about your disability. Talk to others who have a similar disability and ask them about their experiences, especially with health care. Attend workshops or talks that are relevant to your disability and read everything you can find on the subject. In addition, work on establishing a "receptive" relationship with health care providers.

EDUCATING THE EDUCATED

Excellent resources are available. Bring along information that you know will educate.

There is no doubt that health care providers are well educated. Some are experts in their field. This is especially important to remember because you have now entered their field and may be playing their ball game with their rules. However, this does not mean that you can't educate them about you and the nuances of your disability.

While it is helpful to educate your provider, it is not necessary that you be the "guinea pig" when students training in the field are involved. Many people who are disabled have been used as a "good example" or an "excellent case" to illustrate an illness, disease, or disability. If you are not comfortable discussing your concerns with anyone other than a trained, experienced provider, you have the right to refuse to be seen by someone who is still in training. You are not a "case," you are a person. Don't be exploited.

HAVE A PROTECTIVE STRATEGY-FOR EXAMPLE, PUT A TEAM TOGETHER

Have a friend or loved one become part of your health care "team."

It is important to have someone who knows you well—a friend or family member—come with you when you interact with the health care delivery system, or be available to be called upon in an emergency. This may not always be possible, so consider wearing a Medic Alert bracelet or carrying a "Personal Medical Profile" *(see* Figure 30.1*)*.

For me, nothing has been more affirming than my relationships with those who respect my integrity as a woman first, as a woman with a disability second. It has taken time to establish a team of supporters. Sometimes the team members change as my needs change but whenever I am about to interact with the health care delivery system I use certain criteria to determine how comfortable I am

Consider using a comprehensive PERSONAL MEDICAL PROFILE form the next time you visit your doctor. The PERSONAL MEDICAL PROFILE conveys essential information about your condition and underlying chronic disorders. Designed by Linda Crabtree, a woman with a disability who has a chronic illness, this form is extremely useful in providing accurate information to medical personnel, and may be critical in emergency situations. It states, for example, your main medical problems, information on your specialist, the orthotics and/or prosthetics you use, drug sensitivity, personal preferences and any other pieces of information that caregivers should know about you. Let the PERSONAL MEDICAL PROFILE form speak for you! It costs $5.00 (postage included), is printed on light yellow heavy bond, folded in three, and fits into a plastic see-through sleeve. Please write to Phoenix Counsel Inc., One Springbank Drive, St. Catharines, Ontario L2S 2K1.

Payment in advance would be appreciated.

FIGURE 30.1

with my participation in the process. When I am a partner in my own health care, I feel better no matter how serious or debilitating the illness or problem I am currently experiencing.

SPEAKING MY LANGUAGE

If you do not understand the treatment you are receiving, the tests that have been done on you, the medication or therapy prescribed, ask for clarification.

Although over the years I have become very knowledgeable, I almost always have to ask health care providers to speak in a language I can understand. Knowledge is truly a source of personal power. What you don't know really can hurt you. It is also critical that the lines of communication between you and the providers involved in your health care are open.

HAVE A PLAN

Go to an appointment or clinic with a "check off" list of questions, concerns, and other issues to remind you of what ground you want covered during the limited time you have with the health care provider.

Before going to see a health care provider, give some thought to what it is you need from this person. Is it important if this person is male or female? Is his or her office accessible to you? Do you need to arrange for extra time in the appointment or are other accommodations required because you have a disability? Do you want to bring someone with you whom you trust and who will support you if you and the provider have a difference of opinion? Ask friends, relatives or others you trust about people they have seen and trusted. What do you do if your choices are limited and you end up seeing someone who would not necessarily be your first choice?

I've even found it helpful to have a close friend go over my list as she very often thinks of things I have overlooked. The following can help you with your own plan:

- Describe your problem or concern as clearly as you can.
- Ask for a copy of the report before you leave. A file is kept on you and you have the right to read what is written about your visit. Once you get the copy of the report, read it carefully. If you do not understand what has been said or disagree with any of it, let the provider know and ask for clarification.
- Before you leave, briefly go over in your own words what has been said. In this way, you and the provider can both see that you have understood everything.

DAWN Ontario provides a helpful list of suggestions to make the most of any visit to a health care provider, for instance:

- Bringing someone with you for support or help.
- Taking notes or taping the session so you will remember what you are told or what information is provided.
- Signing forms only after you have a clear understanding of them. Maybe a friend could go over these with you.
- Making sure you understand any prescription drugs. Why is it being prescribed? Are there any side effects? Let the doctor know if you have experienced side effects from other drugs.

Taking charge and having a plan can make you feel wonderful. It is a healthy boost to your self-esteem to know that you have had some say in how things went at the appointment. Lack of experience in this is what leads so many women toward a diminished confidence. When you are sick or have a health problem, you will only feel worse if you feel bad about the interaction itself. A low opinion of yourself can lead to self-abusive acts or make you more vulnerable to emotional abuse inflicted by others. In the long term, you will feel better and enhance your self-confidence, if you have a plan of action for taking as much control as possible of the health-related events in your life.

Part VII: *Study Questions and Disability Awareness Exercise*

1. How does AIDS challenge the rehabilitation and health care system to practice what it preaches?
2. Should the care of a person with a severe disability be allowed more resources than a person with a nonsevere disability?
3. Should resources be limited when a person reaches a particular age? At what age and how would that decision be made?
4. Should all families and family members be required to be caregivers for a family member with a disability? How can society decide who should or should not be required?
5. Discuss how alcohol and drugs can be major factors and stressors in the disability experience.
6. Are there any situations you can think of that create a disability experience that is so complex that the right to die could outweigh the right for treatment and rehabilitation?
7. Are the principles of psychosocial rehabilitation and the concept of recovery equally relevant to emotional disability and physical disability?
8. What are the advantages and limitations of a biopsychosocial approach to HIV-AIDS?
9. Discuss the psychosocial implications unique to the treatment and rehabilitation of persons with HIV-AIDS.
10. Identify and discuss a disability that approximates the needs and concerns related to AIDS
11. Can technocratic priorities and spiritual values be complimentary? If so give an example.
12. Do spiritual based therapies have a place in the emerging realm of managed care? Why? Why not?
13. Are the principles of spirituality better suited to some disabilities than others?
14. Discuss the unique problems, issues, and concerns related to a client with dual diagnosis.
15. In your opinion, what is the relationship between psychopathology and substance abuse dependence?
16. How do the goals of traditional treatment relate to persons who are chemically dependent?
17. What are the principles of recovery?
18. Do the principles of recovery related to mental illness apply to physical illness?
19. Discuss loss as it relates to the treatment of people with mental illness.
20. Discuss the health care issues faced by women with a disability.

21. What suggestions are made to empower women?
22. How are empowerment issues for men and women similar? Dissimilar?

IS THE BEST YET TO COME?

Perspective

One way to explore the future is to reflect on the past. When doing this exercise, it may be helpful to consider the many advances and developments that have occurred during the past 20 years e.g., technology and medical rehabilitation.

Goals

1. To consider the potential changes and opportunities that will impact future disability experiences.
2. To explore how the disability experience will be influenced by the future.
3. To personalize the disability experience as part of the normal aging process.

Procedures

1. Project yourself to the year 2010.
2. Choose a severe physical or mental disability that would currently result in significant functional limitations for you.
3. Compare what you believe will be the major medical and rehabilitation advances in relation to your disability by 2010 as compared to now. Write these down and discuss in your group.
4. Discuss your functional levels in 2010 as compared to now.
5. What other changes in the lives of persons with disabilities do you believe may occur by 2010? What factors may contribute to the change?
6. In your opinion, in what ways may the quality of life in 2010 be better and / or worse for you and other persons with disabilities?

APPENDIX A

Representative Books Related to the Psychological and Social Impact of Disability

The following books published since 1990 represent contributions to the understanding of the psychological and social impact of disability. The organization of this listing is based on date of publication, with newer books listed first.

Psychosocial Adaptation to Chronic Illness and Disability, by Hanoch Livneh and Richard F. Antonak, published by Aspen Publishers, Inc., Gaithersburg, MD, in 1997.
> This book focuses on the construct of psychological adaptation to chronic illness and disability and provides information about this construct from theoretical, measurement and historical perspectives. It also provides a review of the research literature relevant to 18 specific chronic illness and disability conditions. It provides a balance between theory, research, and application.

Sexual Function in People with Disability and Chronic Illness: A Health Professional's Guide, edited by Marca L. Sipski and Craig L. Alexander, published by Aspen Publishers in Gaithersburg, MD, in 1997.
> This broadly written book is designed to provide an overview of sexuality and disability as well as information and research specific to a particular topic of interest. Virtually every aspect of sexuality as it applies to persons with disabilities is included in the book's 29 chapters.

Sexuality after Spinal Cord Injury, by S. Ducharme and K. Gill, published by Paul H. Brooks, Baltimore, MD, in 1997.
> This book, according to the authors, is meant as a down-to-earth discussion of sexual questions for people with spinal cord injuries. It provides an introduction to the anatomy of spinal cord injuries, sexuality, and the phases of sexual stimulation, followed by practical information concerning the physical and emotional issues of sexuality after spinal cord injury.

Enabling Romance, by K. Kroll and E. L. Klein, published by Woodbine House, Rockville, MD, in 1995.
> This sensitive and insightful book draws on the authors' intimate experiences to provide an awareness of the special sexual concerns of persons with

disabilities. Practical suggestions as well as resources for use by counselors and individuals with disabilities are provided.

Encyclopedia of Disability and Rehabilitation, edited by Arthur E. Dell Orto and Robert P. Marinelli, published by Macmillan, New York, in 1995.

With more than 150 entries and more than 200 contributing authors, this 820-page book is a reference volume for individuals with disabilities, their families, coworkers, caregivers, and the public. A basic tenet of the book is that a variety of people play an important part in the lives of persons with disabilities with the goal of empowering the individual with a disability to live as independently as possible. Many entries focus on psychosocial issues.

Managing Chronic Illness: A Biopsychosocial Perspective, edited by Perry M. Nicassio and Timothy W. Smith, published by the American Psychological Association, Washington, DC, in 1995.

This state-of-the-art resource focuses on the provision of psychological services to adults with chronic medical conditions from a biopsychosocial model. The 10 chapters focus on central issues in the application of this model rather than focusing upon differing conditions.

Sometimes you Just Want to Feel Like a Human Being: Case Studies of Empowering Psychotherapy with People with Disabilities, by Mary Ann Blotzer and Richard Ruth, published by Brookes Publishing Company, Baltimore, in 1995.

Using case studies taken from their clinical practice the authors provide an overview of their empowering philosophy and practice in providing psychotherapy to persons with disabilities.

Personality and Adversity: Psychospiritual Aspects of Rehabilitation, by Carolyn L. Vash, published by Springer Publishing Company, New York, in 1994.

The author draws on her own experiences as a person with severe disabilities to provide effective strategies to cope with disability. The main theme of this book centers on adversity as central to psychospiritual growth.

Social and Psychological Foundations of Rehabilitation, by Robert A. Chubon, published by Charles C Thomas, Springfield, IL, in 1994.

This book, which the author describes as a "what is" book as compared to a "how to" manual, focuses on the concepts, milieu, and critical issues in rehabilitation as well as the impact of disability. It is intended to promote interdisciplinary education and collaboration with emphasis on client involvement in their rehabilitation.

Counseling Persons with Physical Disabilities: Theoretical and Clinical Perspectives, by Laura E. Marshak and Milton Seligman, published by Pro-ed, Austin, in 1993.

This book draws upon the clinical experiences, research findings, the writings and first person accounts of persons with disabilities, as well as input from colleagues, friends, students and clients. It broadly presents a means of helping persons with physical disabilities who seek psychological intervention, to adjust to the challenges they face.

Perspectives on Disability (2nd Edition), edited by M. Nagler, published by Health Markets Research, Palo Alto, in 1993.

As with the first edition the author focuses on various facets of social change affecting people with disabilities including issues of empowerment, advocacy, integration and diversity. This issue is a balance of classic and more current articles.

Disability in America: Toward a National Agenda for Prevention, by Andrew M. Pope and Alvin R. Tarlov, published by National Academy Press, Washington, in 1991.

This book, which focuses on the prevention of disabilities, has chapters authored by leaders within this field who discuss disability as a result of injuries, developmental conditions, chronic disease and aging, as well as by secondary conditions arising from primary disability conditions. It goes beyond traditional medicine and rehabilitation to present an applied model to prevent disability.

Disability in the United States: A Portrait from National Data, edited by Susan Thompson Hoffman and Inez Fitzgerald Storck, published by Springer Publishing Company, New York, in 1991.

This book is designed as a central source of national data on persons with disabilities. Using national data sources a wealth of information is provided on multiple aspects of disability including employment, independent living, specific impairments, education, institutionalization, and many other topics.

Empirical Approaches to Psychosocial Aspects of Disability, edited by Myron G. Eisenberg and Robert L. Glueckauf, published by Springer Publishing, New York, in 1991.

This text provides a theoretical and empirical perspective in the study of psychosocial factors impairing persons with physical and emotional disabilities. Because many of the topics under consideration transcend one specific type of disability, the editors have structured the book to allow material to be categorized in the widest possible areas.

Medical and Psychosocial Aspects of Chronic Illness and Disability, by Donna R. Falvo, published by Aspen Publishers, Inc. in Gaithersburg, MD, 1991.

This book is intended to provide rehabilitation professionals or professionals in training, who have little or no medical training, with the essential knowledge of the medical, psychosocial and functional aspects of a variety of disabling conditions. General information relevant to all disabling conditions is first presented. This is followed by specific chapters related to both physical and psychological disabilities.

Advances in Clinical Rehabilitation, edited by Myron Eisenberg and Roy C. Greziak, published by Springer Publishing Co., New York, beginning in 1987 with Volume 3 published in 1990.

This series is designed to provide timely and practical information about rehabilitation interventions from a multidisciplinary perspective. Each of three volumes to date covers four topical content areas: advances in clinical assessment, advances in rehabilitation technology, selected topics, and advances in rehabilitation research. Disability topics covered include low-back pain, brain injury, childhood disabilities, spinal cord injury, thermal injury, and cancer in Volume 1, and brain disorders, disabilities in the elderly, pain, feeding disorders, and aphasia in Volume 2. Volume 3 includes clinical electromyography, stroke, cardiac rehabilitation, and low vision and blindness.

Critical Issues in the Lives of People with Severe Disabilities, edited by Luanna H. Meyer, Charles A. Peck and Lou Brown, published by Paul H. Brooks, Baltimore, in 1990.

This book, which is officially sponsored by The Association for Persons with Severe Disabilities (TASH), is designed to provide an analysis of the contemporary values, research and practice as these affect the lives of persons with severe intellectual disabilities. The purpose of the book is to empower persons with severe disabilities as fully participating members of their communities.

Ethical Issues in Disability and Rehabilitation, edited by Barbara Duncan and Diane Woods, published by the World Institute on Disability, Oakland, CA, Rehabilitation International, New York, and the World Rehabilitation Fund, New York, in 1990.

Focusing on decision making as it relates to bioethics, this publication is a report of an international symposium held in 1989 designed to provide a forum for suggestions on how persons with disabilities can become more active and influential in this area. It includes a collection of conference papers and commentary, as well as an annotated international bibliography.

Psychological Aspects of Developmental and Physical Disabilities: A Casebook, edited by Michel Hersen and Vincent B. VanHasselt, published by Sage, Newbury Park, NY, in 1990.

This book provides examples of the types of psychological intervention that can be applied to problems of persons with physical and developmental disabilities. The emphasis is on detailed presentations of 14 individual clients by experts with an emphasis on psychological assessment and treatment. The 14 case studies cover a wide range of physical and mental disabilities.

Psychological Aspects of Serious Illness: Chronic Conditions, Fatal Diseases, and Critical Care, edited by Paul T. Costa, Jr. and Gary R. VandenBos, published by American Psychological Association, Washington, in 1990.

This book, part of the Master Lecturers in Psychology series, highlights some of the major issues in the psychological aspects of serious illness from the perspective of five master lecturers. Diverse in its offerings it includes topics such as psychosocial factors, bioethical issues, stigma, coping, and developmental perspectives.

APPENDIX B

Representative Journals Related to the Psychological and Social Impact of Disability

American Journal of Occupational Therapy, 4720 Montgomery Lane, P. O. Box 31220, Bethesda, MD 20824-1220.

> AJOT is an official publication of The American Occupational Therapy Association, Inc. (AOTA). Articles pertain to the many aspects of occupational therapy.

American Journal of Psychotherapy. Official journal of the Association for the Advancement of Psychotherapy, Inc., Belfer Education Center, 1300 Morris Park Avenue, Room 402, Bronx, NY 10461-1602.

> AJP publishes a wide range of articles relevant to psychotherapists including those who work with people who have disabilities.

Annals of Behavioral Medicine, The Society of Behavioral Medicine, 401 East Jefferson Street, Suite 205, Rockville, MD 20850.

> This publication focuses on a wide range of both theoretical and applied issues relevant to the practice of behavioral medicine including topics important to persons with psychiatric and physical disabilities.

Archives of Physical Medicine and Rehabilitation. Suite 1310, 78 East Adams Street, Chicago, IL.

> *Archives* is the official journal of and is published monthly by The American Congress of Rehabilitation Medicine and the American Academy of Physical Medicine and Rehabilitation. The mission of the *Archives* is to disseminate information about the practice of rehabilitation, particularly rehabilitation medicine.

The British Journal of Medical Psychology, The British Psychological Society, St. Andrews House, 48 Princess Road East, Leicester, LE1 7DR, UK.

> The *Journal* aims to promote theoretical and research developments in the field of medical psychology.

Disability and Society, Carfax Publishing Limited, 875-81 Massachusetts Avenue, Cambridge, MA 02139.

This international journal addresses current issues that impact the lives of persons living the disability experience.

Disability Studies Quarterly, University Affiliated Program, University of Hawaii, 1776 University Avenue, UA4-6, Honolulu, Hawaii, 96822.

This quarterly is a valuable resource that provides a comprehensive overview of current literature, reviews, and events designed to meet the needs of consumers as well as professionals.

Families, Systems, and Health, Inc., The Journal of Collaborative Family Health Care, P. O. Box 20838, Rochester, NY 14602-0838.

A peer-reviewed, interdisciplinary journal that publishes clinical research, and training and theoretical contributions in the area of families and health, with particular focus on collaborative family health care.

Journal of Applied Rehabilitation Counseling is a quarterly journal published by the National Rehabilitation Counseling Association, 8807 Sudley Road, #102, Manassas, VA 20110-4719.

This quarterly is concerned with issues of importance to the practicing rehabilitation counselor. The focus is on implications for practice, with less emphasis on technical and research issues.

Journal of Chronic Diseases is published monthly by Pergamon Press, Maxwell House, Fairview Park, Elmsford, NY 10523.

It explores various aspects of chronic illness for all age groups, including long-term medical and nursing care, the impact of chronically ill persons on the community, and rehabilitation needs.

Journal of Counseling and Development is published six times per year by the American Counseling Association, 5999 Stevenson Avenue, Alexandria, VA 22304.

The official journal of ACA, it includes articles of broad interest to counselors who work in schools, colleges, community, rehabilitation agencies, and the government.

Journal of Head Trauma Rehabilitation is published quarterly by Aspen Publishers, 7201 McKinney Circle, Frederick, MD 21701.

It provides information for practicing professionals on the clinical management and rehabilitation of the person with a head injury.

Journal of Disability Policy Studies is published by the Dept. of Rehabilitation Education and Research, University of Arkansas, 346 N. West Avenue, Fayetteville, AR 72701.

It addresses a broad range of topics on disability policy from the perspectives of a variety of academic disciplines and publishes articles pertaining to both macro- and micro-policy issues.

Journal of Rehabilitation is a quarterly professional publication by the National Rehabilitation Association, 633 South Washington Street, Alexandria, VA 22314.
The journal is concerned with the rehabilitation field in general. Articles cover a broad expanse of interests and are usually nontechnical and nonresearch in nature.

Professional Psychology: Research and Practice, American Psychological Association, 750 First Street, NE, Washington, DC 20002-4242.
This APA journal focuses on topics of interest to the professional practice of psychology including psychologists who serve persons with disabilities.

Psychiatric Rehabilitation Skills, 7230 Arbor Drive, Tinley Park, IL 60477.
A biannual journal for clinicians, administrators, family members, and consumers involved in the day-to-day implementation of psychiatric rehabilitation programs with a focus on practical hands-on information.

Psychiatric Rehabilitation Journal, Center for Psychiatric Rehabilitation, 930 Commonwealth Avenue, Boston, MA 02215.
The purpose of the journal is to encourage the communication of information relevant to the rehabilitation of people with psychiatric disabilities in keeping with the goal of improving the quality of services designed to help the community adjust to people who have a psychiatric disability.

Psychosomatics is the quarterly official journal of the Academy of Psychosomatic Medicine, 5824 North Magnolia, Chicago, IL 60660 and is published by American Psychiatric Press, 1400 K. Street, NW, Washington, DC 20005.
This quarterly explores the role of emotional factors in the daily practice of comprehensive medicine.

Psychosomatic Medicine is a semimonthly journal published by the American Psychosomatic Society, 265 Nassau Road, Roosevelt, NY 11575.
This journal is concerned with fostering knowledge concerning psychosomatic problems.

Rehabilitation Counseling Bulletin is a quarterly journal published by the American Rehabilitation Counseling Association, 5999 Stevenson Avenue, Alexandria, VA 22304.
This journal focuses on articles illuminating theory and practice and exploring innovations in the field of rehabilitation counseling. It contains a substantial proportion of articles related to psychological issues in disability.

Rehabilitation Digest, Easter Seals/March of Dimes National Council, 45 Sheppard Avenue, East, Suite 801, Toronto, Ontario M2N5W9.
It focuses primarily on issues of major concern to consumers providing practical, timely information.

Rehabilitation Education, the official journal of the National Council on Rehabilitation Education is published quarterly by Elliot & Fitzpatrick, Inc., 1135 Cedar Shoals Drive, Athens, GA 30605.

This journal publishes a variety of rehabilitation-focused articles that would be of interest to rehabilitation educators, researchers, and practitioners.

Rehabilitation Nursing is published monthly by the Medical Economic Co., 4700 W. Lake Avenue, Glenview, IL 60025-1485.

This journal includes a variety of articles that would be of interest to the rehabilitation nurse and other allied health specialties.

Rehabilitation Psychology is the official publication of Division 22, Rehabilitation Psychology of the American Psychological Association, 1200 Seventeenth Street, NW, Washington, DC 20036.

It publishes articles on the psychological and behavioral aspects of rehabilitation. Its scope is broadly defined to include scholarly research of a theoretical and empirical nature.

Sexuality and Disability is published quarterly by Human Sciences Press, 232 Spring Street, New York, NY 10013.

The purpose of this journal is to provide a forum for clinical and research progress in the area of sexuality as it relates to a wide range of physical and mental illnesses and disabling conditions.

APPENDIX C

Representative Organizations Serving Persons with Disabilities

AARP Disability Initiative
601 E Street NW
Washington, DC 20049

Access to Respite Care and Help (ARCH)
800 Eastowne Drive
Suite 105
Chapel Hill, NC 27514

Alexander Graham Bell Association for
the Deaf
3417 Volta Place NW
Washington, DC 20007

Alliance of Genetic Support Groups
35 Wisconsin Circle
Suite 440
Chevy Chase, MD 20815

Alzheimer's Association
919 North Michigan Avenue
Suite 1000
Chicago, IL 60611

American Amputee Foundation, Inc.
(AAF)
P.O. Box 250218
Little Rock, AR 72225

American Association for Respiratory
Care (AARC)
11030 Ables Lane
Dallas, TX 75229

American Association of Kidney Patients
(AAKP)
111 South Parker Street
Suite 405
Tampa, FL 33606

American Association of Psychiatric
Services for Children (AAPSC)
1200-C Scottsville Road
Suite 225
Rochester, NY 14624

American Association of the Deaf-Blind
814 Thayer Avenue
Suite 302
Silver Spring, MD 20910

American Burn Association
New York Hospital Cornell Medical
Center
525 East 68th Street, Room L-706
New York, NY 10021

American Cancer Society (ACS)
National Office
1599 Clifton Road NE
Atlanta, GA 30329

American Chronic Pain Association
(ACPA)
P.O. Box 850
Rocklin, CA 95677

American Council of the Blind (ACB)
1155 15th Street NW
Suite 720
Washington, DC 20005

American Diabetes Association, Inc. (ADA)
National Center
1660 Duke Street
Alexandria, VA 22314

American Disability Prevention and
  Wellness Association
18113 Town Center Drive
Olney, MD 20832

American Epilepsy Society (AES)
638 Prospect Avenue
Hartford, CT 06105

American Foundation for the Blind (AFB)
15 West 16th Street
New York, NY 10011

American Heart Association (AHA)
7272 Greenville Avenue
Dallas, TX 75231

American Kidney Fund, Inc.
6110 Executive Boulevard
Suite 1010
Rockville, MD 20852

The American Liver Foundation
1425 Pompton Avenue
Cedar Grove, NJ 07009

American Lung Association (ALA)
1740 Broadway
New York, NY 10019

The American Lupus Society (TALS)
3914 Del Amo Boulevard, Suite 922
Torrance, CA 90503

American Pain Society (APS)
5700 Old Orchard Road
First Floor
Skokie, IL 60077-1057

American Paralysis Association (APA)
500 Morris Avenue
Springfield, NJ 07081

American Parkinson Disease Association
  (APDA)
1250 Hylan Boulevard
Staten Island, NY 10305

American Printing House for the Blind
  (APH)
1839 Frankfort Avenue
P.O. Box 6085
Louisville, KY 40206

American Rehabilitation Association
  (ARA)
P.O. Box 17675
Washington, DC 20041

American Self-Help Clearinghouse
St. Clares-Riverside Medical Center
Denville, NJ 07834

American Sickle Cell Anemia Association
  (ASCAA)
10300 Carnegie Avenue
Cleveland, OH 44106

American Spinal Injury Association
  (ASIA)
345 East Superior Street
Room 1436
Chicago, IL 60611

Amyotrophic Lateral Sclerosis
  Association (ALSA)
21021 Ventura Boulevard
Suite 321
Woodland Hills, CA 91364

Apple Computer, Inc.
Worldwide Disability Solutions Group
Mail Stop 38DS
1 Infinite Loop
Cupertino, CA 95014

Applications of Technology to the
Rehabilitation of Children with
Orthopedic Disabilities
Los Amigos Research and Education
Institute, Inc. (LAREI)
7503 Bonita Street, Bonita Hall
Downey, CA 90242

The Arc
500 East Border Street
Arlington, TX 76010

Architectural and Transportation Barriers
Compliance Board (ATBCB)
1331 F Street NW
Suite 1000
Washington, DC 20004

Arthritis Foundation
1314 Spring Street NW
Atlanta, GA 30309

Assistance Dog Institute
P.O. Box 2334
Rohnert Park, CA 94927-2334

Association for Children with Down's
Syndrome, Inc. (ACDS)
2616 Martin Avenue
Bellmore, NY 11710

Association for Macular Diseases, Inc.
(AMD)
210 East 64th Street
New York, NY 10021

Association for the Care of Children's
Health (ACCH)
7910 Woodmont Avenue
Suite 300
Bethesda, MD 20814

Association of Birth Defect Children, Inc.
(ABDC)
5400 Diplomat Circle
Suite 270
Orlando, FL 32810

Asthma and Allergy Foundation of
America (AAFA)
1125 - 15th Street NW
Suite 502
Washington, DC 20005

Blinded Veterans Association (BVA)
477 H Street NW
Washington, DC 20001

The Candlelighters Childhood Cancer
Foundation (CCCF)
7910 Woodmont Avenue
Suite 460
Bethesda, MD 20814-3015

CDC National AIDS Clearinghouse
P.O. Box 6003
Rockville, MD 20850

Center for Accessible Housing
North Carolina State University
Box 8613
Raleigh, NC 27695-8613

Center for Children with Chronic Illness
and Disability
Division of General Pediatrics and
Adolescent Health University of
Minnesota
420 Delaware Street
Minneapolis, MN 55455

Center for Rehabilitation Technology
(CRT)
490 - 10th Street NW
Atlanta, GA 30332-0156

Charcot-Marie-Tooth Association
(CMTA)
601 Upland Avenue
Upland, PA 19015

Children's Hospice International (CHI)
700 Princess Street
Suite LL
Alexandria, VA 22314

Clearinghouse on Child Abuse and
Neglect Information
P.O. Box 1182
Washington, DC 20013-1182

Cleft Palate Foundation
1218 Grandview Avenue
Pittsburgh, PA 15211

Cooley's Anemia Foundation, Inc.
129-09 26th Avenue
Flushing, NY 11354

Cornelia de Lange Syndrome Foundation
(CdLS Foundation)
60 Dyer Avenue
Collinsville, CT 06022-1273

The Council for Exceptional Children
(CEC)
1920 Association Drive
Reston, VA 22091

Courage Center
3915 Golden Valley Road
Golden Valley, MN 55422

Crohn's & Colitis Foundation of America,
Inc. (CCFA)
386 Park Avenue South
New York, NY 10016

Cystic Fibrosis Foundation (CFF)
6931 Arlington Road
Bethesda, MD 20814

Deafpride, Inc.
1350 Potomac Avenue SE
Washington, DC 20003

Delta Society
Service Dog Center
P.O. Box 1080
321 Burnett Avenue South, 3rd Floor
Renton, WA 98057-9906

Department of Veterans Affairs (VA)
810 Vermont Avenue NW
Washington, DC 20420

Disabled American Veterans (DAV)
P.O. Box 14301
Cincinnati, OH 45250

Dogs for the Deaf, Inc.
10175 Wheeler Road
Central Point, OR 97502

Dysautonomia Foundation, Inc.
20 East 46 Street
Room 302
New York, NY 10017

Epilepsy Foundation of America (EFA)
4351 Garden City Drive
Landover, MD 20785

FacioScapuloHumeral Society, Inc. (FSH
Society, Inc.)
3 Westwood Road
Lexington, MA 02173

Families of Spinal Muscular Atrophy
(SMA)
P.O. Box 1465
Highland Park, IL 60035

The Family Caregiver Alliance (FCA)
425 Bush Street
Suite 500
San Francisco, CA 94108

Fanconi Anemia Research Fund, Inc. (FA)
66 Club Road
Suite 390
Eugene, OR 97401

Gazette International Networking Institute
(GINI)
5100 Oakland Avenue
Suite 206
St. Louis, MO 63110

General Rare Disorder Network
Vanderbilt University
AA3223, Medical Center North
Nashville, TN 37232-2195

Guide Dog Foundation for the Blind, Inc.
371 East Jericho Turnpike
Smithtown, NY 11787

Helen Keller International, Inc. (HKI)
90 Washington Street - 15th Floor
New York, NY 10006

Huntington's Disease Society of America
(HDSA)
140 West 22nd Street
6th Floor
New York, NY 10011

International Association of
Laryngectomees (IAL)
c/o American Cancer Society (ACS)
1599 Clifton Road NE
Atlanta, GA 30329

International Association of Psychosocial
Rehabilitation Services (IAPSRS)
10025 Governor Warfield Pkwy, #301
Columbia, MD 21044

International Center for the Disabled
(ICD)
340 East 24th Street
New York, NY 10010

The International Council for Learning
Disabilities (CLD)
National Office
P.O. Box 40303
Overland Park, KS 66204

International Hearing Dog, Inc. (IHDI)
8901 East 89th Avenue
Henderson, CO 80640

International Lutheran Deaf Association
(ILDA)
1333 South Kirkwood Road
St. Louis, MO 63122

International Polio Network (IPN)
5100 Oakland Avenue
Suite #206
Saint Louis, MO 63110

International Rehabilitation Medicine
Association (IRMA)
1333 Moursund Avenue
Suite A-221
Houston, TX 77030

Job Accommodation Network (JAN)
918 Chestnut Ridge Road
Suite 1
P.O. Box 6080
Morgantown, WV 26506-6080

Job Opportunities for the Blind (JOB)
1800 Johnson Street
Baltimore, MD 21230

Judge David L. Bazelon Center for Mental
Health Law
1101 15th Street NW
Suite 1212
Washington, DC 20005-5002

Juvenile Diabetes Foundation
International (JDF International)
432 Park Avenue South
New York, NY 10016

Klinefelter Syndrome and Associates (KS
and Associates)
P.O. Box 119
Roseville, CA 95678-0119

Leukemia Society of America
600 Third Avenue, 4th Floor
New York, NY 10016-1901

Little People of America (LPA)
P.O. Box 9897
Washington, DC 20016

Lowe's Syndrome Association (LSA)
222 Lincoln Street
West Lafayette, IN 47906

Lupus Foundation of America, Inc.
4 Research Place
Suite 180
Rockville, MD 20850

March of Dimes Birth Defects Foundation
(MOD)
1275 Mamaroneck Avenue
White Plains, NY 10605

Muscular Dystrophy Association (MDA)
3300 East Sunrise Drive
Tucson, AZ 85718

Myasthenia Gravis Foundation (MGF)
222 South Riverside Plaza
Suite 1540
Chicago, IL 60606-6001

Narcotics Anonymous (NA)
P.O. Box 9999
Van Nuys, CA 91409

National Adrenal Disease Foundation
(NADF)
505 Northern Boulevard
Suite 200
Great Neck, NY 11021

National Alliance for the Mentally Ill
(NAMI)
2101 Wilson Boulevard
Suite 302
Arlington, VA 22201

National Amputation Foundation (NAF)
73 Church Street
Malverne, NY 11565

National Arthritis and Musculoskeletal
and Skin Diseases Information
Clearinghouse
Box AMS
9000 Rockville Pike
Bethesda, MD 20892

National Association for Hearing and
Speech Action (NAHSA)
10801 Rockville Pike
Rockville, MD 20852

National Association for the
Craniofacially Handicapped (FACES)
P.O. Box 11082
Chattanooga, TN 37401

National Association for Visually
Handicapped (NAVH)
22 West 21st Street
New York, NY 10010

National Association of Anorexia Nervosa
and Associated Disorders (ANAD)
P.O. Box 7
Highland Park, IL 60035

National Autism Hotline
Prichard Building
605 - 9th Street
P.O. Box 507
Huntington, WV 25710

National Braille Association, Inc. (NBA)
3 Townline Circle
Rochester, NY 14623-2513

National Brain Tumor Foundation
785 Market Street
Suite 1600
San Francisco, CA 94103

National Burn Victim Foundation (NBVF)
32 Scotland Road
Orange, NJ 07050

National Cancer Institute (NCI)
National Institutes of Health
U.S. Department of Health and Human
   Services Bethesda, MD 20892

National Council on Disability (NCD)
1331 F Street NW
Suite 1050
Washington, DC 20004-1107

National Council on Independent Living
   (NCIL)
2111 Wilson Boulevard, Suite 405
Arlington, VA 22201

National Council on the Aging, Inc.
   (NCOA)
409 - 3rd Street SW
Washington, DC 20024

National Diabetes Information
   Clearinghouse (NDIC)
P.O. Box NDIC9000
Rockville Pike
Bethesda, MD 20892

National Digestive Diseases Information
   Clearinghouse (NDDIC)
9000 Rockville Pike
Box NDDIC
Bethesda, MD 20892

National Down Syndrome Society
   (NDSS)
666 Broadway
New York, NY 10012

National Easter Seal Society (NESS)
230 West Monroe Street
Suite 1800
Chicago, IL 60606

National Federation of the Blind (NFB)
1800 Johnson Street
Baltimore, MD 21230

National Foundation for Facial
   Reconstruction (NFFR)
317 East 34th Street
New York, NY 10016

National Fragile X Foundation
1441 York Street
Suite 215
Denver, CO 80206

National Brain Injury Foundation, Inc.
1776 Massachusetts Avenue NW
Suite 100
Washington, DC 20036

National Heart, Lung, and Blood Institute
   (NHLBI) Information Center
P.O. Box 30105
Bethesda, MD 20824-0105

The National Hemophilia Foundation
   (NHF)
The Soho Building
110 Greene Street
Suite 303
New York, NY 10012

National Hospice Organization (NHO)
1901 North Moore Street
Suite 901
Arlington, VA 22209

National Institute for Burn Medicine
   (NIBM)
909 East Ann Street
Ann Arbor, MI 48104

National Institute of Allergy and
   Infectious Diseases (NIAID)
National Institutes of Health
U.S. Department of Health and Human
   Services
Building 31
Room 7A50
Bethesda, MD 20892

National Institute of Diabetes and
  Digestive and Kidney Diseases
  (NIDDK)
U.S. Department of Health and Human
  Services
Building 31
Room 9A04
9000 Rockville Pike
Bethesda, MD 20892

National Institute of Neurological
  Disorders and Stroke (NINDS)
National Institutes of Health
U.S. Department of Health and Human
  Services
Building 31
Room 8A-06
Bethesda, MD 20892

National Kidney and Urologic Diseases
  Information Clearinghouse (NKUDIC)
Box NKUDIC
9000 Rockville Pike
Bethesda, MD 20892

National Kidney Foundation (NKF)
30 East 33rd Street
New York, NY 10016

National Library Service for the Blind
  and Physically Handicapped (NLS)
Library of Congress
1291 Taylor Street NW
Washington, DC 20542

National Mental Health Association
  (NMHA)
1021 Prince Street
Alexandria, VA 22314

National Multiple Sclerosis Society
733 3rd Avenue
6th Floor
New York, NY 10017

National Network of Learning Disabled
  Adults (NNLDA)
P.O. Box 32611
Phoenix, AZ 85064-2611

National Neurofibromatosis Foundation
  (NNFF)
141 Fifth Avenue
Suite 7-S
New York, NY 10010-7105

The National Organization for Rare
  Disorders (NORD)
P.O. Box 8923
New Fairfield, CT 06812

National Organization on Fetal Alcohol
  Syndrome (NOFAS)
1815 H Street NW
Suite 710
Washington, DC 20006

National Osteoporosis Foundation (NOF)
1150 17th Street NW
Suite 500
Washington, DC 20036 1603

National Parent Network on Disabilities
  (NPND)
1600 Prince Street
Suite 115
Alexandria, VA 22314

National Parkinson Foundation
1501 NW Ninth Avenue
Miami, FL 33136

National Rehabilitation Association
  (NRA)
633 South Washington Street
Alexandria, VA 22314-4193

National Rehabilitation Information
  Center (NARIC)
8455 Colesville Road
Suite 935
Silver Spring, MD 20910-3319

National Retinitis Pigmentosa Foundation
1401 Mt. Royal Avenue
Fourth Floor
Baltimore, MD 21217

The National Scoliosis Foundation
72 Mount Auburn Street
Watertown, MA 02172

National Spinal Cord Injury Association
(NSCIA)
545 Concord Avenue
Cambridge, MA 02138

National Stroke Association (NSA)
8480 East Orchard Road
Suite 1000
Englewood, CO 80111-5015

National Stuttering Project (NSP)
4601 Irving Street
San Francisco, CA 94122

National Tay-Sachs and Allied Diseases
  Association, Inc. (NTSAD)
2001 Beacon Street
Suite 204
Brookline, MA 02146

National Therapeutic Recreation Society
(NTRS)
National Recreation and Park Association
2775 South Quincy Street
Suite 300
Alexandria, VA 22206

Neurofibromatosis, Inc. (NF, Inc.)
8855 Annapolis Road
Suite 110
Lanham, MD 20706-2924

Osteogenesis Imperfecta Foundation, Inc.
(OIF)
5005 Laurel Street
Tampa, FL 33607-3836

Paralyzed Veterans of America (PVA)
801 Eighteenth Street NW
Washington, DC 20006

Parkinson's Disease Foundation, Inc.
(PDF)
William Black Medical Research Building
Columbia-Presbyterian Medical Center
650 West 168th Street
New York, NY 10032

The Phoenix Society for Burn Survivors,
Inc.
11 Rust Hill Road
Levittown, PA 19056

Polycystic Kidney Research Foundation
(PKRF)
922 Walnut Street
Suite 411
Kansas City, MO 64106

Prader-Willi Syndrome Association
1821 University Avenue West
Saint Paul, MN 55104-2801

President's Committee on Employment of
  People With Disabilities (PCEPD)
1331 F Street NW
Washington, DC 20004-1107

Recovery, Inc.
The Association of Nervous and Former
  Mental Patients
802 North Dearborn Street
Chicago, IL 60610

Rehabilitation Research and Training
  Center for Substance Abuse and People
  with Disabilities
Wright State University
Projects on Drugs and Disability
School of Medicine
3640 Colonel Glenn Highway
Dayton , OH 45435

Rehabilitation Research and Training
  Center on Personal Assistance Services
World Institute on Disability
510 - 16th Street
Oakland, CA 94612

Sickle Cell Disease Association of
America, Inc. (SCDAA)
3345 Wilshire Boulevard
Suite 1106
Los Angeles, CA 90010

The Simon Foundation for Continence
P.O. Box 835
Wilmette, IL 60091

Society for Disability Studies (SDS)
Department of Sociology
Gallaudet University
Washington, DC 20005

Special Olympics International (SOI)
1350 New York Avenue NW
Suite 500
Washington, DC 20005

Spina Bifida Association of America
(SBAA)
4590 MacArthur Boulevard NW
Suite 250
Washington, DC 20007-4226

Spinal Cord Injury Network International
(SCINI)
3911 Princeton Drive
Santa Rosa, CA 95405-7013

Spinal Cord Society (SCS)
Route 5, Wendell Road
Fergus Falls, MN 56537

Spinal Network
23815 Stuart Ranch Road
Malibu, CA 90265

Stuttering Foundation of America (SFA)
3100 Walnut Grove Road, #603
P.O. Box 11749
Memphis, TN 38111-0749

TASH- The Association for Severely
Handicapped
11201 Greenwood Avenue North
Seattle, WA 98133

Tourette Syndrome Association (TSA)
42-40 Bell Boulevard
Bayside, NY 11361

United Cerebral Palsy Associations, Inc.
(UCPA)
1522 K Street NW
Suite 1112
Washington, DC 20005

Vestibular Disorders Association (VEDA)
P.O. Box 4467
Portland, OR 97208-4467

Well Spouse Foundation (WSF)
P.O. Box 801
New York, NY 10023

Williams Syndrome Association
P.O. Box 297
Clawson, MI 48017

Wilson's Disease Association
P.O. Box 75324
Washington, DC 20013

World Institute on Disability (WID)
510 - 16th Street
Suite 100
Oakland, CA 94612

INDEX

Page numbers in *italic* indicate figures. Page numbers followed by "t" indicate tables.

succumbing, disability with, 232, 330
writings on empowerment, 331
Energy
depletion of, with emotional reactions,
32–42
prenatal, 38
Energy balance, through control of
emotional reactions, 38
Energy model, 32–42
alternative medicine, shift to, 36–37
emotions, health and, 38–40
energy, role of, 37–38
harmony and balance among all types
of matter, 37
relevance to psychology, rehabilitation,
40–42
Enlargement of scope of values, 140
Entelechy, Greek concept of, 334
Environmental barriers, 5
Epilepsy, as childhood chronic illness,
68–69
Epilepsy Foundation of America (EFA),
address, 443
Essay on Population, 20–21
Ethics, 43–54
chronic illness, ethical dilemmas in,
45–50
contractual model, for medical decision
making, 47–48
deliberative model, for medical decision
making, 49–50
dilemmas in rehabilitation, 43–54
educational model, for medical decision
making, 47t, 48–49
empathy, in resolving ethical issues,
50–52
models, ethical, 46–50, 47t
paternalistic model, for medical decision
making, 46–47
psychologists, training, 52–53
rehabilitation, ethical dilemmas in,
45–50
Etiology, in medical model, 4
Eugenics Movement, 20–26
abortion debates, influence on, 22
disability discrimination and, 12–31
domestic relations, disability in, 13–18

marriage, right to, 16–17
parenting, right to, 17–18
relations, domestic, disability in, 13–18
stereotypes, disability and, 18–20
sterilization, 13–16
laws regarding, 13
Existential anxiety, 8
Existential courage, 329–339
alcoholism, as breakdown in courage, 330
alter ego, counselor as, 337
anomie, 335
The Art of Counseling, 330
awareness of consequences, 333
counseling professions, 331–332
courage, conditions present with, 330
defined in existential literature, 334–335
emotional courage, 334
entelechy, 334
existential counseling, 337
fear of spiritual nothingness, 337
free will, 331
giving in, 330
informed consent and, 332
intellectual courage, 334
intentionality, 334
breakdown in, 335
Lustig, Paul, 332–334
meaninglessness, 335
neurotic anxiety, 335
physical courage, 334
in responding to ambivalence, 332
substance abuse, as breakdown in
courage, 330
succumbing, disability with, 232, 330
writings on empowerment, 331
Expectancy, hope and, 153

FacioScapuloHumeral Society, Inc. (FSH
Society, Inc.), address, 443
Families of Spinal Muscular Atrophy
(SMA), address, 443
Family, mental illness in, 340–357
confidentiality, 354–355
family members, impact of mental
illness on, 347
family needs, meeting, 349
interventions, family, 349–353